FUNDAMENTALS OF CLINICAL IMMUNOLOGY

J. WESLEY ALEXANDER, M.D., Sc.D.

Professor of Surgery, Director, Transplantation Division,
and Acting Director, Paul I. Hoxworth Blood Center,
University of Cincinnati Medical Center
College of Medicine, Cincinnati, Ohio

ROBERT A. GOOD, Ph.D., M.D.

President and Director, Sloan-Kettering Institute for
Cancer Research, New York, New York

1977

W. B. SAUNDERS COMPANY • Philadelphia • London • Toronto

W. B. Saunders Company: West Washington Square
                           Philadelphia, PA 19105

                           1 St. Anne's Road
                           Eastbourne, East Sussex BN21 3UN, England

                           1 Goldthorne Avenue
                           Toronto, Ontario M8Z 5T9, Canada

Library of Congress Cataloging in Publication Data

Alexander, J. Wesley, 1934–

Fundamentals of clinical immunology.

1. Immunologic diseases.   2. Immunology.
I. Good, Robert A., 1922–   joint author.

II. Title. [DNLM: 1. Immunology. QW504 A376f]
RC582.A43   616.07'9   77–75530
ISBN 0-7216-1101-X

Fundamentals of Clinical Immunology   ISBN 0-7216-1101-X

Last digit is the print number: 9   8   7   6   5   4   3   2   1

We would like to dedicate this book
to our students,
who are our most effective teachers.

PREFACE

Immunology is a relatively new and rapidly expanding discipline which developed symbiotically with bacteriology during the past century. In its older and classical meaning, immunology was the branch of science that investigated the processes by which individuals defend themselves against infection; early immunologists dealt primarily with studies of antibody and the development of vaccines. It was later found that hypersensitivity reactions resulted from antigen-antibody interactions, and the study of allergic disorders became part of the immunologist's work. More recently, cellular immunity has been recognized as being important in processes that have to do with recognition phenomena, self-characterization, growth, heredity, aging, infection, cancer, and transplantation of tissue and cells.

With this expansion, the term immunology has extended far beyond the limits of its original meaning. In fact, immunology has grown exponentially to embrace every discipline of medicine, with benefit to all. Today, hardly a patient can be treated without involving immunologic principles in some way. It is evident that to provide optimal patient care, clinicians of today must know much about this expanding and exciting discipline. Nonetheless, to learn all of modern immunology would be a formidable, if not impossible, task. Our purpose in writing this book is to provide a short and comprehensive review and condensation of the principles of immunology as they apply to clinical practice. It is hoped that it will serve as a useful aid to both students and practitioners.

J. WESLEY ALEXANDER
ROBERT A. GOOD

ACKNOWLEDGEMENTS

The authors would like to acknowledge their appreciation to Dr. Dwight Stinnett and Mr. Peter Issitt, who reviewed portions of the manuscript for possible omissions, to Mrs. Norma Thornton and Mrs. Rosemary Rahn for their care in typing the manuscript, and to Mr. George Vilk of the W. B. Saunders Company for his editorial assistance.

CONTENTS

SECTION II LABORATORY AND CLINICAL TESTS

SECTION III CLINICAL APPLICATIONS

1

Introduction and Historical Perspectives

The practice of medicine must have evolved from what we would consider today to be witchcraft. Objective evidence of surgical treatment dates as far back as Neolithic times when trephining was practiced, presumably to provide an exit for evil spirits from the minds of the affected. Trephined skulls have been found in widely dispersed areas throughout the world, giving evidence that this was not an uncommon operation of the prehistoric era. The first written evidence of surgical practice was inscribed on a stone near Babylon about 2000 B.C.; it enumerated a series of penalties and regulations, now known as the Code of Hammurabi. The earliest scientific document that has been discovered is the Edwin Smith Papyrus, written about 1700 B.C. This is a surgical treatise describing a series of case histories that provide us with a good insight into the state of practice at that time. The document itself is felt to be a compilation of observations handed down through centuries, beginning with the period between 3000 and 2500 B.C.

By the time of the writings of Hippocrates, about 400 B.C., a great deal of experience and knowledge had accrued concerning certain conditions, notably fractures, dislocations, wounds, and diseases. Like the Egyptians, Hippocrates was well aware of the complications of infection and tetanus, but, in addition, seemed to have a grasp of some of the modern concepts of wound healing and infection. He realized the desirability of primary healing without infection and also appreciated that free drainage of purulent discharges was essential. He preached that oil or greasy remedies were not good for fresh wounds; nevertheless, the practice of treating wounds in this manner continued for many centuries.

Most surgeons up to and including the time of Ambroise Paré (1517?–1590) made their fame by caring for the injured during wartime. Their practices must have been rather depressing, since approximately three out of every four persons injured in battle died, primarily from hemorrhage and sepsis. Even in the Franco-Prussian War, in the latter part of the nineteenth century, the mortality from gunshot wounds of the abdomen approached 100 per cent. The destiny of many wars before modern times was, however, determined by the presence of disease rather than by military strategy. Infection was always the leading cause of disease and death in both peace and war.

Throughout the history of mankind before the beginning of the nineteenth century, advances in the practice of medicine and surgery came pitifully slowly. Immunology was unknown, although the custom of inhaling crusts from smallpox lesions to prevent the development of smallpox infection in later life had been practiced by the Chinese since A.D. 1500. By 1718, variolation (injection of material from crusts or fluids of smallpox blisters) was extensively practiced throughout the Eastern world. The practice was introduced into Western medicine by Lady Montagu, wife of the British ambassador to Turkey, who had her children immunized to smallpox.

By the time the American colonies developed into an independent nation, variolation was extensively practiced and debated. Indeed, clear evidence from what must be considered to be the equivalent of clinical trials showed that variolation was effective and could be practiced with low mortality. The problem remained that the virus used could be transmitted, so protection by variolation was hazardous to the community at large.

Jenner published his monumental work on vaccination for the prevention of smallpox in 1798, and in the following 175 years, both immunology and medicine grew at an increasingly rapid rate. Jenner's recognition that the shiny-faced milkmaids did not develop smallpox because they had previously been infected with cowpox was revolutionary. This discovery provided the first clear evidence that active immunization could be used safely to prevent a dangerous infectious disease, that attenuated viruses could be used for effective active immunization, and that resistance to infection might be associated with inflammatory reactions occurring with greater speed and intensity than in nonimmunized persons. It even suggested the concept of interference of one virus infection by another. From this early beginning in immunology, progress toward the control of infection often led the increasingly common advances in medicine.

By the time of Lister, in the last half of the eighteenth century, the care of patients in Europe had gradually shifted from the home to hospitals, where overcrowding and unclean conditions prevailed. To be hospitalized for a major operative procedure or with a compound fracture meant almost certain death in some hospitals. The situation was not universally dismal, however, as the idea of disinfection and cleanliness had been developing over the preceding hundred years. Both Oliver Wendell Holmes, in America, and Ignaz Semmelweis, a young Hungarian, connected the high mortality from puerperal sepsis to transmission of the disease by the unclean hands of attending physicians. Semmelweis carried out beautifully controlled experiments which showed that simply washing the hands after attending an autopsy could reduce the incidence of puerperal sepsis. Perhaps in part because of the fervor derived from his experimental demonstrations, but more likely because of the resistance of "the Establishment" to his new ideas, he antagonized the leaders in medicine and obstetrics and could not convince those in power of the great benefit to be derived from his new principles of infection and decontamination. He fought so hard to persuade the medical leadership that the practice of medicine must change that he lost his position, his health, and his mental stability. Ironically, he died from blood poisoning in an insane asylum in Vienna in 1865, the same year that Joseph Lister first used carbolic acid as an antiseptic.

Lister, an Englishman, was disturbed by the observation that death from hospital gangrene was much more prevalent for patients treated in a hospital environment than for patients with similar lesions who were treated at home. As a result of studying Pasteur's work, which in 1854 had shown that bacteria caused fermentation, he reasoned that bacteria might likewise cause fermentation in wounds. He was pondering the best way to attack this problem when he had the good fortune to pass a sewage disposal plant and was struck by the fact that the disinfected sewage had lost its characteristic stench. Finding that carbolic acid was used to disinfect the sewage, he applied carbolic acid to the wounds of his patients with dramatic success. After two years of experimenting, he had accumulated indisputable evidence that the treatment had a remarkable effect in preventing hospital gangrene. His first work was published in 1867, but it was not well received, and it took a number of years before wide acceptance was gained.

In 1864, Pasteur had shown that heat would kill bacteria, and from this observation came the term pasteurization. Pasteur, who made all of his great contributions by studying disease, showed that chicken cholera and anthrax in animals could be prevented by vaccination, and later made the outstanding contribution of vaccination against rabies. Koch (1878) observed that different types of bacteria could cause different types of wound infections and disease. As a result of Lister's studies on antisepsis and the early observations of Pasteur and Koch, the period of antiseptic surgery emerged. In 1886, von Bergman introduced the steam sterilizer, and in 1890, Halstead introduced rubber gloves, developed to protect the sensitive hands of his faithful scrub nurse, who later became his wife, from the irritating effects of carbolic acid. Schimmelbusch published his book on aseptic technique in 1892, and Mikulicz introduced the mask in 1896, thus making the concept of aseptic technique almost complete by the beginning of the twentieth century. Surgical infection had by no means been eradicated, but the mortality from injury and operation fell remarkably during this period, and to have an operation no longer meant almost certain death. Partly because of this and partly because the use of anesthesia allowed surgeons to be slower and more precise, technical surgery developed at a rapid rate.

Many other advances were accumulating that formed the basis for understanding the process of infection and immune resistance. Metchnikoff, one of the major pioneers of immunology, whose stature and contributions were exceeded only by Pasteur, elucidated the role of phagocytosis and cellular immunity in the two decades before 1900. Killed vaccines were introduced in 1886 by Solman and Smith. Buchner described complement (alexin) in 1893, and Bordet elucidated the comparative roles of antibody and complement in cell lysis in 1899. Wright and Douglas demonstrated in 1903 that acquired immunity resulted from both humoral and cellular elements, and described opsonization. Thus, soon after the beginning of this century, a basic understanding of immunity to infection had developed.

In 1888, Roux and Yersin discovered the exotoxin of diphtheria, and found that an antitoxin could be produced in animals that would neutralize its toxic effects. Von Behring and Kitasato (1890) showed that active immunization was possible and that immunity to diphtheria and tetanus toxins could be passively transferred to another animal by the injection of serum. The first Nobel Prize in medicine was given to von Behring in 1901 for these great achievements. Roux later used horse antitoxin successfully for the treatment of human diphtheria (1894). Production of tetanus antitoxin was a natural outgrowth of these earlier observations and, in 1914, equine tetanus antitoxin was used with great success for preventing the dreaded and highly fatal disease of tetanus that so frequently followed war wounds. Later (1923), Glenny and Ramon found that toxins could be made to lose their toxic property while still retaining their antigenic property. As a result of their observations, a highly effective immunizing agent was developed that virtually eliminated tetanus in our troops during and after World War II.

Shock was another problem facing physicians of the early twentieth century. It was believed by many that blood transfusions would be helpful in preventing death following hemorrhage, if they could be given with safety. Transfusion of blood from animals to humans was first attempted in the mid-seventeenth century and met with occasional success, but, more often, transfusions were disastrous. Transfusions of blood from one human to another were tried in the early nineteenth century with greater success, but these, too, were sometimes associated with severe and even fatal reactions. Karl Landsteiner, a quiet, brilliant laboratory investigator, discovered the major blood group antigens of human red blood cells in 1900 and described their interactions with agglutinins in the plasma. As a direct result of his experiments, safe blood transfusions became possible after appropriate typing and cross-matching. In 1914, citrate was introduced to prevent clotting. Stored blood was used for transfusions in World War I, but it was not until the period between World War I and World War II that blood banking became safe. The development of modern surgery had to await Landsteiner's monumental discovery of the blood group antigens and adequate means for the safe storage and transfusion of blood, even though most of the technical problems had been solved by the early twentieth century. Landsteiner described the blood groups M and N only a few years after the ABO system was found, but it was not until 1940 that Landsteiner and Wiener discovered the Rh factors.

In a beautiful interpretation of an experiment of Nature that reveals the power of immunology, Levine and Stetson, that same year but independently of Landsteiner and Wiener, discovered that erythroblastosis fetalis was caused by immunization of the mother against the blood cells of her own child. The isoimmunization so produced also resulted in sensitization that led to a severe, nearly fatal transfusion reaction in a mother who was given her husband's red blood cells. The agglutinin present in the mother's blood that was responsible for the death of the child and a transfusion reaction against the father's cells also reacted with the red cells of 85 per cent of the general population, but not with those of the other 15 per cent. This discovery was then linked to the systematic analysis of the Rh system of antigens on red blood cells described by Wiener and Landsteiner, and knowledge of the pathogenesis of Rh disease (erythroblastosis fetalis) was complete. It remained only to be discovered that the sensitization produced by the entry of small numbers of the infant's Rh+ cells into the Rh− mother's circulation after parturition was responsible. Here another important experiment of Nature showed the way. Levine had noticed that erythroblastosis fetalis occurred less frequently when the father was Rh+ and the mother Rh− if the two were also mismatched at the ABO system, with the father being A or B and the mother, O. These observations led to the postulation by Finn et al. and Gorman and Freda that treatment of the mother with antibody directed against the Rh+ cells might prevent erythroblastosis fetalis by preventing sensitization of the mother with these immunogenic cells. This approach was studied first in prison volunteers, leading to the successful prevention of the immunologically based neonatal disease by modulation of the immune response.

Early in this century, it became apparent that immune reactions could be damaging as well as beneficial, and Richet and Portier (1902) showed that anaphylaxis was an immunologic reaction. The Arthus reaction was described the following year. About the same time, von Pirquet and Schick began their studies of serum sickness and showed that disease of the skin, heart, joints, blood vessels, and kidneys, as well as fever, could be caused by the body's immunologic reaction to foreign protein. In 1918, Prausnitz and Küstner, studying Prausnitz' food allergy to boiled fish protein, discovered that local wheal and erythema reactions could be studied in nonsensitive recipients by passive transfer of serum or antibody that became fixed to the skin. From their studies, they discovered not only the immunologic basis of this kind of allergy but also immunization for desensitization against atopic allergy. By 1925, Zinsser showed the differences between immediate and delayed types of sensitivity.

In another direction of inquiry, the great pioneer of immunochemistry Paul Ehrlich was the first to use quantitative measurements in immune reactions. Because of his interest in dyes, he introduced useful methods for examining the cells of blood and tissues, and he developed salvarsan, the first effective chemotherapeutic agent against any microorganism. The antibacterial action of penicillin was first rather accidentally discovered by Alexander Fleming in 1928, but it was several years before the significance of this discovery was realized. In 1932, Gerhard Domagk developed prontosil, which was an effective antibacterial agent against Streptococcus. Later, the active ingredient was found to be sulfanilamide, active against a wide variety of organisms. It was used so enthusiastically that allergic and toxic reactions came to be a significant limiting problem. The tedious process of isolation and purification of penicillin was accomplished in 1941, by Howard Florey and Ernst Chain. Penicillin received its first major trial in World War II during the North African campaign, and it was also at this time that blood transfusions reached a high point of safety and effectiveness. Few clinicians need to be reminded of the usefulness of antibiotic therapy, although these agents are sometimes overused and abused.

Techniques for analysis of immune reactions have significantly improved our understanding of these processes. Some of the milestones include introduction of precise quantitative chemical methods for measurement of antibodies and antigens through precipitin analysis (Heidelberger, 1924–1926), definition of optimal proportioning for quantitation of precipitating antibody (Dean and Webb, 1926), immunoelectrophoresis (Grabar and Williams, 1953), and later a wide array of biochemical and immunochemical techniques.

The discovery by Alexis Carrel that animal cells can be grown in tissue culture and that viruses can be grown in the cultured cells paved the way for development of antivirus vaccines against polio by Enders, Weller, and Robbins, which has further provided the method for development of vaccines against measles, rubella, mumps, rubeola, and many other viruses. Capacity to grow viruses on the chorioallantoic membrane of embryonated eggs, developed by Cox, provided the essential methodology for development of antivirus vaccines against influenza and yellow fever, and the modern rabies vaccine.

Studies of the association of increased serum globulin levels with plasmacytosis by Bing and Plum in 1937, followed by Kolouch's study of plasmacytosis in subacute bacterial endocarditis and the subsequent demonstration that antigenic stimulation caused the development of both plasma cells and antibody, opened the modern approaches for study of the cellular basis of immunity. These investigations, followed by Bjoerneboe and Gormsen's demonstration of the intimate relationship of plasmacytosis and hypergammaglobulinemia through studies of hyperimmunization, led to Fagraeus' beautiful experiments, which proved that plasma cells synthesize and secrete antibody, and Coon's demonstration, using immunofluorescent techniques, that plasma cells synthesize immunoglobulins. Kunkel's study of the chemistry of myeloma protein and Edelman and Porter's incisive chemical studies of purified antibody and myeloma proteins led to the now virtually complete definition of the chemistry of immunoglobulins and antibody.

One recent milestone was the discovery of hypogammaglobulinemia by Bruton in 1952, which opened the door for studies of immunodeficiency and structure-function relationships in the lymphoid system. Good et al. soon showed that agammaglobulinemic patients could not produce antibodies, but could develop delayed allergy—a clinical demonstration that agreed with Chase and Landsteiner's earlier findings in experimental animals: that antibody could passively transfer immediate type sensitivity, but only lymphocytes could transfer delayed allergy. These fundamental analyses permitted dissection of the immunity system into two separate arms, now called the T and B cell systems.

The classic studies of Medawar and his colleagues in 1944 and 1945 initiated a flurry of interest in the problems of transplantation. These investigations established that immunologic processes are clearly involved in allograft rejection of normal organs. Further, they showed that cell-mediated immune processes could be analyzed and manipulated experimentally. These approaches led directly to clinical transplantation and to better understanding of tumor immunity.

This discussion now brings us to the doorstep of modern immunology, where contributions are not only too numerous to credit here, but form the basis for the rest of this book. It may be of interest to the reader to review the background of some of the pioneers who were destined to change the face of medicine through immunology. Jenner and Koch both started their careers as country doctors. Landsteiner was a pathologist who devoted his full efforts to research on immunologic problems, but made his major contribution, that permitted blood transfusions, while studying a clinical problem. Pasteur was a chemist who always studied disease. Metchnikoff, about whom we will say more later, was a Russian biologist. Paul Ehrlich was both a physician and chemist; Heidelberger, a chemist; Fleming, a bacteriologist; Medawar, a zoologist; and Coombs, a veterinarian. Our society owes a great debt to these pioneers. One of the great strengths of immunology as a contributor to human welfare is that its contributions have derived in large part from application of the most basic scientific approaches to issues of disease.

IMMUNOLOGY IN MODERN MEDICINE

It is apparent from the foregoing brief historical review that the fundamental discoveries in immunology have profoundly influenced the development of every branch of medicine and surgery. Today, immunology has an even greater impact on all medical disciplines. Growing numbers of patients are recognized who have immunologic deficiencies or abnormal immune responses as the sole basis for their disease. The principles of immunology are used in the treatment and prevention of infection, and in understanding the processes of inflammation and tissue repair. Chemotherapeutic agents and other treatment modalities may modify the capacity of an individual to respond to infection or to an immunologic stimulus. Drugs, themselves, may cause severe allergic reactions. Major operative procedures depend upon the availability of blood which is selected by immunologic methods. A whole new area of therapeutic practice, organ transplantation, is now beginning to be made feasible through histocompatibility matching and manipulation of the immune response. Other major areas of disease, such as cancer and degenerative diseases, are closely linked to immunologic changes. Nephrologists must be applied immunologists as much as they are applied physiologists. Rheumatology is essentially modern immunology applied to the clinic. Most of the important diseases addressed by modern hematology must either be analyzed with immunologic methods or involve immunologic processes in their pathogenesis or treatment. Dermatologic disorders and neurologic problems are very much in the immunologic arena these days, and almost all gastrointestinal diseases have central issues of an immunologic nature. Even the modern revolution in endocrinology is based on radioimmunoassay, one of the powerful new tools of modern immunology. Much of clinical chemistry, in fact, may soon be based on very sensitive and discriminating immunologic tests, which can be fully automated. In short, practically all of modern medicine and surgery find immunologic principles and applications essential for understanding and analysis of their problems.

PROSPECTS FOR THE FUTURE

It is difficult to predict the future, but the rate of progress and accumulation of basic knowledge in immunology ensure that exciting and almost unbelievable advances will make many phases of current clinical practice obsolete. Within the foreseeable future, we predict that it will be possible to transplant most organs with a high rate of success and to correct most types of immunodeficiency, whether inherited or acquired. We will be able to enhance resistance to infection, and treat and prevent many of the troublesome infections now resistant to antibiotic therapy. It seems virtually certain that we will be able to diagnose cancer earlier and more accurately by immunologic means. In the future, we should be able to effectively treat increasing numbers of types of cancer by combinations of immunotherapy, surgery, and chemotherapy, and immunology will be used to prevent some and perhaps many cancers.

Since failing of the immunologic functions, autoimmunity, and infection underlie so many of the diseases of aging, it seems probable that important control of the diseases of aging will be achieved by immunologic manipulations. By actively altering the immune process through the development of immunopharmacology, we should be able to ease the allergic patient at long last and immunization against unwanted immunity is a distinct possibility.

We have great confidence that most, if not all, of these predictions will come to pass in this century by the application of the fruits of basic research in immunology, directed pragmatically at the interface between clinical medicine and the fundamental laboratory. Perhaps no body of knowledge is at present more important for clinicians to learn than the fundamentals of the immune process.

SECTION I
THE BASICS OF IMMUNOLOGY

The immune response does not often involve a single process.
Lymphocytes, phagocytic cells, the vascular system, antibody,
complement, and other components of the body have complex
interactions, which cannot be understood by studying only
one or two facets of this intertwining maze. In this section, it
is our purpose to present a background of basic facts and
concepts of immunity, which together will allow interpretation
of immunologic disease and the application of immunologic
principles to clinical practice.

2

Development of the Immune Response

Immunity usually implies resistance, not only to infectious agents, but also to foreign particles, toxins, living cells, and cancer. A destructive process is almost always involved, and the success of the immune process is based upon the ability of living organisms to recognize, by various means, the foreignness of complex molecules which are unrelated to their own normal structure. Immunity may be acquired as a result of prior experience with the chemical structure of a foreign substance, or it may be nonspecific, in which case it is genetically determined.

The genetic control of resistance to foreign substances encompasses an exceedingly broad body of knowledge that deals with basic cellular function, but since it is not our purpose to expound on the more esoteric aspects of cellular biology, we will confine our discussion to those features that we feel may relate directly to clinical practice, while realizing that what seems to be of practical significance to one individual is often deemed worthless by another. The basic concepts of nonspecific immunity are best exemplified by innate resistance to microbial infection (Chapter 13).

In contrast to nonspecific or innate immunity, acquired immunity is an adaptive response to an antigenic stimulus, which results in the acquisition of immunologic memory, the synthesis of specifically reacting antibody and the development of specifically reactive lymphocytes. Adaptive immunity is related to the phylogenetic and ontogenetic development of the lymphoid system and, when fully expressed, it is a characteristic possessed only by vertebrate animals. Although most clinicians infrequently have a direct concern with developmental problems involving the lymphoid organs, a brief review of the growth and maturation of these systems will promote a better understanding of the concepts more directly applicable to clinical immunology.

EVOLUTION OF ADAPTIVE IMMUNITY

Phylogenetic Development

Invertebrate animals maintain an effective defense against invasion of microorganisms, but the precise mechanisms by which this defense is effected are not well understood. Many attempts have been made to demonstrate a specific adaptive immune response to antigenic stimuli in invertebrates, but none have been convincingly successful. Allografted skin can be rejected by earthworms, but it is not clear whether these responses have been specific or nonspecific. Even corals seem to have capacity for distinguishing between self and nonself which has a cellular and genetic basis, but the cellular or molecular mechanisms, or both, have not yet been elucidated. Many of the invertebrates have humoral substances that agglutinate or combine with soluble or cellular antigens from genetically dissimilar species, including pathogenic bacteria, and these, in fact, may be produced in greater quantities following stimulation with the foreign material. However, the increased production of these substances appears to be a biochemical adaptation rather than an immunologic one, since no immunologic memory is developed.

Extensive studies have been done to demonstrate adaptive immunity in the cyclostomes (primitive vertebrates). In the hagfish, the most primitive true vertebrate, no truly organized lymphoid tissue is present, but evidence has now been presented that these animals can slowly reject skin allografts, and there seems to be specific memory for the experience. Further, it has been found by some but not others that antibodies of high molecular weight may be found to certain antigens. In the lamprey, transplantation immunity is already well developed, and the ability to produce humoral antibodies definitely exists, although there is antibody response to only a few among many antigens. In the lamprey, one immunoglobulin migrates electrophoretically as an alpha globulin and sediments in the ultracentrifuge as an 11-14S component. High and low molecular weight antibodies have been described, and it has been claimed that the immunoglobulins have both heavy and light chain polypeptides, as do the immunoglobulins of higher vertebrates. Much more work is needed to more completely define the immunoglobulin molecules of the primitive fishes.

Studies with other primitive fishes, such as the guitarfish, primitive sharks (for example, the horned sharks and more modern elasmobranches), cartilaginous freshwater fishes, chondrostean fishes, and primitive bony fishes, reveal a progressive complexity of lymphoid structure and increasing immunologic vigor and adaptability which parallel the ascent on the phylogenetic scale. As the thymic and splenic tissues became better developed, so did the ability to express both cellular and humoral immunity as distinct immunologic processes. In paddlefishes, sharks, and higher fishes, not only is there more organized lymphoid tissue, but also antibody-producing plasma cells can be found that are much like mammalian plasma cells. The immunoglobulins produced, although variable in polymer size, seem molecularly very similar to IgM. Only one kind of immunoglobulin with a single heavy chain is found in these species. The production of IgM type of antibody occurs phylogenetically before the development of IgG antibody. The ability to produce a second immunoglobulin which may be homologous to IgD or even IgG appears first in the lungfish and is well developed for amphibians and reptiles.

Amphibians and reptiles both have a well-developed adaptive immunity, but the response to an antigenic stimulus is somewhat temperature dependent. Birds and mammals have fully developed mechanisms for adaptive immunity and fully developed primary and secondary lymphoid organs which consist of the thymus, spleen, lymph nodes, and characteristic lymphoid tissues along the gastrointestinal tract. In all species having a thymus, this organ seems to govern differentiation of the T lymphocyte population. The bursa of Fabricius is the primary lymphoid organ in birds that governs differentiation of the B lymphocyte population. All birds and mammals possess germinal centers in their peripheral lymphoid tissues that seem to be associated with the development of ability to produce the IgG type of antibody, sites for rapid expansion of lymphoid cell populations, and vigorous forms of immunologic memory.

The most important point to be made in this short review is that the ability to express adaptive immunity parallels the development and elaboration of organized lymphoid structures. Figure 2-1 and Table 2-1 illustrate the key phylogenetic steps in the development of immunity.

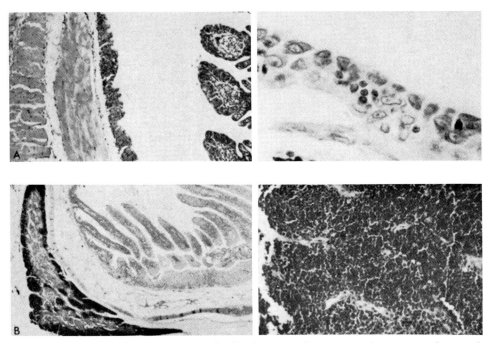

Figure 2-1.   Key evolutionary steps in the development of immunity. The primitive thymus of the lamprey *(A)* consists of a few lymphocytes in the gills. In the guitarfish *(B)* the thymus has become independent.

Illustration continued on the following page

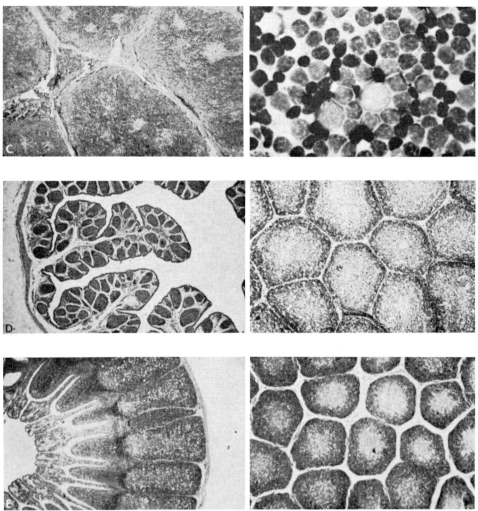

Figure 2–1 *Continued.* The paddlefish *(C)* has a lobular thymus with many varied cells. In addition to the thymus, the chicken *(D)* has a bursa of Fabricius, and the rabbit *(E)* has Peyer's patches which are microscopically similar. (From Good, R. A., Hosp. Prac., 2:40–41, 1967. Photos show two levels of magnification.)

Ontogenetic Development

Like the phylogenetic development of adaptive immunity, ontogenetic development parallels the formation, differentiation, and maturation of lymphoid tissues. The degree of lymphoid maturation at the time of birth may vary widely, depending upon the species. For example, the opossum and mouse are exceedingly immature when born, have only vestiges of a thymus, and have not developed a lymphoid spleen or lymph nodes. In the chicken, both the thymus and bursa of Fabricius (see text to follow) are well developed at the time of hatching, but secondary lymphoid organs are poorly developed. In man and in the dog, "peripheralization" of lymphatic cells has occurred

TABLE 2–1. PHYLOGENETIC DEVELOPMENT OF ADAPTIVE IMMUNITY

	DEVELOPMENT OF ORGANIZED LYMPHOID TISSUE	PRODUCTION OF HUMORAL ANTIBODY AND IMMUNOLOGICAL MEMORY	TRANSPLANTATION (CELLULAR) IMMUNITY
Invertebrates	Not demonstrated	Not demonstrated	May be present
Hagfish, a cyclostome, the most primitive of the true vertebrates	Not demonstrated	May be present	May be present
Lamprey (Petromyzon) also a cyclostome; next step in vertebrate evolution	Primitive; collections of lymphocytes in gills. Epithelial thymus and splenic organization without lymph follicles	Primitive, but present; responses to few antigens	Present and vigorous
Lower cartilaginous fishes (guitar fish, primitive sharks, paddlefish)	Independent thymus and spleen	Well developed to some antigens, poor response to others	Present and vigorous
Higher fishes	Well developed	Better developed	Fully developed
Amphibians	Well developed	Well developed for most antigens; temperature dependent; two immunoglobulins	Developed, but temperature dependent
Reptiles	Well developed	Well developed for most antigens; temperature dependent; at least two immunoglobulins	Developed, but temperature dependent
Birds	Well developed. Clear separation of thymic and bursal functions	Fully developed; multiple immunoglobulins	Fully developed cell system
Mammals	Well developed. Separation of thymic and gut-dependent lymphoid functions demonstrated in those species studied	Fully developed; five classes of immunoglobulins	Fully developed T cell system; multiple subclasses of T cells

well before the time of birth, and the spleen and lymph nodes are well developed. In keeping with the maturational development of their lymphoid structures, the opposum, the mouse, and the rat are considerably more deficient in adaptive immune responses at the time of birth than is man or the dog.

In man, the first lymphoid organ to develop is the thymus, and the epithelial elements are formed first (by the sixth to eighth fetal week). Some authorities have felt that lymphoid cells arise subsequently by direct transformation of epithelial cells under the influence of the mesenchymal stroma, but better evidence indicates that the thymus is a site for differentiation of yolk sac, fetal liver, and, ultimately, bone marrow–derived mesenchymal stem cells to lymphocytes. Circulating lymphocytes are soon found, and lymph nodes are developed by the fourth month of gestation. Lymphopoiesis is found in the spleen at four to five months' gestation. In birds, the entire antibody-producing system of cells develops in a hindgut derivative, the thymus-like bursa of Fabricius. As in the thymus, mesenchymal cells come to the bursa where they undergo differentiation to cells that can produce Ig and antibodies. No other animal species has been found to have a bursa, and development of the antibody- and Ig-producing cells in mammals seems to begin in the fetal liver or other gut-associated lymphoid structures, which then function like the bursa for development of B lymphocytes.

Regardless of the species of animal, each has a similar ontogenetic pattern of immunologic maturation. This has been studied particularly well in the lamb, which has a gestation period of 150 days. The fetus is totally unresponsive to antigens prior to the 35th day of gestation, but between the 35th and 41st day, it develops the capacity to produce antibodies to certain viruses. By the 66th day, the fetus can produce antibodies to ferritin, but the ability to produce antibody to egg albumin is not developed until the 125th day. Full immunologic capacity, however, is not present at the time of birth, and there may be no response to antigens such as *Salmonella* or BCG even as long as six weeks after birth. In humans, some antibody responses develop long before birth, although significant antibody production to many other antigens may not appear until after birth. Meaningful antibody response to a few antigens, may not appear until ten weeks after birth.

Although more recent experience using techniques with increased sensitivity has proved that immunoglobulins are produced by a fetus, the amount of antibody production is very little compared to that produced by an adult, largely because of the relative protection of the fetus from antigenic stimulation. In all species, there remains the need for providing immunoglobulins to the immunologically immature newborn. The method for doing so varies somewhat with the species and with the number of layers of placental tissue between maternal and fetal circulation. Pigs and cows have five to six complex cellular layers separating maternal and fetal circulation, and none or only minuscule amounts of the maternal immunoglobulins are transferred transplacentally to the fetus. These newborn animals therefore have insufficient antibody to protect them from common pathogens, and their survival depends upon absorption of intact antibody from the maternal milk. Man, on the other hand, has only two placental layers, and immunoglobulins of the IgG variety are transferred transplacentally to the fetus. IgA and IgM are not transferred. The ability for transplacental transfer of IgG is not a function of the size of the IgG molecule, but seems to be an active transport process requiring the Fc portion of the immunoglobulin molecule. (See Chapter 6 for definition of terms.)

In keeping with the observation that poorly differentiated lymphoid cells produce primarily macroglobulins, the first antibodies to be synthesized by the developing fetus or newborn are of the 19S type (IgM). As the individual matures, IgD production develops, then IgG is produced, and still later in ontogeny, the ability to produce IgA develops. A few circulating and tissue lymphocytes of the human fetus have been shown to produce either IgM or IgG molecules as early as the eighth week of gestation. At this time, small lymphocytes have been shown to be able to produce only IgM; larger lymphocytes may produce IgD or IgM and then IgG. IgA molecules are not produced until later, generally after birth.

ADAPTIVE IMMUNITY AND AGING

Immunologic competence develops in an orderly manner in the very young, and it gradually improves to reach a peak of responsiveness about the time of puberty. With increasing senescence, however, immunologic responsiveness begins to wane, and the increase in susceptibility of aged individuals to infections undoubtedly results in part from this diminution in the immune processes. The mechanisms for the decline are becoming clearer with recent investigations, and thymic involution may be the most important controlling factor in involution of the peripheral lymphoid tissues. Immunity based on thymus-derived lymphocytes wanes earlier and more completely than does that based on B lymphocytes. Accelerated immunologic aging has been demonstrated in neonatally thymectomized animals, but wasting following neonatal thymectomy can be prevented by a germ-free environment, by transplantation of mature peripheral lymphoid cells, by the transplantation of thymic tissue, and to some extent by thymus implanted in a millipore chamber. The aging process in the lymphoid tissue in older animals can be stopped temporarily by forming a parabiotic union with genetically identical young animals or by injecting large numbers of lymphocytes from a younger animal. Experiments showing reconstitution of neonatally thymectomized mice with thymus fragments implanted in cell-impermeable millipore chambers, and experiments showing reconstitution of lymphoid tissue and immunologic function by injection of certain extracts of thymus both argue that the thymus elaborates an important hormone, thymopoetin, capable of inducing differentiation of precursors and probably expanding the numbers of lymphoid cells in the peripheral lymphoid tissues. Studies with a functional stromal epithelial tumor which seems to produce such a factor lend substantial support to this view. However, thymus alone or thymic hormones alone cannot completely forestall the waning of immunologic vigor with age. To date, the most impressive correction of the immunodeficiency of aging has been transplantation of both thymus and stem cells from the bone marrow.

The synthesis of circulating antibody as a response to a wide variety of antigenic stimuli has been shown to be relatively deficient in old age, the major deficiency being in the IgG fraction with the IgM antibody response relatively unchanged. This suggests that the immune mechanism gradually reverts to the more primitive form seen in very young individuals. In the very aged, antibody response may be minimal, although in some individuals it is quite well maintained. In contrast, increase in antibody production to endogenous antigens (antinuclear antibodies and other autoantibodies) occurs with great frequency during senescence (see Chapter 16). In a variety of species, aged animals exhibit a diminished capacity for the expression of both immediate and delayed hypersensitivity reactions, especially the latter and, with the waning, autoimmunity and cancer occur.

The immunodeficiency of aging can be estimated to be about 10 per cent dependent upon the environment in which the cells find themselves and about 90 per cent due to cellular, largely T cell, deficiencies. Even the declining antibody production with aging can in large part be explained on the basis of deficiencies in the T cell helper population.

EVOLUTIONARY ADVANTAGES OF ADAPTIVE IMMUNITY

We do not wish to comment on the reasons for evolutionary changes or the origin of the species of man, but merely point out that evolutionary changes do occur and that new species have emerged when mutational events have been advantageous. The development of a lymphoid system undoubtedly has been of importance to the survival of vertebrate animals, not only as protection from microbial invasion but also possibly providing a mechanism for surveillance to remove mutated clones of cells that bear antigenic differences from the host. This may be a major line of defense against virus invasion and even against cellular invasion. With an increasing complexity of genetic information being coded in the genome and with the increasing specialization of the individual cells of vertebrates, there has been a much greater opportunity for mutational events to occur. Many mutational events are lethal to the cell, but others lead to autonomy and neoplasia. One theory proposes that mutational events resulting in neoplasia probably occur repeatedly in normal individuals, and that these new cells may be recognized as being foreign and are destroyed by cellular surveillance mechanisms (Chapters 3, 4, and 14).

Perhaps not as evident is the overall advantage of replenishing older members of the species with younger and more vigorous ones. It is probable that programmed immunologic events play a significant role in the removal of effete individuals of the species as well as effete cells within the individual. By programmed involution of the lymphoid tissues, the individual becomes more susceptible to infection, less resistant to neoplastic change, and more prone to the development of fatal illness, including heart, vascular, renal, and autoimmune diseases.

ANTIGENS

Antigens may be defined as those molecular structures having chemical determinant groups capable of stimulating the elaboration of antibodies which have high specificity for combination with the reactant groups of the foreign molecule. The determinant groups of antigens may be as diverse as the possible variations in chemical structure, but the reaction site is usually exceedingly small and may involve as few as seven amino acids of the antibody molecule. The specificity of the reaction may be highly developed, and variations as minor as a change in the steric structure of a haptenic group can be recognized by specific antibody. Since a small change in size or shape may alter reactivity, most antigenic sites are relatively rigid.

While the chemical reactant sites determining the specificity of the antibody are relatively small, they must be part of a much larger molecule to be an effective antigen. Molecules having a molecular weight of less than 5000 rarely stimulate antibody production except as haptens. Haptens are chemicals of small molecular weight which themselves cannot elicit an antibody response, but which can provide antigenic specificity when they are conjugated with larger molecules. The larger molecule need not itself be immunogenic. Usually, as a molecule becomes larger and more complex, it becomes more effective an an antigen. Molecules of high molecular weight (500,000 or greater) with complex polypeptide-carbohydrate or protein structures and those with repeating structural units are among the best antigens and may even stimulate B lymphocytes directly. Pure proteins and pure carbohydrates may be strongly antigenic, but pure lipids are usually poor antigens. As the chemical structure of an antigen becomes more unlike the chemical structures of the animal into which it is injected, it becomes more likely to stimulate antibody production. Some antigens are extremely potent, eliciting antibody responses when given in nanogram quantities, while others can be effective as antigens only when given with adjuvants (see Chapter 10). Some antigens, such as endotoxin, stimulate primarily IgM production, whereas others stimulate primarily IgG or IgE.

With every antigenic stimulation, there are undoubtedly many effects on lymphoid cells. In the same animal, tolerance, immunologic memory, the development of delayed hypersensitivity, and the production of circulating antibody may occur. One important factor in the kind of response elicited by an antigen is the route of administration. Immunization by the intravenous or intraperitoneal routes tends to stimulate the production of circulating antibody to a greater degree than delayed hypersensitivity, but intravenous injection is also the route most likely to produce tolerance. Intradermal injection usually provides a much stronger stimulus than does subcutaneous or intramuscular injection. When antigen is given mixed with complete Freund's adjuvant, very high levels of circulating antibody may be produced, and delayed hypersensitivity is also strongly stimulated. Injection of antigen with Freund's adjuvant in the footpads is the most likely route to produce delayed hypersensitivity in animals. Antigen processing is discussed in Chapters 3 and 4.

3

Lymphocytes and Their Function

The origin of lymphocytes can be traced to pleuripotent stem cells, first found in the embryonic yolk sac, then the fetal liver, and lastly in the bone marrow. Evidently, this stem cell can give rise to slightly more committed stem cells which are precursors for either lymphocyte series or the hematopoietic series (Fig. 3–1). While lymphocytes are ultimately derived from the same type of stem cell, there is clear evidence that lymphocytes mature into two separate and distinct lymphoid systems under the influence of signals derived from their local microenvironment in early development (Fig. 3–2). It was later found that the cells of the two systems have very complex interactions with one another within each system and between the two sys-

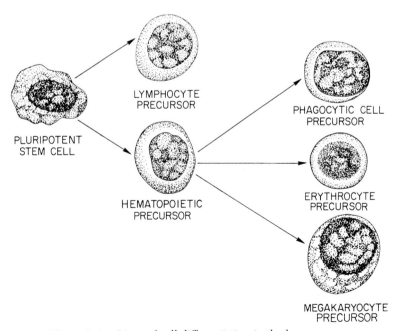

Figure 3–1. Lines of cell differentiation in the bone marrow.

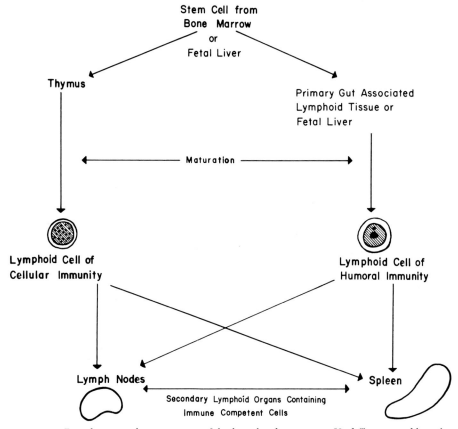

Figure 3–2.   Developmental organization of the lymphoid structures. Undifferentiated lymphoid precursors which develop in the yolk sac, liver, or bone marrow are released into the circulation and populate either the thymus or gut-associated primary lymphoid structures. Under the influence of these primary lymphoid organs, the cells undergo a process of maturation and become committed to being the type of lymphocyte that is effective in expressing either cellular immunity or the production of specific immunoglobulins. After release from the primary lymphoid organs, they circulate and populate the secondary lymphoid organs, the spleen, and lymph nodes.

tems. These interactions involve both helper and suppressor influences, and the full consequences of these cellular interactions in health and disease are just now being understood.

ORGANIZATION OF THE LYMPHOID SYSTEM

THE DUAL SYSTEM

The first evidence for a dual system of lymphoid cells came from studying genetic and acquired immunodeficiencies in clinical medicine. However, the most conclusive evidence of a division within the lymphoid system came from analysis of the differential influences of the thymus and bursa of Fabricius in chickens. The bursa of Fabricius is a small lymphoid organ derived from an outpouching of the hindgut of birds. If thymectomies are done in chickens at the time of hatching, and the chicks are irradiated to destroy lymphoid cells that have already peripheralized, the birds develop a profound deficiency of cellular immunity, i.e., the ability to express allograft rejection, graft versus host responses, and delayed hypersensitivity. If, instead, a bursectomy is done, and the chicks are irradiated or treated with cyclophosphamide shortly after hatching, they become totally agammaglobulinemic and fail to respond to an antigenic stimulus by producing circulating antibody. On the other hand, they readily reject homografts and develop delayed allergic reactions. Examination of the peripheral lymphoid structures in these two experimental models shows that ablation of the thymus causes a diminution in circulating lymphocytes and small lymphocytes of the thymic-dependent areas of the lymphoid organs (Fig. 3–3). Very few small lymphocytes can be found in the spleen and lymph nodes, but germinal centers are intact, and plasma cells are numerous. When the bursa has been destroyed or removed, the opposite is true. Many small lymphocytes may be found and circulating lymphocyte levels are normal, but germinal centers disappear and no plasma cells can be found. These findings have clearly demonstrated that there are two primary systems of lymphoid tissues in the chicken, one being dependent upon maturation of T lymphocytes under thymic control and the other dependent upon maturation of B lymphocytes in the bursa of Fabricius. The control of maturation appears to be exercised by epithelial cells derived from ectodermal-entodermal interaction that provide a specialized environment.

It has been possible to remove the bursa of the developing embryo while it is still in the egg, and these studies show that the bursa of Fabricius in the chicken is the only site where lymphocyte differentiation to antibody-producing cells occurs. They also prove that differentiation of cells with the

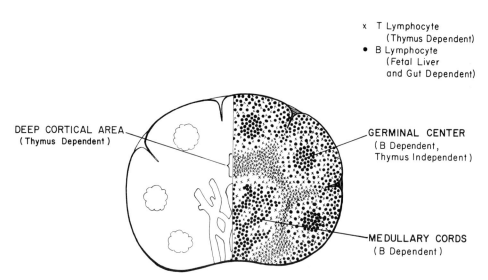

Figure 3–3.   Diagrammatic sketch of a lymph node showing the T dependent and B dependent areas.

capacity to synthesize IgM occurs within the chicken bursa before the differentiation of the capacity to synthesize IgG and IgA. The synthesis of IgM by the bursal lymphocyte precursors begins about the 12th day of embryogenesis, and IgM is expressed on the surface of the cells by the 14th day. Rapid proliferation of the bursal cells leads to formation of small follicles. Release of the bursal cells to populate the secondary lymphoid structures occurs about the 17th day, and bursectomy before this time will usually render the chicken totally and permanently agammaglobulinemic. The developmental ability to produce IgG and to release IgG-producing cells follows a tempo similar to that for IgM. Bursectomy at 19 days of development will result in a chicken that can produce IgM but not IgG or IgA. Bursectomy at hatching often results in a selective deficiency of IgA.

The epithelial thymus develops from the branchial clefts, whereas the epithelial bursa develops from an epithelial outpouching of the proctodeal plate of the dorsal cloaca at the posterior end of the intestinal tract. Prior to hatching, the thymus is also populated by undifferentiated cells which mature under the influence of the epithelial components to become populations of lymphoid cells committed to performing functions of cell-mediated immunity. After maturation, they begin to circulate and populate the secondary lymphoid organs (spleen and lymph nodes).

Since mammals have no organ similar to the bursa of Fabricius, it was thought for some time that the findings in the chicken had little to do with the development of active immunity in humans. However, it has recently been shown that functions equivalent to those of the bursa of Fabricius can be attributed to the fetal liver, and most investigators now feel that later in life, the bone marrow can exert an influence similar to that of the bursae in fowls. Some evidence seemed to link the appendix, intestinal tonsil (sacculus rotundus), and Peyer's patches in rabbits and dogs, the so-called gut-associated lymphoid tissue (GALT), to an equivalent of bursal function. However, the best present evidence is that GALT serves as a major expanding site for certain T and B lymphocyte populations. In mice, it is argued that the lymphoid cells of the B system develop in either the bone marrow or the liver. Lymphocytes developing commitment under influence of the thymus are commonly known as T cells, and lymphocytes developing commitment for immunoglobulin synthesis under influence of the bursa or its mammalian equivalent are known as B cells.

A spectrum of immunologic deficiency diseases in man has been described that supports the concept of an independent development of T cells and B cells. The three human diseases that closely parallel the experimental models produced by extirpation of the bursa or both thymus and bursa in neonatal chickens are the Bruton type of agammaglobulinemia, the DiGeorge syndrome, and the Swiss type of agammaglobulinemia.

In the Bruton type of agammaglobulinemia, the thymus and T lymphocytes are normal, but there is a deficiency of the development of B cell components of the lymphoid tissues. Clinically, cellular immunity in these patients is normal, but there is an almost complete absence of circulating immunoglobulins, and a lack of germinal centers and plasma cells. The number of lymphocytes in the circulation is normal, as is lymphocyte development in the areas of the lymphatic tissues that have been shown in experimental animals to be thymus dependent.

In the DiGeorge syndrome, there is a failure of development of the epithelial anlage of the third and fourth pharyngeal pouches, with consequent absence of the thymus and parathyroid glands. The gut-associated lymphoid tissues are normal in their development and appearance, and B lymphocytes predominate in blood and lymphoid tissues. By contrast, T lymphocytes are absent or present in very small numbers. Clinically, patients having this syndrome exhibit marked deficiencies of cellular immunity, but have normal levels of immunoglobulins. These patients can produce antibodies well to many antigens, although a diminished response to some is seen, and they have well-developed plasma cells. In the third type, severe combined immunodeficiency (Swiss type), there are marked developmental abnormalities of both the B lymphoid tissues and thymus-derived lymphoid tissues. Children with this disease have striking deficiencies of both cellular and humoral immunity, and they usually die before two years of age.

These and other related syndromes will be discussed in greater detail in Chapter 19. They are mentioned here as substantial support for the concept of the development of two lymphoid systems in man: one which requires the thymus for the maturation of lymphoid T cells having to do with the cellular type of immunity, and the other which may depend upon the gut-associated lymphoid tissues or bone marrow for maturation of lymphoid B cells which produce immunoglobulins.

Population of the peripheral lymphoid organs (spleen and lymph nodes) by T and B cells from the central lymphoid structures occurs in mice and chickens at or around the time of birth. Neonatal extirpation of the central lymphoid organs has a profound effect on immunological development in those species in which the population of the secondary lymphoid tissues has not occurred, but has little effect in those species in which population of the secondary lymphoid tissues takes place well before birth. If, for example, population of the secondary lymphoid structures occurs before the time of birth, as in the dog and man, neonatal thymectomy has little effect on the development of subsequent immune responses. If peripheralization has not occurred or is incomplete, as in the chicken, rat, and mouse, removal of the primary lymphoid tissues may have a profound effect on the development of immune responses. Neonatally thymectomized mice may be restored to normal by transplantation of a syngeneic thymus or by injection of large numbers of lymphocytes from the spleen, lymph nodes, or thymus, but not by bone marrow cells.

LYMPHOCYTE RECIRCULATION

In the adult animal, there is a continuous circulation of lymphocytes from the blood to the tissues and lymphoid structures, and back to the blood stream. Lymphocytes may enter peripheral tissues and be carried to the first draining lymph node, but a far more important mechanism is entry directly from the blood stream. Lymphocytes may exit from the circulation through

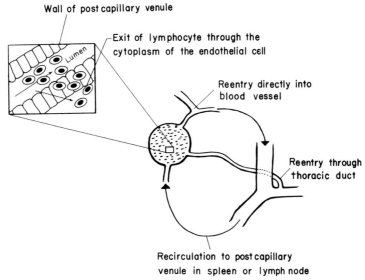

Figure 3-4. Diagrammatic sketch of the circulatory cycle of lymphocytes. The lymphocytes which circulate in this fashion are primarily of thymus dependent origin. In the spleen, reentry into the blood vessels occurs directly, while lymphocytes from lymph nodes reenter the circulation via the thoracic duct.

morphologically specialized endothelial cells of the postcapillary venules of the lymph nodes, but they also exit through capillaries, small vessels in spleen, and other sites. After a variable period of residence in the lymph nodes or spleen, they may reenter the circulation directly (spleen) or via lymphatic channels and the thoracic duct (lymph nodes) (Fig. 3-4). This concept of repopulation and recirculation by lymphocytes is important in understanding the effector mechanisms of committed lymphocytes.

Both B cells and T cells may recirculate, but B cell recirculation is slower and B cells tend to be more sessile in the hematopoietic and lymphoid tissues. In thoracic duct lymph, about 85 per cent of the cells are T cells.

SECONDARY (PERIPHERAL) LYMPHOID STRUCTURES

The secondary or peripheral lymphoid structures perform exceedingly important functions, being the home of both T and B cells. In these structures occur antigen processing, induction of the immune response, differentiation and maturation of cells, and release of effector substances. Most of these processes are reviewed later, but the general structure is discussed here.

Lymph Nodes. The structure of a lymph node is shown diagrammatically in Figure 3-3. It can be divided into three general areas: the outer cortical lymphoid concentration containing the germinal centers, the deep cortical areas, and the medulla which contains the cords. Both B and T lymphocytes enter the node through the peripheral sinuses by exiting into

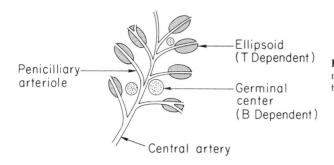

Penicilliary arteriole — Ellipsoid (T Dependent)

Germinal center (B Dependent)

Central artery

Figure 3–5. Diagrammatic representation of the white pulp of the spleen of a mouse.

the cortex via the postcapillary venules. For undetermined reasons, the B cells find their way to the follicles and the T cells "home" to the deep cortical areas. The medullary cords contain mostly B cells, including many plasma cells, and it is there that antibody formation occurs. Phagocytic cells or macrophages line the sinusoids and are scattered throughout the node. Highly specialized dendritic "macrophages" are located in the sites where germinal centers develop and in the deep cortical areas as well. Recent evidence from ultrastructural study has shown that these dendritic cells are different in the T and B dependent regions of the lymphoid tissues.

Spleen. The spleen is composed of white pulp and red pulp. The white pulp (Fig. 3–5) is represented by dense collections of lymphocytes located about arterioles after they leave the trabeculae. These vessels later divide into penicilliary arterioles having a characteristic spindle-shaped sheath, and then form capillaries and sinuses. The red pulp is composed of cords and long sinuses lined by elongated spindle-shaped cells. B cells are found in the follicles, which are typically located between bifurcating penicilliary arteries and in the red pulp (plasma cells). T cells tend to collect in perivascular lymphoid sheaths around the central and penicilliary arterioles, but are also found in smaller proportion in the red pulp and in the mantle zone about germinal centers. Unlike lymph nodes, lymphocytes from the spleen exit back directly into the circulation, although a few leave via lymphatics.

Gut-Associated Lymphoid Tissues. In mammals, these are represented by the tonsils, Peyer's patches, appendix, sacculus rotundus (in some species), and lamina propria. While they may play a central role, they also clearly have secondary roles especially involved in expansion of the local antibody synthesis and cellular immune systems. Indeed, there is evidence that they are especially involved local domains of immunologic function, which include entero-enteric and apparently an entero-pulmonic and entero-mammomic lymphoid cell circulation.

T LYMPHOCYTES

Lymphocytes can be divided generally into small, long-lived cells and larger, short-lived cells. T cells and B cells may be of either type and cannot be differentiated by this criterion, although circulating small lymphocytes

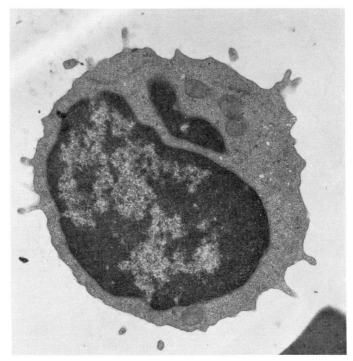

Figure 3–6. Electron micrograph of a normal human small lymphocyte. (Courtesy of Drs. J. G. White and C. C. Clawson.)

(Fig. 3–6) are most often T cells, accounting for about 75 per cent of blood lymphocytes. Morphologic criteria also do not separate T cells from B cells, even when the electron microscope is used. However, by scanning electron microscopy, B cells usually can be seen to have a more "hairy" surface, with numerous cytoplasmic projections, whereas T cells tend to have a smoother surface. Both form blast cells when stimulated by either antigen or nonspecific mitogens. The best means for differentiating these two populations of lymphocytes are by surface markers and studies of function of purified cells and of functional defects of immunity in animals or patients lacking a specific kind of cell (Table 3–1). The last technique was discussed above.

SURFACE MARKERS OF T CELLS

Specific Antigens

In the mouse, where studies are most complete, several well-defined differentiation antigens located on the cell membrane have been characterized by alloantisera (Fig. 3–7). The θ or Thy-1 antigen is perhaps the best known and is also expressed on brain cells. Certain alloantigens called Ly antigens are restricted to the T lymphocytes (Ly 1,2,3), while others are found on both B and T cells or only B cells. The Ly $1+2-3-$ phenotype cells contain the cell populations that are capable of exerting helper cell func-

TABLE 3–1. DISTINGUISHING CHARACTERISTICS OF HUMAN T
AND B LYMPHOCYTES

	T Lymphocytes	B Lymphocytes
Maturation of precursor cells	Thymus	Fetal liver Gut-associated lymphoid tissue (?) Bone marrow (?)
Location in lymph nodes	Deep cortical region	Germinal centers and medullary cords
Electrophoretic mobility	High	Low
Surface by scanning electron microscopy	Tends to be smooth	Tends to be more hairy
Forms rosettes with sheep erythrocytes	Yes	No
Specific antigens by absorbed heteroimmune sera	Yes – raised against thymus	Yes – raised against chronic lymphatic leukemia or other B cell sources
Surface receptor for Fc of IgG	No in most; yes for small sub- population	Yes
Surface receptor for C3b	No	Yes
Presence of surface immuno- globulin	No	Yes
Responsiveness to: PHA and Con-A Pokeweed mitogen *E. coli* lipopolysaccharide	 High High Low	 Low High, in presence of T lymphocytes High
Basis of surface specificity and capacity to combine with antigen	V region Ig on cell surface constituents	IgM or IgM and IgD, other immunoglob- ulins

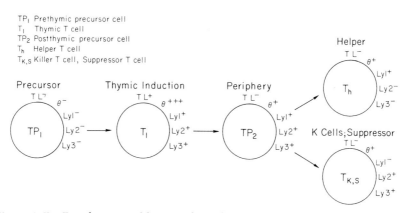

Figure 3–7. Development of functional subclasses of T lymphocytes of the mouse.

tions. The Ly 1−2+3+ phenotype is associated with the killer cell functions for allogeneic tumor cells and also the suppressor T cell functions thus far defined in the mouse. Cells with an Ly 1+2+3+ phenotype seem to be a more labile population of cells, that can act as precursors of the stable Ly 1+2−3− or Ly 1−2+3+ phenotypes. Ly 1+2−3− cells comprise some 30 per cent of the circulating and peripheral lymphoid cells in the mouse, Ly 1−2+3+ approximately 10 per cent, and the Ly 1+2+3+ phenotype, 50 to 60 per cent.

In some strains of mice a so-called TL surface alloantigen is found on the thymocytes, but this antigen is lost when the cells enter the peripheral compartments. The TL+ phenotype on peripheral lymphoid cells, however, may be present on leukemic lymphocytes that are derived within the thymus from thymus lymphoid cells or their precursors. These cells, like those of certain human leukemias, may also possess the enzyme terminal transferase (Tdt), which can serve as an additional marker of the cells.

In humans, alloantibodies with specificity for T cells can be found in the sera of some patients with lupus erythematosus, infectious mononucleosis, or other diseases. Specific antisera to T cells can be made by the immunization of animals with thymocytes and cross-absorption with the purified B lymphocytes to remove common lymphocyte antigens. Alloantibodies that recognize antigen specifically on all or some T lymphocytes have recently been discovered in serum of some grand multiparae. Such antisera may very well form a basis for the dissection of the T lymphocyte subclasses in man parallel to that so characteristic of the mouse. Recently, C4 has also been demonstrated on the surface of lymphocytes which are presumably T cells.

Erythrocytes and Other Receptors. Human T cells have surface receptors that react with sheep erythrocytes, forming rosettes with red cells about a central T lymphocyte. T cells from other species rosette with heterologous erythrocytes of different specificity. For example, guinea pig T cells rosette with rabbit erythrocytes. The receptors involved are not immunoglobulin in nature, and T cells do not react with antisera to immunoglobulins. Some human T cells also have receptors for the Fc portion of IgG, but this is also possessed by B cells. As cells age or become activated, some receptors are less well expressed. By a rosetting method, using as indicators ox red blood cells coated with purified IgM or IgG antibodies to the ox erythrocyte, it has been shown that human T lymphocytes can be divided into two populations that have receptors either for μ or γ heavy chain components. These two populations of human T cells seem to exert differing roles in immune reactions. The T cells with receptors for μ determinants seem to act as helper cells in the differentiation of B cells to immunoglobulin synthesizing and secreting cells. By contrast, the T cells with IgG (γ) receptors permit only proliferation after stimulation and may act to inhibit development of plasma cells and immunoglobulin synthesis.

Those characteristics by which the members of T cells and B cells and third population lymphocytes can be enumerated are summarized in Table 3–2.

Response to Mitogens. T lymphocytes respond to phytohemagglutinin (PHA) in solution with a brisk mitogenic response and the production of

TABLE 3–2.   SURFACE MARKER AND RESPONSE CHARACTERISTICS
OF CIRCULATING LYMPHOCYTES

T LYMPHOCYTES	B LYMPHOCYTES	THIRD POPULATION OF LYMPHOCYTES
Rosette spontaneously with sheep RBC	Do not rosette with sheep RBC	Do not rosette with sheep RBC
Lack readily demonstrable surface membrane Ig	Have readily demonstrable surface membrane Ig	Lack surface membrane Ig
Respond by proliferation to PHA, Con-A, and pokeweed mitogens	Respond by proliferation after stimulation with pokeweed mitogen	Do not respond to mitogens by stimulation
Activated cell develops receptors for Fc portion if IgG	Have relatively low affinity receptors for Fc for Fc portion of IgG.	Have high avidity receptors for Fc portion of IgG Revealed by rosetting with RhD antisera (Ripley rosettes)
Proliferate in response to allogeneic cells	Do not proliferate in response to allogeneic cells	Do not proliferate in response to allogeneic cells
Proliferate in response to antigen in solution. Have specific antigens on their surface which can be recognized by allo- or heteroantisera. Θ or Thy 1, Ly 123 in mouse, HTLA in man	Do not proliferate when stimulated by most soluble antigens. In presence of T cells, proliferate and differentiate to plasma cells after stimulation with pokeweed mitogen	Do not proliferate when stimulated by soluble antigens to which host is immunized. May act as antibody dependent cytotoxic lymphocytes

lymphokines. Similarly, T lymphocytes respond by proliferation to the plant lectin concanavallin A (Con-A), and both T and B lymphocytes respond by proliferation to pokeweed mitogen (Table 3–2).

INDUCTION OF IMMUNITY IN T CELLS

When antigen is presented to the peripheral tissues, it may reach the lymph nodes via the afferent lymphatics as soluble or free antigen, or be engulfed by macrophages. The unprocessed antigen is either taken up by macrophages or becomes localized on the processes of dendritic reticular cells within the follicles. The role of macrophages in antigen processing and transfer is discussed in Chapter 4. The thymus dependent areas rapidly differentiate many blast cells, which can soon be detected in the circulation (three to four days). The blast cells divide to produce a progeny of small lymphocytes that mediate cellular immune responses and may be considered to be immune T cells or antigen-reactive T cells. Some of them surely have the property of immunologic memory. Memory T cells later appear as small lymphocytes in the thoracic duct and, as long-lived lymphocytes, they circulate and recirculate through blood and lymph lymphoid tissues. For reasons that are poorly understood, perhaps because of different types of processing by macrophages, immunity to certain antigens tends to stimulate T cell responses more than B cell responses. These antigens include histoplasmin, antigens of other fungi, tuberculin, certain viruses, and histocompatibility antigens.

ANTIGEN RECEPTORS OF T LYMPHOCYTES

The precise nature of the antigen receptor on the surface of T lymphocytes remains a matter of considerable debate. However, there are compelling reasons to believe that it is very much like an immunoglobulin in its specificity. A hypothetical scheme that we advanced in 1970 seems to remain the most plausible explanation (Fig. 3–8). Several observations support this hypothesis: (1) The immunoglobulins are synthesized in segments and later united to form the intact molecule. Variable and constant portions are under different DNA instruction; (2) Antisera to Fab, especially the antigen combining site (as with antiidiotype antibody), inhibits mixed lymphocyte cultures, graft versus host reactions, and antigen binding to T cells; and (3) Specificities of receptors for antigens are identical to those for immunoglobulin antibodies, with only a few exceptions.

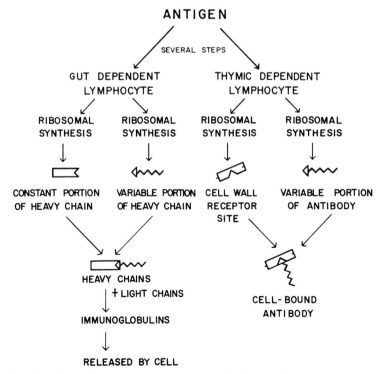

Figure 3–8. Hypothetical similarities between antibody synthesis by gut dependent (B) lymphocytes and thymus dependent (T) lymphocytes.

Since the antigen receptor of T lymphocytes is cellbound, the cell-mediated reactions of delayed hypersensitivity and graft versus host cannot be transferred with serum. The T cell surface antibody may be composed of cell surface components besides the combining site.

When an antigen is introduced into a sensitized individual, it localizes, at least in part, in the lymphoid tissues. Antigen reactive T lymphocytes seem to be recruited to areas of antigen localization and soon exhibit a brisk proliferative response. Localization, however, may not be specific except in the direct vicinity of the antigen.

Transfer Factor

Several investigators have now presented evidence to support the existence of a previously controversial material, transfer factor, which can be extracted from the lymphocytes of humans who express defined delayed hypersensitivity reactions. Administration of transfer factor to nonsensitized individuals facilitates development of delayed sensitivity and the presence of specific receptors on T lymphocytes. Transfer factor is dialyzable (MW < 10,000, perhaps nearer 2000 D), stable at 37°C for six hours, and resistant to treatment with DNase, RNase, and trypsin. For unknown reasons, transfer factor has been poorly demonstrable in animals that express delayed hypersensitivity reactions very well, or in any animal other than man. Although there no longer is any serious question that transfer factor exists, many of the phenomena attributed to it remain controversial, and its ability to confer specificity has been questioned. Evidence now indicates that the low molecular dialysate of lymphocytes contains a material that greatly enhances the T cell–mediated responses to complete antigens and even haptenes like 2-4 dinitrochlorobenzene (DNCB), which can couple to the body's proteins as a carrier. If transfer factor is, indeed, acting nonspecifically, we may have been wrong in trying to require it to act specifically in precisely controllable animal systems.

In spite of this new evidence of its lack of specificity, clinical evidence in man shows that transfer factor can beneficially influence some of the most recalcitrant of human diseases. These include chronic mucocutaneous candidiasis and certain of the immunodeficiency diseases, such as the Wiskott-Aldrich syndrome.

Functions of T Cells

Immunologic reactions that require the participation of living lymphocytes have been recognized for many years, but our understanding of cell-mediated immunity, including so-called delayed hypersensitivity and transplantation immunity, has only recently been great enough to formulate meaningful and definitive concepts. Cell-mediated immune reactions are of profound importance in antimicrobial defense, autoimmune diseases, certain acquired allergies — especially to chemicals and drugs, transplantation rejection, and defense against cancer. These are discussed in detail in later chapters. Complete inability to develop and express this important defense mechanism is not compatible with long life.

Delayed hypersensitivity skin reactions typify the biological changes that accompany cell-mediated immune reactions. When tuberculin or some other appropriate antigen is injected intradermally in a suitably sensitized individual, an erythematous, indurated lesion develops slowly, reaching its maximum size in 48 to 72 hours. These changes then regress slowly over a period of several days. The early lesion is characterized microscopically by a mild neutrophilic inflammatory cellular response, with the accumulation of only a few lymphocytes within the first few hours, but, during the subsequent 48 to 72 hours, the injection site becomes densely infiltrated with interstitial mononuclear cells resembling both lymphocytes and macrophages.

The migration of lymphocytes into an inflammatory lesion is an expected consequence following almost any type of stimulus that causes an initial accumulation of neutrophils. In sensitized individuals, binding of antigen to specific receptor sites on T lymphocytes provides the stimulus that initiates a number of biologically important events, including direct cytotoxicity by the activated cell and the elaboration of substances known as lymphokines. While T lymphocytes are the source of some lymphokines, it is likely that other cells produce many of them. The role of these activated cells and lymphokines is discussed in more detail in several subsequent chapters (8, 13, 14, 15), but a brief description of the lymphokines seems warranted here.

LYMPHOKINES

Macrophage Migration Inhibiting Factor.   When cells from a peritoneal exudate of an animal are put into capillary tubes and placed into an appropriate viewing chamber containing tissue culture medium, the macrophages migrate radially from the end of the tube. If one adds to the medium minute quantities of an antigen to which the animal expresses a delayed hypersensitivity type of reaction, the macrophages fail to migrate from the capillary tube. Antigens that do not cause delayed hypersensitivity reactions in that animal do not cause an inhibition of macrophage migration when added to the medium. This test, therefore, provides a highly specific in vitro correlation of delayed hypersensitivity in the intact animal (see Fig. 11–7).

It was soon found that sensitized lymphocytes in the peritoneal exudate were responsible for this phenomenon. Within six hours after specific antigen reacts with the receptors of sensitized lymphocytes, the cells actively begin to synthesize and release a glycoprotein which is known as macrophage migration inhibitory factor (MMIF). MMIF has a molecular weight approximating 50,000, is destroyed by trypsin and neuraminidase but not by DNase or RNase, and does not lose activity when heated at 56°C for 30 minutes. Lymphocyte transformation is not required for the synthesis of MMIF, but MMIF itself has mitogenic properties and may cause blast formation. It has now been convincingly separated from macrophage activating factor (MAF), which can increase activity and aggressiveness of macrophages. It has not been proven to be significantly cytotoxic. Small numbers of lymphocytes can produce enough MMIF to inhibit the migration of a great many macrophages, and the biological effect of MMIF on macrophages is not species specific.

MMIF has not been isolated in an entirely pure form, but injections of relatively pure preparation into the skin will cause the development of lesions that are entirely similar to typical delayed hypersensitivity reactions, except that the evolution of the lesion is accelerated by about 24 hours. From these observations, it seems likely that at least one biological effect of MMIF is to promote the delivery of mononuclear phagocytes to sites of inflammation mediated by hypersensitivity reactions that involve T lymphocytes.

LMIF.   Distinct from MMIF is a substance that is liberated by T lymphocytes on contact with PHA, Con-A, antigens to which the host has been sensitized, and allogeneic cells. This glycoprotein has a molecular weight of 70–80,000 D and acts selectively to stimulate migration of purified populations of polymorphonuclear leukocytes. LMIF and the LMIF response can be precisely quantified and this test is used as one of the most reliable in vitro indices of cell-mediated, T cell dependent immune responses.

Chemotactic Factors.   A chemotactic factor for macrophages and another for neutrophils have been described. There is also possibly a lymphokine chemotactic for lymphocytes.

Mitogens.   Lymphokines have been partially purified that will stimulate the division of lymphocytes, being both antigen dependent and antigen independent.

Interferon.   This is an inducer of an antiviral state in cells. It is produced by T lymphocytes, among other cells, and is released by these cells upon stimulation of lymphocytes by antigens to which the host has been sensitized. There may be several forms of interferon (discussed in more detail in Chapter 13).

Others.   Cytotoxic factors, growth inhibitory factors, maturation factors, skin-reactive factors, and several other lymphokines have also been described. It is likely that some of these are identical to others and have several biologic functions.

B LYMPHOCYTES

Surface Markers and Receptors

Unlike T Cells, B cells do not form rosettes with unmodified erythrocytes from sheep. However, recent studies indicate that a subset of human B lymphocytes forms rosettes with mouse erythrocytes. B lymphocytes also have receptors for the Fc portion of IgG and for C3b (Fig. 3–9). Therefore, erythrocytes reacted with specific IgG antibody, or whose surface has been coated with C3b by any mechanism, will form rosettes with B lymphocytes. Various classes of immunoglobulin may be expressed on the surface of B

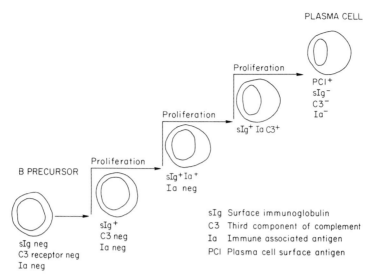

Figure 3-9. Surface markers in differentiation of B lymphocytes.

lymphocytes, but any one cell generally expresses only one type of Ig. A notable exception is that IgM and IgD are both present on the surface of many B cells. Most of the B cells in circulating blood possess IgM surface immunoglobulin and a large proportion possesses both IgM and IgD immunoglobulins. This finding raises important questions concerning the function of IgD in the body economy. By studying the surface Ig and markers on cells in human embryos, it has been established that IgM is the first Ig that appears on the surface of B lymphocytes. In embryos of 10 to 12 weeks, it is the only Ig at the surface of the cells. IgD next makes its appearance, followed later by a switch of some cells to IgG and IgA. Capacity to rosette with mouse red blood cells appears at least as early during development of B lymphocytes as ability to produce surface IgM.

RESPONSES TO MITOGENS

Both T and B cells can respond by proliferation to most mitogens when the latter are presented properly to them, but there are differences in the degree of responsiveness. B cells are much more specifically stimulated by lipopolysaccharide and poorly stimulated by PHA or Con-A when the latter is in solution. However, if PHA or Con-A is placed on the surface of latex beads, B lymphocytes can be made to respond to these T cell mitogens. The biological significance of their responsiveness is not yet clear, even though responsiveness to these lectins is useful for assessing lymphocyte functional status in disease.

INDUCTION OF IMMUNITY IN B LYMPHOCYTES

The specificity of antibody molecules for greatly diverse types of antigens with seemingly endless variations has been a subject of great interest and considerable controversy. Incredibly, in 1900 Ehrlich advanced a theory of antibody formation which supposed that antigen molecules combined with preexisting sites on the surface of cells, stimulating the cells to synthesize specific antibody. Because of the very large number of possible antigenic specificities to which animals can respond by specific immunization, it was later felt that antibody formation was antigen-instructed, perhaps by a template, either directly or indirectly.

Abundant evidence to the contrary, however, has now been gathered, and most authorities support the view that an expansion of a population of genetically precommitted cells, as first proposed by Jerne in 1955, is the basis of both cell-mediated and humoral immunity and the most plausible explanation for antibody specificity. Burnet formalized this view into the concept of clonal selection in 1957. This theory presupposes that the initial recognition of an antigen occurs by interaction with antibody receptors that have arisen spontaneously in the absence of antigen and are present on few among many lymphocytes. Therefore, the role of antigen is to stimulate a specific clone of lymphocytes to expand, and to synthesize immunoglobulin that reacts to that antigen. As yet, it is unclear how so many diverse clones of lymphocytes are produced. Some favor a germ line theory of development of this heterogenicity and others favor some form of rapid somatic mutation. To our view, however, most studies support the clonal selection hypothesis and the germ line theory of development of antibody diversity.

Most compellingly, experiments in animals have shown that B cells have antigen-reactive receptors on their cell surface that will bind to antigen. These cells are often called antigen-reactive cells or antigen-binding cells. In nonstimulated or nonimmunized animals, approximately 1 of 10,000 to 1 of 100,000 B lymphocytes are reactive cells for a given antigen. Antigenic stimulation may increase the number of antigen-reactive cells as much as 1000-fold, or up to 1 to 3 per cent of the total lymphocytes. Experiments using the technique of passing lymphocytes through a column in which an antigen is linked to an inert substance, such as a glass bead, have shown that antigen-reactive cells can be depleted by a specific antigen. By injecting cells from one animal, which have been depleted by adsorption to a specific antigen, into an irradiated recipient, it is possible to show that, after recovery from irradiation, the recipient remains unable to react to that particular antigen by producing antibody whereas he may react normally to the injection of other antigens. Experiments using radioactive antigens to kill antigen-binding cells have similarly shown that reaction to specific antigen can be selectively abolished.

The antigen-reactive sites of B cells are clearly immunoglobulin in nature. In man, blood lymphocytes predominantly have both IgM and IgD on their cell surface. A few have exclusively IgD or IgM and about 2 per cent have exclusively IgG, predominantly IgG2. A very small number carry exclusively IgA or IgE. It has been determined that in the nonimmunized animal, antigen-reactive cells contain IgM on their surface and not IgG. In this regard, antibody against the μ heavy and light chains, but not against the γ heavy chain, will block the induction of an immune response.

PATCHING AND CAPPING

Surface immunoglobulin on B lymphocytes has been investigated using fluorescinated or radiolabeled antiimmunoglobulin reagents. When first reacted, the antiimmunoglobulin is uniformly distributed over the surface of the cell. However, after reaction with antibody, it soon forms a patchy distribution as small immune complexes form on the cell surface. These spots soon agglomerate on the end of the cell opposite the Golgi apparatus to form a polar cap, an active membrane movement requiring metabolic activity. The cap is soon internalized by endocytosis and the cell surface remains devoid of immunoglobulin for 15 to 30 minutes. However, surface immunoglobulin is fully restored within 6 to 8 hours. This precise phenomenon occurs when multivalent antigen reacts with specific immunoglobulin receptors on the cell membrane. It is this process of patching, capping, and internalization of the antigen-antibody complex that seems to trigger proliferation of the cell, initiation of further differentiation under appropriate circumstances, and the formation and secretion of a specific antibody. The clonal selection theory of antibody synthesis is further supported by the observation that individual lymphocytes form only a single antibody when stimulated, and it is of one heavy chain isotype and one allotype. Also, a single cell expresses only one receptor specificity. It has a single idiotype.

On the other hand, it is clear that single cells may switch from IgM synthesis to IgG synthesis and probably synthesis of IgA and IgE in certain instances. The role of IgD on the surface of lymphocytes is uncertain at the present time. Once stimulated to proliferation by specific antigenic stimulus, the B cells may give rise to the memory B cells or, upon further differentiation, plasma cells which are highly specialized for antibody synthesis and secretion (pumper cells).

The important interactions of lymphoid cells of different classes with one another and with macrophages to achieve differentiation, plasma cell development, Ig synthesis, and secretion of antibodies are discussed later in this chapter.

FUNCTION

From the above discussion, it is apparent that B cells function primarily to form a recognition unit capable of the elaboration of specific antibody when primed by an antigenic challenge. As discussed later, this antibody primarily functions to provide specificity for an amplification process leading to powerful defense against foreign invaders, immunologically mediated injury, or even protection from immunological injury.

K CELLS, NULL CELLS, OR THIRD POPULATION LYMPHOCYTES

Besides the T and B cells, a third major population of lymphocytes in the peripheral blood exists, some of which are called K cells because they can participate in antibody dependent cytotoxicity phenomena. Sometimes they are referred to as null cells because they lack the markers characteristic for T cells or B cells. The best surface marker for these cells is that they form rosettes with human RhD+ cells that have been coated by apparent monovalent antibodies against RhD antigen. Such antisera were originally identified in a patient whose name was Ripley, and the rosettes formed with the third population cells are sometimes called "Ripley rosettes." This third population of lymphoid cells lacks readily demonstrable surface Ig, but the cells carry highly avid membrane receptors for C3 and the Fc portion of the IgG molecule, and may kill target cells sensitized with IgG antibody (antibody dependent cell-mediated cytotoxicity). They are not phagocytic.

CELL INTERACTIONS

A decade ago, the lymphoid system seemed to be falling nicely into two broad categories of cells that dealt with completely independent functions. T cells were involved with cell-mediated immune reactions, including delayed hypersensitivity and allograft rejection, and B cells dealt solely with the synthesis and secretion of immunoglobulins. While it is clear that these two populations of cells do develop differently and have highly specialized and individualized functions, their interrelationships are seen to be increasingly complex, and these interactions now represent one of the most important components of modern immunobiology. At the present time, it is clear that important interactions occur between macrophages and T cells, macrophages and B cells, T cells and B cells, T cells and T cells, and all three types of cells acting synergistically to cooperate in an immune response.

T cell and B cell interaction has been of particular interest in this regard, and T cells can act either as helper cells or suppressor cells for B cell activity. The role of suppressor T cells will be discussed further in Chapter 9. In efforts to encompass the meaning of these complex cellular interactions, Jerne has proposed that the immune responses, like responses of the central and peripheral nervous systems, be visualized as a network of interacting cells and processes and considered in terms of theories that deal with the behavior of networks. It seems that many experiments and analyses in years to come will be designed and interpreted in this perspective.

Experiments in T cell–deficient animals with a normal B cell system have shown a poor response of antibody production to stimulation with the majority of antigens. However, certain antigens do seem to elicit a good response in the absence of T lymphocytes, and the antigens that stimulate B cells directly have usually been found to be polymeric in nature. Lipopolysaccharide endotoxin is an example of such an antigen. Such antigens are usually referred to as T independent antigens. T cells and B cells also often require the participation of macrophages, as evidenced by the observation that pure populations of lymphocytes have a markedly reduced or absent mitogenic response to the presentation of antigen. If mononuclear phagocytes are added to these purified populations of lymphocytes, restoration of the antigenic response is observed. Indeed, macrophages that contain antigens can induce antibody formation when injected into a nonimmunized recipient animal. The relationship of antigen transfer, however, is at best confusing since other investigations indicate that antigen-reactive T cells release a cytophilic mediator that becomes attached to macrophages. This leads to an arming of the macrophages which will then permit B cells to be stimulated by interaction with antigen. Thus, it appears that antibody formation by the B cells' response to a T dependent antigen may require three cells (the macrophage, T cell, and B cell) and that the B cells respond to a double signal.

Many experiments support the fact that hapten specificity is found in B cells, whereas the carrier determinants are present on T cells. Whether this results in a concentrating of antigen on the B cell surface or is essential to the two signal stimulation is not known with certainty.

Both in vitro and in vivo experiments have shown that the response of B cells can be enhanced by T cells, even when the T cell recognizes antigen that is on a molecule separate and distinctly different from that which stimulates the B cells. In this situation, it is likely that T cells release a mediator after reacting with an antigen, and that this mediator enhances the response of B cells to T dependent antigens by a nonspecific means. Support for the soluble nature of the mediator has come from experiments which indicate that cell-free supernatants of T cells activated by antigen have increased the response of B cells to an unrelated antigen. Macrophages may be important in the elaboration of some of these soluble mediators. How the mediators work has not been determined at this time.

Since T cell and B cell interactions are so important in the immune process, the reasons for the relatively clear formation of T cell and B cell dependent areas in the peripheral lymphoid tissues remain a puzzle. Perhaps the interaction takes place in the afferent lymphatics and sinuses entering the node. Studies of injection of antigen into chickens have shown that further interaction of B cells with macrophages may occur in the germinal centers. After the injection of human serum albumin, antibody appears in the circulation on about the fifth day, concurrent with a rise in plasma cells. Associated with the formation of antigen-antibody complex, there is localization of antigen first in and on macrophages around the penicilliary arterioles. Later, these antigen-bearing dendritic cells form clusters at the angles between the penicilliary arterioles, and this is associated with the formation of germinal centers (see Fig. 3–5). Within the germinal centers, there is intensive cellular proliferation of B cells. Presumably, this proliferation occurs because of a cloning of antigen-reactive cells within the germinal center. How the B cells migrate to the circulation or to the medullary cords in lymph nodes is still not clear. What is clear is that the dendritic cells present antigen on their surfaces to the B cells within the germinal center, and aid in the expansion of a B cell population reactive to that antigen. It has been postulated that the germinal centers are involved in expanding the B lymphoid systems, providing the site for quantal proliferation of lymphocytes that permits further differentiation to IgG- rather than IgM-producing cells. They may also be involved in some way in terminating responses to a particular antigen.

As mentioned, it appears that two signals are necessary for the elaboration of antibody by antigen-reactive B cells. The first signal involves interaction with antigen receptors on the cell membrane of the B cell, whereas the second signal is generated by T cells and/or macrophages interacting with the B cell when the involved T cells have been specifically stimulated by antigen. It is interesting that the IgG response to soluble antigen is usually more sensitive to T cell cooperation than the IgM response. Binding of T dependent antigens to B cell receptors occurs, but is insufficient to activate the cell to differentiation and antibody production. The cooperative factor may be either nonspecific or specific for T-B interaction.

It has been suggested that the second signal to B lymphocytes could be produced nonspecifically by the binding of activated C3 to the receptor on B cells. Development from precursor cells to fully differentiated B lymphocytes appears, in the mouse, to require a series of differentiation steps, each of which must stem from the former in the sequence. These relationships are indicated in Figure 3–9. This series of differentiations can be driven by the hormone ubiquitin which has been purified and fully defined chemically.

The molecular basis for the specific suppressive influence of T lymphocytes has recently been defined as including (a) the combining site with activity identical to that of specific immunoglobulin antibody, (b) the antigen toward which the specific suppressor response is directed, and (c) cell surface components that possess antigenic determinants of Ia.

4

Mononuclear Phagocytes

Mononuclear phagocytic cells are an essential component in all animal species, from man to the amoeba; in the latter instance, they are represented by the entire organism. The mononuclear phagocyte is a digestive cell throughout the animal kingdom, and the processes of phagocytosis and intracellular digestion by these cells have strong similarities among all animal species. They are derived from undifferentiated mesenchymal cells early in embryonic life, but their source may vary in adult life and also may vary from species to species. The mononuclear phagocytes of the blood are monocytes, but there are widely distributed tissue macrophages throughout the body, being particularly concentrated in the liver (Küpffer cells), spleen (littoral cells), lymph nodes (reticular cells), lung (dust cells), bone marrow, pituitary, and loose connective tissue. Specialized tissue macrophages are also found in the brain (microglia). Together, these mononuclear phagocytes constitute the reticuloendothelial system (RES). The fixed tissue macrophages of the RES are located primarily in the organs with a large blood supply, and one of the predominate functions of these cells is to remove particulate matter and effete cells. They also synthesize and release complement components, detoxify poisons, and process antigenic material.

ORIGIN AND DEVELOPMENT

The blood monocyte is the best studied of the mononuclear phagocytes in man and other higher vertebrates. It is the intermediate cell in the line that arises in the bone marrow and ends with a tissue macrophage (Fig. 4–1).

BONE MARROW PRECURSORS

Monoblasts are morphologically similar to myeloblasts, and it is uncertain whether these represent different cell lines or reflect common origin in pleuripotential precursors. Abundant evidence now indicates that the granu-

41

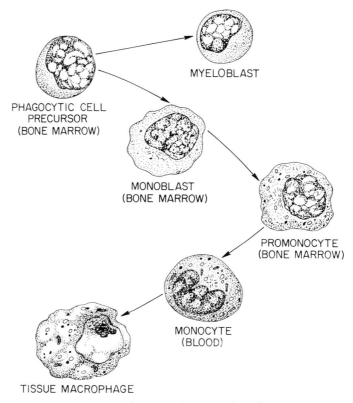

Figure 4–1.   Development of mononuclear phagocytes.

locytic series and mononuclear phagocytes share common stem cells in the bone marrow. In monocytic leukemia, cells presumed to be monoblasts are found in the marrow in increased frequency. These cells show little avidity for glass surfaces, are poorly phagocytic and have slow motility. In a later stage of development, cells designated as promonocytes are found to be glass adherent. They are relatively large (10 to 20 microns in diameter), have a high cytoplasmic-nuclear ratio, and a basophilic cytoplasm. They have developed a conspicuous Golgi complex, numerous azurophilic granules, and prepolysomes. These cells appear to be capable of endocytosis, but phagocytosis occurs poorly if at all.

THE BLOOD MONOCYTE

Monocytes are large mononuclear cells that account for 3 to 5 per cent of the leukocytes in the peripheral circulation of man. In infants, both relative and absolute numbers are increased. The cells range in size from 10 to 18 microns in diameter and have a centrally located, indented nucleus with a grayish blue cytoplasm when stained by Wright's stain. They contain variable numbers of azurophilic granules. When studied by electron microscopy, the Golgi apparatus is well developed and mitochondria are evenly distributed through the cytoplasm (Fig. 4–2). These cells are actively phagocytic

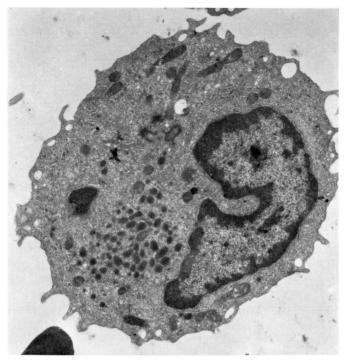

Figure 4–2. Electron micrograph of a normal monocyte. (Courtesy of Drs. J. G. White and C. C. Clawson.)

and have specific and avid receptors at their surface for both IgG and complement (C3). Some cells in the circulation appear to have structures intermediate between monocytes and large lymphocytes, and these must be characterized by functional criteria. Monocytes have a relatively short circulation time in the blood with a clearance time of about three days. There is both a circulating pool and a marginated pool of cells located at the surface of blood vessels throughout the body. The marginated pool is about three times as large as the circulating pool. Removal from the vascular space occurs at an exponential rate with a T 1/2 of 8.4 hours. It has been estimated that the normal monocyte turnover rate in man is approximately 7×10^6 cells per hour per kilogram of body weight. The absolute monocyte count in an adult ranges between 300 and 500 cells per cubic millimeter. This figure is perhaps half again as large in children.

MACROPHAGES OF THE INFLAMMATORY LESION

By the use of tritiated thymidine labeling experiments, it has been possible to show that the macrophages accumulating at the focus of an acute inflammatory process are derived almost entirely from the circulation. Studies using the skin window technique of Rebuck (see Chapter 11) have shown that many of these phagocytes are morphologically indistinguishable from lymphocytes when they first migrate into the lesions. Some of the macrophages in inflammatory lesions undoubtedly arise from preexisting tissue histocytes. The monocyte is morphologically different from tissue macrophages and macrophages found within inflammatory exudates. Transitional forms between the two are found frequently, however, and change from the characteristic blood monocyte to a characteristic tissue macrophage has been observed repeatedly, both in tissue culture and by using in vivo techniques, such as the rabbit ear chamber. The tissue macrophages are larger than monocytes. They measure 20 to 80 microns in diameter and contain one or more vesicular nuclei and numerous inclusion bodies or large cytoplasmic granules. Current evidence suggests that lysosomal enzymes of these cells are synthesized in the endoplasmic reticulum and form in the Golgi apparatus into primary lysosomes (Fig. 4–3). Cell division has been observed among mononuclear phagocytes in chronic inflammatory lesions and even in relatively acute inflammatory processes in which T cell based cell-mediated immunity plays a role. Multinucleated giant cells may be formed by the fusion or incomplete division of mononuclear macrophages. Macrophages may also form typical epithelioid cells upon further maturation. Tissue macrophages appear to be able to live for very long periods, possibly several years, and they may replicate or become dormant.

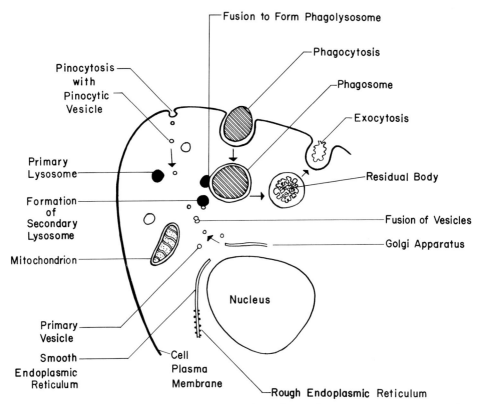

Figure 4–3. Diagrammatic sketch of the vesicular and granular structures of a mononuclear phagocyte.

ALVEOLAR MACROPHAGES

Evidence is now quite definitive that alveolar macrophages originate, at least in part, from blood monocytes. Three types of mononuclear phagocytes derived from lavage preparations taken from human lungs have been described morphologically. The most common type (type A) accounts for approximately 95 per cent of the cells. These cells are large, with a mean diameter of 20 to 30 microns. They contain numerous mitochondria and lysosomes and have abundant granular endoplasmic reticulum. These cells are metabolically active, phagocytic, and adhere readily to glass. Type B cells account for approximately 5 per cent. They also average about 30 microns in size, but differ from type A cells by having a smaller nuclear-cytoplasmic ratio, fewer cytoplasmic granules, and large green-staining inclusion bodies. Type C cells comprise less than 1 per cent when macrophages are washed from normal lungs, but may be the major cell in patients with lipoid pneumonia. These cells are large, averaging 40 microns, may have a foamy cytoplasm, and occasionally contain intact phagocytized cells. Type C cells adhere to glass whereas type B cells do not.

OTHER TISSUE MACROPHAGES

Numerous studies have presented evidence that macrophages in the liver and peritoneal cavity may arise from monocytes that derive from bone marrow. Indeed, this is the prevailing view of the origin of macrophages in all locations. However, studies using tritiated thymidine labeling in one partner of a histocompatible parabiotic pair of rats seem to indicate that this view may not be entirely correct, and it is likely that both local origin and derivation from bone marrow precursors via the blood monocytes contribute to these populations of cells.

METABOLISM AND INTRACELLULAR PHYSIOLOGY

Glycolysis is the principal source of energy for monocytes and tissue macrophages, except the alveolar macrophage, which appears to utilize aerobic metabolism. The latter cells have a rate of oxygen consumption several times greater than that of the peritoneal macrophage or blood monocyte. For them, the process of phagocytosis is markedly dependent upon the oxygen content in the environment.

LYSOSOMES

Lysosomes are membrane-bound, phase-dense cytoplasmic inclusions containing enzymes. The lysosomal enzymes of the macrophages appear to be synthesized by the endoplasmic reticulum and formed into primary lysosomes by the Golgi apparatus. These primary lysosomes fuse to form secondary lysosomes, which may be the equivalent of azurophilic granules. After phagocytosis, the latter fuse with the phagosomes to form phagolysosomes, which are the cell compartment in which digestion of ingested foreign material or debris takes place (Fig. 4–3). Both the number of lysosomes and the amount of lysosomal enzymes may be increased in vitro by increasing the amount of serum in the culture medium. The types of materials digested by pinocytosis or phagocytosis apparently influence the enzymatic composition, probably by means of precursor substances, released into the cytoplasm by the digestive process, that act as inducers of facultative enzyme synthesis. Soluble proteins inbibed by macrophages with pinocytic vesicles are hydrolyzed to amino acids or small peptides, which diffuse readily into the cell sap. Carbohydrates are metabolized by a similar mechanism.

Both the lysosomal numbers and enzymatic content of individual lysosomes increase progressively with cellular maturation. The enzymatic activity may also be influenced by thyroid hormones and by location of the cell. Hyperthyroidism increases specific activity of hydrolytic enzymes in macrophages of affected animals, and enzymatic activity is distinctly higher in alveolar macrophages than in either peritoneal macrophages, blood monocytes, or Küpffer cells. A variety of lysosomal enzymes has been detected in the lysosomes of various species. These include cathepsins and various proteases, peroxidases, arylsulfatase, acid phosphatase, esterases, beta glycosidase, beta glucuronidase, lysozyme, hyaluronidase, myeloperoxidase, and a variety of lipase activities. Human mononuclear phagocytes contain relatively small amounts of lysozyme.

Metabolic Changes with Activation (The "Angry" Macrophage)

Through the interaction with lymphocytes, other macrophages, or a variety of immunopotentiators, macrophages may become activated. Such macrophages may form aggressor cells, which have increased levels of hydrolytic enzymes, increased numbers of mitochondria and lysosomes, greater membrane activity with increased endocytosis, and a greater ability to kill both intracellular bacteria and tumor cells, as will be discussed in subsequent chapters. The moving of macrophages to higher levels of metabolism seems to be an important component of the bodily defense associated with T cell–mediated immunities.

Changes with Endocytosis

Endocytosis represents the process of ingestion or internalization of a part of the external environment by invagination of the plasma membrane. Phagocytosis, a form of endocytosis, is used to designate the ingestion of particulate matter, whereas pinocytosis is used to designate inbibing fluid droplets in vacuoles. Pinocytosis requires oxidative metabolism, whereas phagocytosis for most cells depends largely on glycolytic metabolism. Pinocytosis is dependent upon ATP and does not stimulate cell metabolism to the degree that phagocytosis does.

Monocytes derive the energy for phagocytosis from glycolytic pathways, but alveolar macrophages are dependent upon the availability of oxygen at a tension of at least 25 mmHg. In monocytes, there is a postphagocytic burst of oxygen consumption, hexose monophosphate shunt stimulation, and hydrogen peroxide generation. Peritoneal macrophages show a similar pattern, but on the other hand human alveolar macrophages have been said to show little increase in oxygen consumption following phagocytosis. Recent studies raise questions about the interpretation of this finding. It may be that the high level of activation already existing in pulmonary macrophages is caused by their having regularly been activated by phagocytosis of organisms or particles in the air.

FUNCTION OF MONONUCLEAR PHAGOCYTES

DIRECTED MOVEMENT

Mononuclear phagocytes are often classified as being either fixed or wandering; the latter are mobile, whereas the former are not. The mobile leukocytes are exemplified by blood monocytes and peritoneal macrophages. Upon arriving at an inflammatory focus, directed movement may occur, which is sometimes referred to as a leukotactic response or chemotactic response. An in vitro assay of this chemotactic response is the measurement of directed mobility through membrane filters in modified Boyden chambers. The chemotactic response has been best studied using neutrophils, and the process is more completely discussed in following chapters. However, it is well to point out here that the by-products of complement activation, C3a and C5a, are potent chemotactic substances for monocytes as well. Also, activated kallikrein and plasminogen activator have been described to be chemotactic. Enzymes released from cells that can cleave C5 or C3, or preformed chemotactic substances, such as eosinophil chemotactic factor and monocyte chemotactic factor released from stimulated lymphoid cells, may be important. Two inhibitors of chemotaxis are found in human serum, a chemotactic factor inactivator (CFI) and cell-directed inhibitor (CDI). The former has the activity of an aminopeptidase. The chemotactic factors appear to act on the cell membrane, apparently by altering the plasma gel-sol state so that the phagocytic cell rolls in the direction of the chemotactic gradient. Random motion of a mononuclear phagocyte may cease when the cell is in the vicinity of an attractive particle. With cessation of random motion, directed motion follows. This powerful directed motion appears to act over distances of 100 microns or less.

RECEPTORS ON THE CELL MEMBRANE

Recognition of "foreignness" or non-self is an intrinsic characteristic of phagocytic cells. Macrophages can recognize not only chemically foreign matter, but also altered normal cells or even malignant cells. The mechanism for recognition is probably multifactorial and as yet is not very well understood. Since amoebae and the amoebocytes of even the most primitive invertebrates appear to be able to distinguish self components from non-self, it seems likely that these cells possess self-recognition mechanisms of the most primitive type. Recognition may involve alterations in surface charge or other physical characteristics of cell membranes, but more often it seems to be mediated by recognition (receptor) sites on the macrophage surface, which interact biochemically with chemical sites on the particle, causing attachment. Recognition is also dependent in part upon the physical and chemical environment and is strikingly dependent in many cases upon specific and nonspecific opsonic factors in serum and tissue fluids, notably immunoglobulin and complement. Interestingly, attachment of a particle to a macrophage surface is not necessarily followed by ingestion. Recognition, then, apparently involves sensing by fine chemical sites on the plasma membranes of macrophages. Chemical moieties which may be recognized are carbohydrates, phospholipids, glycoproteins, lipids, proteins, and possibly others.

The recognition region on the cell membrane of macrophages is often called the receptor site. The two types of receptor sites that have been best studied are those for IgG and C3. Most of the studies have been performed using appropriately coated erythrocytes. Human macrophage surface receptors have specificity only for IgG1 and IgG3 immunoglobulin. The immunoglobulin binds to the foreign particles or material via its $F(ab)_2$ region, whereas the receptor on macrophage membranes has specificity for the Fc region. The receptor site is probably the same site that binds cytophilic antibody. Aggregated IgG and immune complexes are more avidly bound to the macrophage surface than is IgG that has not reacted or is not aggregated. Interestingly, monocytes and macrophages do not have receptor sites for IgM antibody bound to erythrocytes. Using experiments with complement-coated erythrocytes, it is apparent that the C3b fragment of the C3 molecule can also be actively bound to macrophage membranes and that the receptor site is distinct from that for the Fc component of the IgG molecule. It is of interest that C3-coated erythrocytes seem to be preferentially cleared from the circulation by the liver and, at certain densities, IgG-coated erythrocytes seem to be preferentially cleared by the spleen.

There are other serum proteins that may aid in particle recognition. One of these that has been more extensively studied is humoral recognition factor (HRF), the presence of which seems to increase particle uptake by liver macrophages via opsonization.

PHAGOCYTOSIS

Phagocytosis is an extensively studied but incompletely understood process by which the phagocytic cells ingest particulate matter, ranging from antigen-antibody complexes, cell components, and virus particles to intact mammalian cells. Phagocytosis of bacteria and erythrocytes has been most studied, and it appears that the phagocytosis of other particulate material takes place by mechanisms similar to those discussed above. For phagocytosis to occur, there must first be recognition that the matter to be phagocytized is foreign to the host, effete, or damaged. Accumulating experimental evidence indicates that the last two categories may be recognized as having foreignness because previously hidden surface determinants on the cell are exposed as a consequence of cellular or molecular aging or as a result of damage. Regardless of the reason, it is apparent that the cells of the reticuloendothelial system can recognize and destroy normal cellular constituents of the body that have expended their usefulness.

Once the phagocyte recognizes the foreignness of a particle, engulfment occurs by a process somewhat similar to pinocytosis, which involves an alteration of the gel-sol state of the cytoplasmic membrane (Fig. 4–3). The cytoplasmic membrane flows around the object, which is eventually engulfed by this invagination, resulting in complete enclosure of the particle by the cytoplasmic membrane of the cell. This structure, which contains the phagocytized particle, is known as the phagocytic vacuole or phagosome. Microtubules and microfilaments may play important roles in the internalization process, but the precise biochemical mechanisms have not been well defined. Unlike neutrophils, macrophages can expulse undigested residual material by a process called exocytosis. A number of factors can influence phagocytosis markedly, including the physical and chemical nature of the environment, the functional integrity of the cell, the presence of opsonins, and the chemical surface characteristics of the foreign particle. Energy for phagocytosis (except for alveolar macrophages) is derived from glycolysis, and the process requires divalent cations. Engulfment proceeds efficiently over a pH ranging from 6 to 8 and occurs readily in hypotonic as well as isotonic solutions.

Phagocytosis is comparatively inefficient when the macrophages are suspended in a liquid medium, and the process is significantly promoted by the presence of fibrillar or membranous structures, such as fibrin or erythrocytes, which aid the trapping of bacteria against surfaces. This phenomenon of efficient phagocytosis against surfaces has been called surface phagocytosis. Attachment of the cells also seems to make them more active in phagocytosis.

The chemical composition of the foreign particle markedly influences the ability of a phagocyte to ingest it. It is well recognized that many bacteria, such as the encapsulated pneumococcus, successfully resist phagocytosis in the absence of specific antibody and complement, and often bacteria actually seem to repel the phagocytes. At other times, there may be a positive attraction of phagocytes to a microorganism by directed chemotaxis. The physicochemical characteristics responsible for these phenomena have not been entirely defined, but it is apparent that the phenomena are real and that the capsule of certain organisms plays an important role in their defense against phagocytosis.

Specific antibody is undoubtedly the most important of the opsonins. Its effect in vivo, however, is always combined with the effect of activated complement, making its own relative effectiveness somewhat difficult to determine. However, phagocytosis in vitro may be markedly enhanced for some particles but not others by specific antibody in the absence of detectable complement. The exact mechanism underlying this process remains unclear, although it obviously involves an alteration of the surface characteristics of the foreign material, resulting from absorption of the antibody to the surface of the particle. It seems likely that for IgG antibody, the receptors on the macrophage for the Fc component are utilized. Opsonic antibodies for bacteria are directed toward somatic antigens rather than flagellar antigens. If the particles are present in sufficient concentration so that aggregation occurs, particle clearance is further enhanced, since phagocytosis is more efficient when particle size is optimal and the optimal particle size may be quite large.

"Natural antibody" is that apparent antibody activity in the serum of individuals who have had no known contact with the specific antigen. The occurrence of a natural antibody need not be the result of genetic determination, but may occur by immunization to substances in the diet or to the microbial flora of the host. Such substances may have antigenically reactive groups in their structure similar to that of the particle or cell to be phagocytized. The specificity and avidity of the antibody in such instances is not as high as that of antibody produced as a result of specific immunization. It is apparent from a number of studies with germ-free animals that natural antibodies to bacteria usually occur as a result of specific experience with a particular bacteria or to immunochemically closely related organisms and not spontaneously.

The opsonic effect of antibody is greatly enhanced by complement system activation by the antigen-antibody reaction. In the case of microorganisms and cells, activated complement damages or alters the cell wall, but complement will also influence phagocytosis of inert particles, such as starch. It has been reported that the uptake of certain bacteria can be enhanced by the presence of serum from newborn piglets which contains no detectable antibodies, suggesting that complement will promote phagocytosis in the absence of antibody. This supposition may or may not be true, but is probably of little consequence in the actual process of opsonization in vivo. What is of importance is the demonstration that removal of complement from phagocytic systems may markedly depress the process of phagocytosis. Recent studies have indicated that complement is essential for full phagocytic activity in almost all test systems in mammals. One form of reticuloendothelial blockade is accomplished by the removal of heat labile serum components absorbed to the surface of the particles inducing the blockade, and the blockade can be reversed by the addition of fresh serum. The component or components removed during reticuloendothelial blockade have been thought to be complement, although this has not been proved, and it could well be that they are natural antibodies. Inhibition of phagocytosis will occur even in the presence of specific immunoglobulin when antibodies to complement in phagocytic systems are employed to decrease the efficiency of immune serum. A number of substances have been found to be anticomplementary, and many of these have been used for many years as an adjuvant to promote the development of infection by microorganisms injected into experimental animals. Usually, the difference between virulent and avirulent organisms depends upon the degree to which opsonization and phagocytosis occur. It has recently been demonstrated that the capsular material of many virulent organisms has an anticomplementary activity. The role of complement in infection will be discussed in greater detail in Chapter 13, and the complement system and its intimate relation to phagocytosis is discussed in Chapter 7.

Other heat labile serum components that behave differently from complement and promote phagocytic activity have been described. These substances have not been characterized, however, and it is possible that they may represent components of complement or even natural, heat labile antibodies.

Eli Metchnikoff, a Russian-born biologist, in addition to his many other basic observations in immunology prior to 1900, demonstrated the role of phagocytic cells in the defense of animals against invasion by microorganisms. Because his work was not well received among the medical scientists of his day, he wrote a book, published shortly after the turn of the century, that summarized his lifetime of work which had been accomplished primarily at the Pasteur Institute in Paris. For the interested reader, this compendium presents a wealth of information and interpretation that frequently approaches and sometimes exceeds our current concepts. Much of his work was forgotten, however, and it is easy to find publications of investigations in recent years that describe experiments and reach conclusions surprisingly similar to those carried out and developed by Metchnikoff and his coworkers in the nineteenth century. To demonstrate the current applicability of his works, we quote an experiment from Binnie's English translation of Metchnikoff's book Immunity in Infective Diseases. In this experiment, Metchnikoff describes the sequence of events following the injection of nucleated goose erythrocytes into the peritoneal cavities of guinea pigs. Guinea pig serum has no morphological effect on the erythrocytes.

"Immediately after the injection, the lymph of the peritoneal cavity begins to show important changes. The white corpuscles which in the normal condition are fairly abundant disappear almost completely. Some small lymphocytes presenting their ordinary aspect may be found, but the few macrophages and microphages [neutrophils] remaining show signs of very grave lesions. They lose their mobility, run together into clumps, and become incapable of ingestion of foreign bodies. At this moment, the phagocytes undergo a critical change which we have designated the name of phagolysis. This condition lasts for about one hour. Some of it continues longer according to the case and circumstance. But after this, the peritoneal fluid becomes filled with leukocytes that have newly come on the scene. These cells make their way by diapedesis through the walls of the congested vessels of the peritoneum. A true aseptic inflammation is produced which induces an exudation of a large number of white corpuscles amongst which are found microphages and still more numerous macrophages. Soon after their appearance, that is to say two or three hours after injection of the blood, macrophages send out very small protoplasmic processes and affix them to the surface of the red corpuscles. There follows an aggregation of the macrophages of the guinea pig with the red corpuscles of the goose, and characteristic masses are produced in which can be recognized both kinds of cells. This union with the very small pseudopodia is the first stage in the ingestion of the red corpuscles by the macrophages. The red corpuscle seized by amoeboid processes passes into the interior of the macrophage. This macrophage seldom is contented with a single red corpuscle. Usually, it devours a large number, and sometimes enormous macrophages may be filled with a score of red corpuscles.

"If the quantity of goose's blood injected into a guinea pig is large (5.0 to 7.0 cc), the ingestion of red corpuscles by the macrophages continues for a considerable period, often for three or four days. In the whole of this time, a number of the red corpuscles remain free in the peritoneal plasma. In spite of this prolonged stay, none of them undergo extra-cellular solution.

"The red corpuscles anchored by the amoeboid processes of the macrophages first present a normal appearance. Later their membrane begins to wrinkle, but as soon as they have passed within the phagocytes the wrinkles disappear and the corpuscles regain their normal aspect. If a little neutral red solution is added to the peritoneal exudation, we observe that the nucleus of the ingested red corpuscle and even its contents are stained red, but the red corpuscles adherent to the surface of the phagocytes retain their normal yellow color. The hemoglobin (of ingested cells) diffuses into the contents of the macrophage through the stroma which has become permeable. The body of the red corpuscle is pretty soon digested, but the nucleus impregnated with hemoglobin persists for a much longer period. It divides into several fragments recognizable by their yellow color, and in certain cases the remnants of red corpuscles may be met within the interior of the macrophage. These macrophages do not remain permanently in the peritoneal fluid. Some three to four days after ingestion, the lymph in the peritoneum contains only leukocytes that have newly come and which contain neither red corpuscles nor their remains. We must open the guinea pig to find any macrophages that devoured red corpuscles. They are to be met with in large numbers in the glandular portion of the omentum, the mesenteric glands, and in the liver and spleen. They are fairly easily recognized by the characteristic aspect of the debris of the red corpuscles. Having devoured the red corpuscles, the macrophages leave the peritoneal fluid and the digestion [is] completed in the positions just mentioned. In the liver they are seen as large mononuclear cells, often with highly developed processes. In this condition, they remind one of Küpffer's stellate cells—a fact that suggested to me the idea that these elements are nothing but white corpuscles which have emigrated to the vessels of the liver.

"Following up the fate of the macrophages that have resorbed the red corpuscles, we find them in the large hepatic vessels, in the vena cava, and even in the blood of the heart, but in these latter situations, they contain merely a few scarcely recognizable remnants of their prey. These phagocytes which left the blood during the inflammation that followed the injection of red corpuscles of the goose re-enter it having fulfilled their function in the final period of the resorption. This resorption must undoubtedly be regarded as an intracellular digestion."

Metchnikoff's observation that the peritoneal macrophages which had phagocytized the goose erythrocytes were found in the liver and closely resembled the Küpffer cells may be a clue concerning the origin of the Küpffer cells, a point still of considerable contention, as discussed earlier. Recent studies using isotopically labeled cells indicate that at least some of the Küpffer cells are derived from lymphocyte-like precursors in the bone marrow that are similar to, if not identical with, the precursors of monocytes and tissue macrophages.

INTRACELLULAR DIGESTION

Once microorganisms or cells have been phagocytized, they are destroyed in most instances by a process of intracellular digestion. Microbial killing, however, does not always follow phagocytosis, and certain microbes will survive for prolonged periods of time within phagocytic cells, either because of the nature of the microbe or because of an abnormality of the phagocyte. Macrophages are characteristically thought not to kill most bacteria as rapidly as neutrophils. However, when human monocytes are obtained under conditions comparable to those used to obtain neutrophils, as in cyclic neutropenia when large numbers of monocytes are present in the circulation and neutrophils are absent, the killing of bacteria seems to be as efficiently accomplished by monocytes as by neutrophils, on a cell for cell basis.

Degranulation of phagocytic cells, which is normally a sequel to the ingestion of microbes, has been observed for many years, but the significance of this process has been appreciated only recently. A bacterium which has been ingested by a phagocytic cell is confined to a vesicular structure whose wall is composed of the invaginated plasma membrane (Fig. 4–3). For reasons which are as yet unclear, the membranes of the cytoplasmic granules (lysosomes) in the region of the phagocytic vacuole (phagosome) fuse with the membrane of the phagocytic vacuole, resulting in emptying of the enzymatic contents of the lysosome into the phagosome to form a digestive vacuole (phagolysosome). It is within this stricture and by this process that some destruction and most of the degradation of the microbe or other particle occur.

The exact role of each of the lysosomal enzymes in antimicrobial defense has not been determined, but purified preparations of some of them have been shown to have direct antibacterial activity. Lysozyme is an enzyme of low molecular weight which causes destruction of bacteria by lysis of the cell wall. Phagocytin is a group of heat stable proteins which have been found to be bactericidal for a wide spectrum of organisms. Other enzymes have also been described which have antibacterial activity, but the combined effect of all the enzymes is undoubtedly more important than the effect of any one. The majority of lysosomal enzymes have a pH optimum that is distinctly acid, usually around 5.0. Acidity in itself kills many microbes and facilitates killing of still others. A group of polypeptides having distinctive antibacterial activity but no detectable enzymatic activity has been isolated from the granules of neutrophils but these do not seem to be present in macrophages. Myeloperoxidase does not seem to be essential for normal killing by macrophages. Another important system is related to H_2O_2 generation within the cell following ingestion. It is now clear that abnormalities of degranulation, metabolism to generate H_2O_2, and deficiencies in lysosomal enzyme activity impair the intracellular killing of microbes by macrophages. Each of these abnormalities may occur on a genetic basis or through physiological alterations.

The processes of intracellular digestion of microorganisms by neutrophils and mononuclear phagocytes are similar, although important differences exist. Mononuclear phagocytes do not contain phagocytin or the antibacterial basic polypeptides and possess relatively small amounts of lysozyme when compared to neutrophils, indicating that the exact enzymatic processes by which antibacterial action is mediated may not be the same for mononuclear phagocytes and neutrophils. In fact, no distinct bactericidal property has yet been identified in extracts of isolated mononuclear phagocytes, with the exception of lysozyme. Enzyme content may vary considerably with the type of mononuclear phagocyte, as mentioned before. Alveolar macrophages contain considerably greater concentrations of lysosomal enzymes than do peritoneal macrophages. The slower rate of bacterial killing sometimes observed for mononuclear phagocytes may reflect, in part, the lower enzyme content of their cytoplasmic granules.

The rate of intracellular destruction of phagocytized bacteria has been variously reported to be increased, unchanged, or decreased by the presence of specific antibody, the difference in the results probably reflecting differences in the effect of the antibody upon the cell wall of the bacteria. Complement increases the rate of intracellular destruction as well as the rate of phagocytosis. Killing of catalase-negative bacteria by the H_2O_2-halogenation pathway and by the toxicity of superoxide (O_2^-), singlet ($'O_2$), and hydroxyl radicals by oxidative metabolism in monocytes and neutrophils seems to be the explanation for at least some of the bactericidal activity of phagocytes.

The host-parasite relationships between microbes and phagocytic cells are the critical determinant of the outcome of microbial invasion. Many bacteria are killed within a few minutes after they have been ingested, and the process may continue progressively to fragmentation and complete digestion with susceptible bacteria. Nondigestible material remaining within the phagosome morphologically forms a residual body (Fig. 4–3). This undigested material may remain for the lifetime of the phagocyte or may be extruded by exocytosis, a process which seems to be the reverse of phagocytosis.

Several types of microorganisms may successfully resist intracellular destruction and reside as intracellular parasites. This group of organisms typically includes several types of fungi, mycobacteria, salmonella, brucella, and *Listeria*. These organisms have been termed facultative intracellular bacterial pathogens. In addition, a number of other pathogenic organisms may survive intracellularly, for example, staphylococcus and *Pseudomonas*, depending upon the characteristics of the bacterium and the functional state of the phagocytic cell. Multiplication of the microbe is often inhibited by phagocytosis even when killing does not occur. Successful, prolonged, intracellular parasitism usually leads to the development of inflammatory lesions and granulomas characteristic of chronic infectious processes.

Antigenic Processing and Transfer to Immune Competent Cells

Lymphocytes and plasma cells are the functional units of antibody production, but are not phagocytic. On the other hand, neutrophils and monocytes are actively phagocytic, but produce no antibody. How, then, are the immune competent cells stimulated to produce antibody to particulate antigens? Neutrophils in inflammatory foci are relatively short-lived and, for the most part, die there, to be phagocytized and removed by macrophages. Both macrophages and neutrophils phagocytize and kill bacteria, and possibly both may process antigens. It has been shown, however, that extracts from neutrophils that have killed certain strains of bacteria no longer possess antigenic properties characteristic for that organism, whereas extracts from mononuclear phagocytes which have killed the same strains of bacteria retain characteristic antigenic properties of the bacterium when injected into nonimmunized animals. It has also been shown that mononuclear phagocytes produce a substance that is sensitive to the action of ribonuclease, which will induce the formation of specific antibody immune competent cells. The best studies seem to indicate that this material contains fragments of antigen coupled to RNA. Direct contact between lymphocytes and macrophages with cytoplasmic bridging between these cells has been observed on numerous occasions, and it has been postulated that lymphocytes and macrophages may interact to achieve active transfer of processed antigenic material or specific ribonucleic acid to the lymphocyte. At least some antigens may remain on the surface of macrophages for prolonged periods of time.

Whether antigenic material is transferred in some instances as part of a complex with ribonucleic acid has not been determined with certainty for all antigens; nevertheless, the vital importance of the macrophage in the processing and transfer of antigenic information to lymphocytes has been established beyond a reasonable doubt. In this regard, transfer of macrophages that have processed antigen to intact animals or to cultures containing only lymphocytes can initiate a specific immune response. Also, pure populations of lymphocytes containing no macrophages have a reduced antigenic response to specific antigens, which can be restored by the addition of macrophages. The exact mechanisms by which antigen is processed by the macrophage are not understood at the present time. Small lymphocytes are present at sites of acute inflammation as well as in the regional lymph nodes, and it is reasonable to assume that the transfer of antigenic information may take place at either side. Once this information has been obtained by the lymphocyte, the processes of specific immunologic adaptation are set into motion (Chapters 3 and 6).

REGULATORY FUNCTIONS OF MACROPHAGES

In addition to regulation of the immune response by processing of antigens, there is recent evidence that macrophages may play important helper and suppressor roles, especially by the elaboration of soluble mediators that may activate lymphocytes or depress their function, sometimes by cytotoxicity.

That monocytes play a crucial positive feedback role in regulation of granulopoiesis by elaboration of a colony-stimulating factor (CSF) has been suggested by many experiments, especially the experiments analyzing cultures of colony-forming cells in a soft agar system in vitro. In fact, the growth of human bone marrow in vitro is made possible by the use of a feeder layer containing monocytes or conditioned media containing CSF derived from adult peripheral leukocytes. Recently, it has been demonstrated that the monocyte and macrophage normally produce CSF and this has led to the concept of feedback regulation of granulopoiesis by mononuclear phagocytes.

The important role of macrophages in infection, tumor immunity, graft rejection, and autoimmune diseases is discussed in subsequent chapters.

5

Granulocytes

Granulocytes represent a type of phagocytic cell different from mononuclear phagocytes. However, both apparently develop from common precursors in the bone marrow, which subdifferentiate to myeloblasts and monoblasts although these cannot be separated by morphologic criteria. The myeloblast then may give rise to neutrophilic promyelocytes, eosinophilic promyelocytes, and basophilic promyelocytes (Fig. 5–1), each differentiating further into a distinct form of granulocyte, i.e., neutrophils, eosinophils, and basophils. The morphogenesis of each of these cell lines is similar, but, for purposes of clarity, they will be discussed individually. As might be suspected by the late phylogenetic appearance of granulocytes, they are more specialized phagocytic cells than macrophages and their relative importance

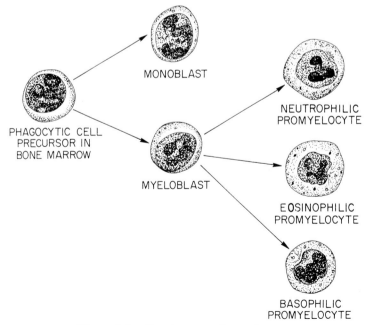

Figure 5–1. Development of granulocytes.

in immunological defense mechanisms appears to increase with phylogenetic ascendancy.

NEUTROPHILS

Neutrophils are also known as neutrophilic granulocytes and polymorphonuclear leukocytes (PMN). Sometimes, the term granulocyte is also used, incorrectly, as a substitute for the neutrophilic cell, which, of course, is the most common and important of the granulocytes.

DEVELOPMENT OF NEUTROPHILS

Development of the neutrophilic series normally occurs only in the bone marrow. Myeloblasts that give rise to neutrophils do not have distinguishing characteristics to differentiate them from myeloblasts giving rise to other types of granulocytes. However, the promyelocyte begins to collect primary (azurophilic) granules in its basophilic cytoplasm. As in the myeloblast, there is a large oval nucleus with one or more prominent nucleoli. The Golgi apparatus is well developed and typically is located adjacent to the indentation in the nucleus. There are extensive granular reticulum and free

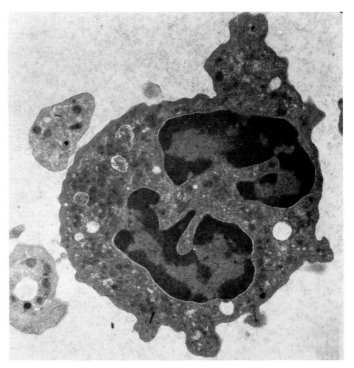

Figure 5–2. Electron micrograph of a normal human neutrophil. (Courtesy of Dr. J. G. White.)

polyribosomes. Further maturation of the cell is characterized by nuclear chromatin being marginated along the inner aspect of the nuclear membrane with progressive disappearance of the nucleoli. The nuclear-cytoplasmic ratio first decreases, then the cytoplasm becomes progressively lost, and the cells become smaller with maturation. The mitochondria become smaller and fewer in number, as do the polyribosomes. A second population of granules then appears, which is known as the secondary or specific granules. At about this stage of the metamyelocyte, production of primary granules ceases or decreases markedly, and the cell becomes committed to the production of secondary granules. As the primary granules become divided among producing cells with cellular division, they become less numerous in each cell, and the secondary granules eventually predominate.

The functionally mature forms of the granulocyte are the band (stab) and multilobed (usually three or four lobes) cells. In these more mature forms (Fig. 5–2), there is progressive lobation of the nucleus with increasing condensation and margination of nuclear chromatin. The Golgi apparatus becomes atrophic and granulogenesis ceases. There are few mitochondria, a decrease in endoplasmic reticulum and ribosomes, and a progressive accumulation of cytoplasmic glycogen. A third (tertiary) population of granules may exist, but may represent simply altered primary granules, since they contain myeloperoxidase.

GRANULES OF THE NEUTROPHIL

Primary granules develop in the neutrophilic progranulocytes by coalescence of dense-cored vacuoles arising from the inner cisternae of the Golgi apparatus. This coalescence forms multicored vacuoles; the core material aggregates and eventually mixes with the less dense material to produce a uniformly dense mature granule of about 0.6 micron in diameter. These large, electron-dense granules contain myeloperoxidase, which serves as a good cytologic marker since this enzyme is located exclusively in the azurophilic granule. In addition, the primary granules have been shown to contain enzymatic activities of acid phosphatase, beta glucuronidase, beta galactosidase, N-acetyl beta glucosaminidase, arylsulfatase, 5′ nucleotidase, alpha mannosidase, arginine-rich cationic proteins, and sulfated mucopolysaccharides. Approximately one third of granule-associated lysozyme is to be found in the primary granules.

As mentioned earlier, production of the primary granule ceases in an intermediate stage of maturation, and the cell begins to produce secondary (specific) granules. These are formed similarly to the primary granules except that they arise from budding of the outer cisternae of the Golgi apparatus. The small granules containing finely granular material form larger and finally mature granules, measuring approximately 0.3 to 0.4 micron in diameter. In the mature neutrophil, there may be smaller forms and even some that are rod-shaped or elliptical. The secondary granule has a distinctive enzymatic marker, alkaline phosphatase. Aminopeptidase occurs at about the same time in the secondary granule, and about two thirds of the lysozyme of the cell is located in secondary granules.

A third type of granule, the tertiary, may be noted in mature neutrophils, but it is uncertain whether this represents a new kind of granule or an alteration of a primary or secondary granule. Other enzymatic activities have been found within the granules of neutrophils. These include ribonucleases, deoxyribonucleases, cathepsins, lipases, proteases, phosphatases, esterases, glucosidases, glucosaminidases, hyaluronidases, collagenases, elastases, phospholipases, kinogenases, histamine, and antibacterial or bactericidal proteins.

DISTRIBUTION AND REGULATION

Normally, only band and mature forms of neutrophils are found in the blood of man. Some of these are free in the circulation and others are adherent to the walls of the blood vessels. The latter is known as the marginated granulocyte pool whereas the former is known as the circulating granulocyte pool. Together, these form the total blood granulocyte pool. Using various techniques, it has been demonstrated that the circulating granulocyte pool contains approximately 22 billion neutrophils in an 80 kg man. A slightly greater number, 27 billion, is normally present in the marginated granulocyte pool, and the two together total almost 50 billion neutrophils. There is free turnover between the two pools, but the mechanisms that involve sequestration and release from the marginated pool are unknown. The time required for clearance of half of the granulocytes from the blood pool is approximately 6.5 hours, and the granulocyte turnover rate is an estimated 114 billion per day for a 70 kg man. In other words, the total number of neutrophils circulating at any one time is completely replaced approximately five times per day. For each circulating neutrophil there are approximately 30 granulocytes in the bone marrow reserve. Thus, there is about a six day supply of neutrophils in the bone marrow reserve, and the transit time from differentiated marrow granulocyte to blood neutrophil is about six days. However, in patients with severe infection, this may be considerably shortened, e.g., to only 48 hours.

From this discussion it is apparent that many variables may influence the number of neutrophils in the blood. Neutrophilia may result from a shift from the marginated to the circulating pool, from increased production, decreased destruction, or increased release from the bone marrow pool. On the other hand, neutropenia may occur with increased destruction, as with infection or hypersplenism, decreased production (as seen following therapy with cytotoxic drugs), a shift to the marginating pool, or decreased release from the marrow.

Not too much is known about the regulation of granulopoiesis in vivo. However, it is clear that precursor cells are injured or destroyed by x-irradiation and drugs which will interfere with DNA synthesis. Much new evidence concerning granulocyte regulation has been obtained in recent years from both in vitro studies and studies of patients following marrow transplantation. In vitro, precursor cells can be stimulated to differentiate during culture by a variety of substances, one of which is a colony-stimulating factor (CSF) present in serum. Colony-stimulating factors have also been ob-

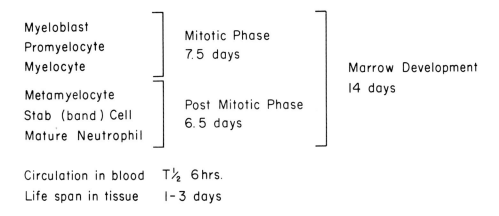

Figure 5–3. Life cycle of neutrophils.

tained from monocytes, macrophages, thymus glands, kidneys, embryonic tissues, and urine. Several lines of investigation, including in vitro culture of marrow cells in soft agar culture, suggest that there is a positive feedback loop from mature macrophages that produce CSF and a negative feedback loop from granulocytes that regulate granulocytosis.

The life span of the mature neutrophil is relatively short – approximately three days once it enters the circulation from the bone marrow reserve. These cells emigrate through the vascular endothelium into the tissue spaces and rarely, if ever, return to the circulatory system. They end their life there and are subsequently removed by macrophages. Figure 5–3 shows the life cycle of the neutrophil.

METABOLISM

The morphologic observation that mature neutrophils have decreased numbers of mitochondria and increased glycogen suggests that much of the energy of these cells may be derived from anaerobic metabolism. This is certainly true, since many important functions, such as phagocytosis and chemotaxis, can progress well in the absence of oxygen. However, particle ingestion can increase oxygen consumption of neutrophils by as much as tenfold or more. This abrupt increase in oxygen uptake is sometimes referred to as a "respiratory burst"; it is characterized by the observation that it is not inhibited by cyanide, indicating that it is not mediated by the mitochondrial pathway. Energy for phagocytosis, and probably for degranulation, is derived by glycolysis under both aerobic and anaerobic conditions. However, the inhibitors of glycolysis have no effect on killing of ingested bacteria once phagocytosis has occurred. Hexose monophosphate shunt activity is also strikingly stimulated by phagocytosis.

CHEMOTAXIS

Migration of neutrophils to an infective focus has been observed by investigators for nearly a century, but the process is still not completely understood. Neutrophils appear to move randomly in normal tissues, but when they are presented with a chemotactic stimulus, they discontinue random motion and can move directly towards the stimulus. This process of directed movement caused by stimulus is called chemotaxis. Like chemotaxis of the mononuclear phagocyte, this process involves an alteration in the cytoplasmic flow in the gel-sol state of the membrane. Undoubtedly, there are cell surface receptors which influence this directed movement. Low molecular weight compounds generated by activation of the complement sequence are among the best defined and best studied of the chemotactic substances, and it is not surprising that the presence of serum will often increase the chemotaxis of neutrophils when studied in vitro. Both C3a and $\overline{C5a}$ have potent chemotactic activity, and the trimolecular complex of $\overline{C567}$ has also been found to be an active stimulant. Bacteria will often activate the complement sequence when placed with serum, and endotoxin and casein are often used for in vitro studies to generate chemotactic factors from complement in serum. In addition, many bacteria will elaborate chemotactically active products in the absence of serum. Tissue products, including damaged leukocytes and other injured tissues, may also have chemotactic activity. The chemotactic influence of these factors is usually enhanced by serum. Finally, there are some chemically well defined substances, such as prostaglandin E_1, that seem to have chemotactic activity.

Chemotaxis by neutrophils has been most often studied in vitro using a modified Boyden chamber technique (Chapter 11). This allows semiquantitation of the response, but it may be considerably different from in vivo events. The precise role of abnormalities demonstrated by this technique has yet to be defined. There is no clear relationship between a decreased ability of neutrophils to ingest and kill bacteria and the chemotactic activity of isolated neutrophils. However, septicemia in humans is often accompanied by poor chemotactic response. Chemotaxis has been studied in vivo by skin window (Rebuck) tests, which are more qualitative than quantitative. However, decreased deposition of neutrophils at sites of inflammation and diminished chemotactic response in vitro both seem to be associated with septic complications. Whether this is cause or effect remains to be determined.

RECOGNITION AND PHAGOCYTOSIS

Recognition and phagocytosis of foreign particles are similar to those of macrophages. Adherence and ingestion are somewhat dependent upon divalent cations. Some microorganisms may be recognized and ingested in media that do not contain serum factors. However, serum opsonins markedly influence recognition and ingestion of the vast majority of microorganisms. IgG with specificity for the microorganisms will often aid in recognition and ingestion because receptors for the Fc fragment of the IgG molecule are present on the membrane of the neutrophil. However, some IgG-coated organisms are not recognized and phagocytized by neutrophils, and various components of the complement pathway may be needed to effect opsonization. For some species, this involves heat stable factors whereas for others, heat labile factors may be important. As mentioned, one of the products of complement activation by either the classical or alternative pathway, C3b, is a potent opsonin. When it has been deposited upon the surface of microorganisms, receptors on the cell surface of neutrophils are enabled to effect recognition and initiate phagocytosis.

The process of phagocytosis by neutrophils is very similar to that described for macrophages (Fig. 5–4). It first involves attachment of a particle or microorganism to the plasma membrane, which induces invagination by a poorly understood mechanism involving the microtubules. This invagination continues until the microbe is surrounded and the external portion of the invagination fuses to internalize the phagocytic vacuole. In this process, a small amount of extracellular fluid is invariably internalized with the phagocytized particle. By an equally poorly understood process, degranulation begins to occur almost as soon as the plasma membrane begins to invaginate. This process results in discharge of the contents of the lysosomal granules into the phagocytic vacuole, also now called a phagolysosome. Usually, some of the contents of lysosomes escape into the surround-

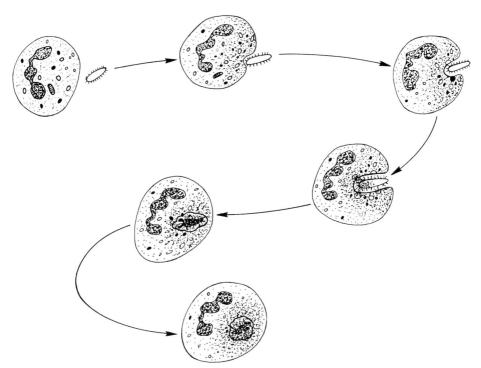

Figure 5–4. Diagrammatic representation of phagocytosis of a bacterium by a neutrophil. Degranulation begins before ingestion is completed.

ings of the cell during this process, and at least some of the abundant digestive materials present in the fluids at inflammatory sites are derived in this
way. Concurrent with the phagocytic process is an increase in glycolysis, an
increase in the hexose monophosphate shunt activity, increase in oxygen
utilization and hydrogen peroxide generation, and an increase in the synthesis of RNA and lipids.

INTRACELLULAR DIGESTION AND MICROBIAL KILLING

Intracellular killing begins with the discharge of lysosomal contents into
the phagocytic vacuole, even before phagocytosis is complete. With ingestion, there is a lowered pH within the vacuole, which provides for optimum
activity of the discharged acid hydrolases. The role of specific antibody
(including IgM) and complement components in intracellular killing, once a
microbe has been ingested, remains to be definitively studied; it is likely that
they continue to be important. Also the relative importance and roles of the
demonstrated lysosomal enzymes and antibacterial substances are not well
defined at the present time. Possibly, a conjoined effect of several of the enzymes is critical. There are obvious differences in the mechanisms involved
in killing of different types of organisms, as will be discussed in Chapter 13.

Studies with the neutrophils from patients with chronic granulomatous
disease of childhood (CGD) have indicated that still other mechanisms may
play a crucial role in the killing of certain classes of bacteria. With particle
ingestion, there is normally a respiratory burst and stimulation of the hexose
monophosphate shunt. The oxidative pathways associated with this are
shown in Figure 5–5. It is apparent that NADH and NADPH dependent ox-
idases and glutathione are key components of these pathways for the production of the intracellular hydrogen peroxide that is actively involved in bacterial killing. In an anaerobic environment, the production of hydrogen
peroxide may be impaired and the killing of many microorganisms may
not occur, H_2O_2, superoxide (O_2^-), singlet ($'O_2$), and (OH^-) radicals are important in intracellular killing. These diffuse into the phagocytic vacuole
and act with halide and myeloperoxidase to kill microorganisms. Some
catalase-positive organisms, such as *Staphylococcus aureus* 502A, obviously
require this pathway for intracellular killing whereas others, such as *Streptococcus viridans*, which is catalase-negative, do not. Such organisms can be
killed both by neutrophils in an anaerobic environment and by the neutrophils of patients with CGD. The killing of the streptococcus by the neutrophils of the patients with CGD may involve H_2O_2 and/or an activated
oxygen generated by the microorganism itself while it is in the phagolysosome—a microbial suicide. Even those organisms that require participation of
oxidative pathways seem to be handled differently, and the neutrophils may
kill one type of organism well on the same day that they kill another type of
organism poorly.

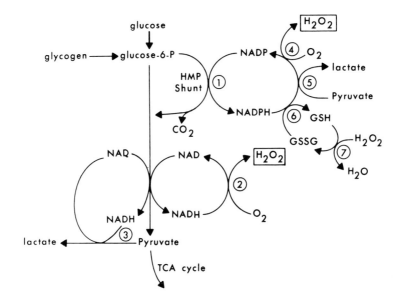

KEY ENZYMES

① glucose 6-phosphate dehydrogenase
② NADH oxidase
③ NADH-linked lactic dehydrogenase
④ NADPH oxidase
⑤ NADPH-linked lactic dehydrogenase
⑥ GSSG reductase
⑦ GSH peroxidase

Figure 5–5. Oxidative pathways of the human neutrophil. (Reproduced by permission from Cline, M. J., The White Cell. Cambridge, Mass., Harvard University Press, 1975, p. 78.)

EOSINOPHILS

Human eosinophils (Fig. 5–6) are characterized by having a bilobed nucleus and many large eosinophilic cytoplasmic granules which have characteristic large electron-dense rectangular or square crystalline bodies within their structure that can be demonstrated by electron microscopy. The granules of eosinophils are formed from the Golgi apparatus in a manner similar to that responsible for granule formation in neutrophils. Azurophilic granules are formed first in the promyelocyte stage. The eosinophilic or definitive granules begin to be produced late in the promyelocyte stage, but for the most part they are produced in the myelocytic and subsequent stages. Immature eosinophils at first lack crystalloid material in their granules, but later, crystalloids form in some of the granules that are composed of parallel lamellae.

In the mature eosinophil, two forms of granules are seen: (1) spherical, homogeneous and dense, and (2) crystalloid-containing. The homogeneous dense granules contain acid phosphatase activity and PAS reactive material.

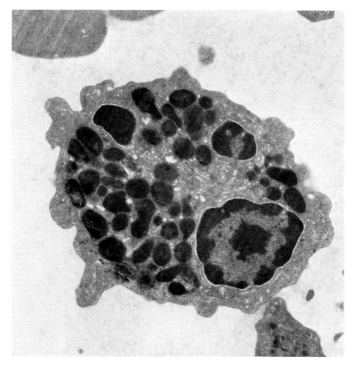

Figure 5-6. Electron micrograph of a normal human eosinophil. The electron-dense crystalline bodies are not apparent in this section. (Courtesy of Dr. J. G. White.)

The crystalloid-containing granules have peroxidase activity and large amounts of zinc and basic proteins. In man, the crystalloids have periodic structure. A variety of enzymes has been found within the eosinophil granules, which include beta glucuronidase, arylsulfatase, cathepsins, ribonuclease, deoxyribonuclease, acid phosphatase, and large amounts of kininase. However, the granules do not contain lysozyme.

The peripheral blood normally has only 100 or so eosinophils per cubic mm, but for each circulating cell there are 100 to 300 eosinophils in a bone marrow reserve and another 100 to 300 in the tissues. Eosinophils spend 3 to 6 days in the bone marrow before being released into the blood, but once there have a very short half-life of some 30 minutes. They marginate on vessel walls and emigrate from them in a manner similar to that employed by neutrophils. Also, they respond to many of the same chemotactic influences, and phagocytize particles in a similar way.

Unlike neutrophils, they accumulate in small numbers at sites of acute inflammation, but are often numerous in association with chronic inflammation. They tend to accumulate at sites where antigen-antibody complexes are present, and histamine and other products of mast cells may act as a chemotactic stimulus. Certain vasoactive mediators, such as serotonin and bradykinin, do not seem to have such activity. Because of the chemotactic effect of histamine, eosinophils accumulate at the site of its release by mast cells. Eosinophils avidly phagocytize certain antigen-antibody complexes, especially those which precipitate at equivalence or slight antigen excess, but nonprecipitating complexes are much less well ingested. Eosinophils also accumulate in areas of repeated injection of antigen. It is interesting that eosinophils may form rosettes in vivo around macrophages that contain antigen.

While phagocytosis by eosinophils resembles that of neutrophils, the process of intracellular digestion is much less efficient for most particulate matter, and it is apparent that eosinophils play a very minor role, if any, in defense against most bacteria. Extracts from eosinophils have been shown to have histamine, serotonin, and bradykinin neutralizing properties, suggesting that these cells might perform a homeostatic function of controlling the duration and severity of an inflammatory lesion. This seems especially true for lesions of allergic inflammation where the products of mast cells or basophils are so prominent. Indeed, "cleaning up" after release of mediators from mast cells in allergic inflammatory reactions has been postulated to be the primary function of this cell. Eosinophils accumulating in an inflammatory site rarely return to the circulation, but they may accumulate in draining lymph nodes where they are engulfed by macrophages. It is possible that eosinophils play a role in the transport of antigenic information to immune competent cells, but this function has not been clearly established. The association of both blood and tissue eosinophilia with certain allergic disorders (especially atopic diseases with increased levels of IgE), parasitism, drug reactions, certain types of malignancy, and certain types of intracellular infection has been known for many years. Until recently, the biological significance of this eosinophilia has been obscure. However, eosinophils have recently been demonstrated to terminate certain processes set in motion by mast cells and basophils and thus they may provide a definitive regulatory role in inflammation.

BASOPHILS AND MAST CELLS

Because the basophilic leukocyte and tissue mast cell serve similar functions, they will be considered together. However, there is no evidence that they share a common origin, and their granules have conspicuous differences, as basophils lack the hydrolytic enzymes and peroxidases found in mast cells.

The site of origin of the basophil, as in neutrophils and eosinophils, is the granulocytic precursors of the bone marrow. Many authorities feel that tissue mast cells arise in the connective tissue from primitive mesenchymal precursors, but this point is unproven, as is the question of whether or not circulating basophilic leukocytes can become tissue-fixed mast cells capable of mitotic division. Morphologically, basophils are easily identifiable, being characterized by a large lobulated nucleus, which is usually round or oval but infrequently lobed. The cytoplasm contains numerous, large, evenly distributed, metachromatic granules (Fig. 5–7). In Wright's stained material, the dark opaque granules usually obscure nuclear configuration. Differentiation

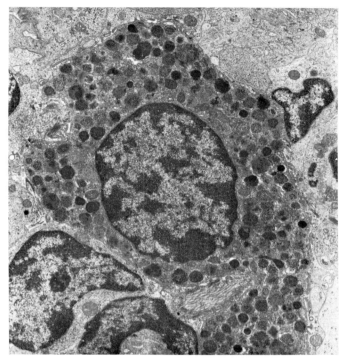

Figure 5–7. Electron micrograph of a normal human mast cell. (Courtesy of Dr. C. C. Clawson.)

of the basophil in the bone marrow is similar to that of neutrophils and eosinophils. Mast cells can be easily identified in tissue sections by staining with toluidine blue, and a characteristic microvillous appearance of the plasma membrane has been demonstrated by electron microscopy. The granules have an unusual structure, characterized by a honeycombed pattern, repeat parallel lamellae, and a hexagonal pattern of banded structures, possibly from a hexagonal arrangement of microfilaments. Heparin and histamine are important components of the granule, and a number of enzymes have been demonstrated to be present within the granule, including some peroxidases and a variety of dehydrogenases. Basophils characteristically lack acid hydrolases, but the latter are present in mast cells.

There is little information about the production and distribution of basophils. The numbers of circulating basophils are relatively high in the newborn and decrease with age. Treatment with adrenocortical steroids will decrease the numbers of circulating basophils, as will thyroid hormone and progesterone. On the other hand, treatment with estrogen increases their numbers. Treatment with nitrogen mustard results in degranulation of tissue mast cells in rats.

Certainly, the functions of basophils and mast cells must be similar since both release granules containing pharmacologically active compounds in response to similar stimuli, including mild mechanical trauma and the presence at their surface of antigen-antibody complexes. IgE binds selectively to the surface of these cells via the Fc portion of the molecule, and interaction of basophil surfacebound IgE antibody with its corresponding antigen triggers the release of histamine and other vasoactive mediators via degranulation. Tissue basophils or mast cells are found in increased numbers in many types of chronic inflammatory responses and in the vicinity of many malignant tumors. In these instances, their significance, if any, has not been established. An intimate relationship between basophil activation and degranulation with tissue eosinophilia has recently been defined, as discussed above.

6

The Immunoglobulins

The specific interaction of antibody with antigens has been observed for nearly a century, and it has long been recognized that antibodies were synthesized as an adaptive response to a stimulus possessing unique properties. In 1938, antibody activity was shown to occur in the gamma globulin fraction of serum. However, it was subsequently demonstrated that not all antibodies are gamma globulins and, as protein structure was further defined, the term immunoglobulin was adopted to designate all types of protein with antibody activity. For convenience, immunoglobulin is usually abbreviated to Ig. As discussed earlier, Ig is synthesized and released only by B lymphocytes. The great bulk of Ig is a product of plasma cells that have nuclear and cytoplasmic properties which especially equip them for synthesis and secretion of antibody and immunoglobulin molecules.

BASIC STRUCTURE OF IMMUNOGLOBULIN

Five distinct classes of immunoglobulins occur in man, with characteristically different chemical structures and biological functions. However, all are similar in molecular structure, having two light (L) polypeptide chains, which may be either the κ or λ variety, and two heavy (H) polypeptide chains, which are different for each class of immunoglobulin (Table 6–1). IgM normally consists of a pentamer of this basic four peptide chain antibody unit, and IgA may occur either as a monomer, dimer, or trimer. IgG, IgE, and IgD occur in the natural state only as four peptide chain monomers (Fig. 6–1). To form the basic immunoglobulin unit of two heavy chains and two light chains, the H chains are linked together by disulfide bonds as well as noncovalent bonds, and each light chain is linked to an adjacent heavy chain by disulfide linkages (Fig. 6–2A). Each pair of heavy and light chains is identical to the other in structure and specificity of its combining site. Each Ig molecule has either κ or λ chains, and hybrids containing both types of light chain do not occur.

Insight into the molecular structure of the immunoglobulins was aided

69

TABLE 6–1.   SUBUNITS OF IMMUNOGLOBULINS

H chains	Five classes of heavy chains exist in man: γ. μ. α. ε. and δ. which determine the type of immunoglobulin. Constant region structure determines the class. μ and ε chains have five domains instead of four. Constant regions contain allelic forms (Gm and Am markers). Variable regions contain the antigen-combining site and idiotypic specificities.
L chains	Two types are found in man: κ and λ. Constant and variable regions about equal in size. Variable region contains antigen-combining site. Ratios of κ to λ in man are about 2:1. L chains are the Bence Jones protein of myelomas.
Fc fragment	Obtained by papain digestion. Contains region that fixes to skin and region for complement fixation. Necessary for placental transfer.
Fab fragment	Obtained by papain digestion. Consists of a light chain and a portion of the H chain. Contains antibody-combining site.
Fab₂ fragment	Obtained by pepsin digestion. Same as intact molecule except that portions of the Fc region of heavy chains above the linking disulfide bond have been removed.
J chains	Secreted by immunoglobulin-producing cells and associated with polymeric IgM and IgA. Molecular ratios may determine units of polymer size. MW 15,000.
Secretory component	In external secretions, the IgA dimer carries a secretory piece having a MW of 60,000, which is synthesized by epithelial cells and attached during secretion of the IgA molecule.

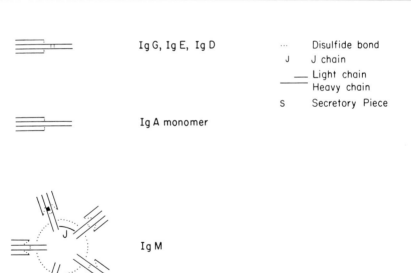

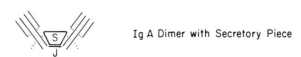

Figure 6–1.   Schematic structures of the immunoglobulin classes. Disulfide bonds may differ from those shown for individual subclasses.

by careful analysis of enzymatic digestion products of the intact molecule and by studies of the myeloma proteins. In both the heavy chains and the light chains, there are constant and variable regions of amino acid sequence. The antigen-binding sites of the antibody are found in the variable region of the molecules. Both the heavy chain and the light chain may contribute to the specificity of the antibody, but of the two, the heavy chain seems to contribute more to the reaction with antigen. The combining sites for the two heavy chains and the two light chains are probably identical. Isolated heavy chains usually bind quite firmly to specific antigen, whereas light chains usually do not bind as firmly. The combination of light and heavy chains from specific antibody is much more effective in binding antigen than are heavy or light chains alone.

Studies of the amino acid sequence show that there is a region of extreme variability in the first 110 residues of both the heavy and light chains as counted from the N terminus. The remaining 110 residues in the light chain and approximately 330 residues in the heavy chain vary much less and comprise the so-called constant regions. Intrachain loops of about 60 residues are found in both the heavy chains (4) and light chains (2), which are stabilized by intrachain disulfide bonds. Certain portions of the variable region display greater variation than others and marked variability (hypervariability) is found in three or four positions on the variable portions of both heavy and light chains. Each hypervariable region is composed of about ten amino acid residues. These represent so-called binding sites and are considered crucial to the specificity of the antibody molecules. The hypervariable regions on the H and L chains are characteristically juxtaposed when the antibody molecule is folded in its natural state. These hypervariable regions seem to contribute greatly to the specificity of the antibody, and the unfolded molecule loses its ability to react strongly with antigen.

If Ig molecules are digested with papain, the polypeptide structure divides into three parts of approximately equal size (Fig. 6–2A): two Fab fragments, each of which contains an antibody-combining site with a light chain and an N terminal half of an H chain, and an FC fragment, which contains the two carboxy terminal halves of the H chains. If, instead, digestion of the molecule is performed with pepsin, the Fc portion is degraded, leaving the two Fab portions linked by a disulfide bond. This fragment is called F(ab)$_2$. The hinge region joins the Fc and Fab portions of the H chain.

IgA and IgM polymers each have one J chain associated with the entire molecule (Fig. 6–1). The J chain is rich in cysteine and has a molecular weight of about 15,000. J chain is secreted by all lymphoid cells producing Ig of all types. The best evidence seems to indicate that the J chains determine polymer size and seal the polymer. IgA of secretory fluids carries an additional polypeptide, the secretory piece, which is synthesized by epithelial cells rather than lymphoid cells. It is attached during transport of the Ig dimer across the epithelial membrane and probably protects the IgA molecule from degradation. Association of J chains, light chains, and secretory components of the IgA molecules is illustrated in Figure 6–2B.

Studies of Ig structure using electron microscopy and x-ray crystallography have helped to reveal its three-dimensional structure. The basic Ig

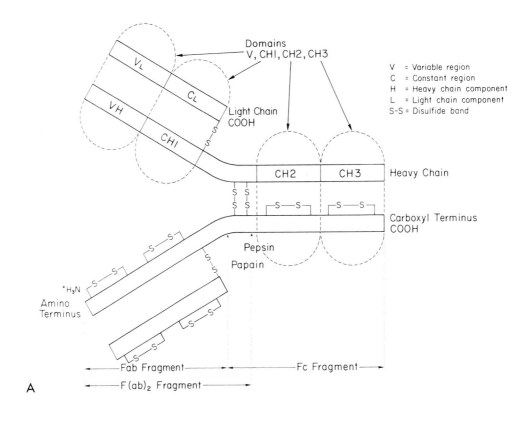

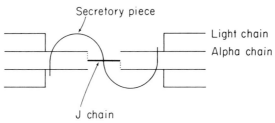

Figure 6–2. *A,* Four-chain structure of an IgG molecule. *B,* Model for combination of J chain and secretory (transport) piece associated with dimeric IgA.

molecular unit appears to consist of symmetrical parts 80 to 120 Å wide and 34 Å thick. When it is reacted with divalent haptens, the molecule assumes a Y shape with the flexibile hinge region apparent about the center of the H chain. The hinge can open to varying degrees. Studies of IgM show a spider-like shape with the Fab portions of the molecule extending outward. X-ray crystallographic studies show that the V_L and V_H regions form a globular domain, and the C_L and C_H regions form another globular domain. Similar domains are found in the Fc portion. However, the interaction between V_L

and C_L and between V_H and C_{H_1} occur at nonhomologous regions on the polypeptide chains. The conformational structure remains basically unchanged after binding to a hapten, but may be significantly changed after binding to a complete antigen.

ANTIGENIC MARKERS OF IMMUNOGLOBULINS

The antigenic specificity of the immunoglobulins is determined by their molecular structure. The antigens of immunoglobulins can be divided into three classes: (1) isotypic antigens, which differentiate major groups and subgroups; (2) allotypic antigens, which are genetically controlled; and (3) idiotypic antigens which are directed against the variable regions of the molecule and may be unique for a given antibody.

Allotypic antigens are characteristically located on the Fc portion of the molecule. The allotypic marker Km (formerly InV) is found on the kappa chain. Km(1) κ chains have valine at position 153 and leucine at position 191, Km(1.2) κ chains have alanine at position 153 and leucine at position 191, and Km(3) κ chains have alanine at position 153 and valine at position 191. Allotypic markers for H chains are called Gm (for gamma marker) on IgG heavy chains and Am (for alpha marker) on IgA. The heavy chain Gm markers are associated with specific subgroups of IgG1, IgG2, and IgG3, but none have yet been described for IgG4. Usually, these markers are structurally represented by single amino acid substitutions.

STRUCTURE-FUNCTION RELATIONSHIPS OF THE IMMUNOGLOBULINS

The major biological activity of the immunoglobulin molecules is to bind to specific antigens, but many other activities, sometimes related to antigen binding, are important (Table 6–2). IgD has not yet been shown to have antibody activity.

IgG

Of the major classes of immunoglobulins, IgG is the most plentiful and undoubtedly the most important in man. Antibodies to most of the bacteria, virus neutralizing antibodies, precipitating antibodies, hemagglutinins, and incomplete hemolysins are among the types of antibody found in IgG. Divalency of the molecular structure permits binding to two antigen molecules at the same time with the formation of a lattice structure with polyvalent antigens, but steric relationships may not permit lattice formation with a few antigens. In humans, IgG is actively transported across the placenta and plays an important role in the defense of newborns against infection since little IgG is synthesized by the fetus in utero. This active transport requires the Fc component of the heavy chain. IgG is formed late in the primary response, and seems to have a regulatory effect on the synthesis of IgM.

TABLE 6–2. SELECTED PROPERTIES OF THE
HUMAN IMMUNOGLOBULINS

	Serum Concentration Mg/Ml	MW	Approximate Sedimentation Constant	MW of H Chain	Electrophoretic Mobility	T½ (days)	Biological Properties
IgG	8–14	150,000	7S	55,000	γ	23 (2 for IgG3)	Activates complement, reacts with rheumatoid factor, sensitizes guinea pig skin, active placental transport. Produced as a late response to antigens.
IgM	0.6–2.0	900,000	19S	65,000	β_{2M}	10	Fixes complement. No placental transfer. Produced as early response to antigens.
IgA	1–3	160,000	7S (9, 11, 13S)	57,000	β_{2A}	5.8	Does not activate complement. Secreted by excretory organs (e.g., saliva, mucus, and colostrum) with transport piece. No placental transfer.
IgE	0.00004	190,000	8S	72,000	γ	2.3	Reaginic antibodies. Sensitizes human skin, leukocytes, and other cells. No placental transfer. May have important defense role in respiratory tract.
IgD	0.03	180,000	7S	63,000	γ	2.8	No known biological function.

Maximal production of IgG can be obtained during immunization by giving the second injection of antigen 30 to 35 days after the first, to allow for maximal differentiation of IgG-producing memory cells. Expansion of the germinal centers is in some way related to increased numbers of IgG-producing cells, possibly by allowing maximal exposure of the cells to antigen on the surface of the dendritic macrophages. The active synthesis of IgG is predominantly by plasma cells in the medullary portions of lymph nodes and in the red pulp of the spleen.

There are four distinct subclasses of IgG, which have different antigenic properties and structures. One of these (IgG4) does not fix complement and IgG2 does so poorly. IgG1 and IgG3 bind to the surface membrane of macrophages and neutrophils. IgG2 does not sensitize guinea pig skin whereas the other subgroups do. The relative concentration expressed as a percentage of serum IgG is as follows: IgG1, 70 per cent; IgG2, 20 per cent; IgG3, 7 per cent; and IgG4, 3 per cent.

IgM

This immunoglobulin is the first to appear after a primary antigenic stimulus, the first to appear in phylogeny and ontogeny, and the last to decrease during senescence. During a primary response, synthesis of IgM characteristically diminishes as the concentration of IgG increases. The regulatory function of IgG on IgM is further suggested by the observation that active IgM synthesis proceeds for a prolonged time when IgG production is inhibited by immunosuppressive treatment.

IgM is a powerful activator of the complement system and is considerably more effective in serologic reactions on a molar basis than is IgG. It is often the predominant antibody formed as a response to gram-negative bacteria, and this probably explains the relatively short period of effective immunity against these bacteria, since IgM is not produced for long periods of time and has a shorter half-life than IgG. Other antibodies characteristically included in this class of immunoglobulins are the Wassermann antibodies, heterophile antibodies, rheumatoid factor, cold agglutinins, hemolysins, and isohemagglutinins. Rheumatoid factors are peculiar among the IgM molecules in that they generally do not fix complement and can interfere with the complement-fixing properties of other IgM and IgG antibodies. The plasma cells that synthesize IgM are found predominantly in the red pulp of the spleen and in zones about the germinal centers and medullary cords of lymph nodes.

IgA

In contrast to IgG and IgM, synthesis of this immunoglobulin occurs in plasma cells located predominantly in the submucosal areas of the mucous epithelial surfaces of the respiratory tract and intestine and in nearly all excretory glands. Approximately 85 per cent of the antibody-producing cells of the lamina propria of the gastrointestinal tract produce IgA. A large proportion of these plasma cells appear to develop in Peyer's patches after intestinal stimulation. There is, then, an enteroenteric system for generating IgA-producing cells that is ultimately deployed in the plasma cells located in the submucosa, especially in the ileal region. Similarly, cells develop in Peyer's patches that give rise to IgA-producing cells in spleen and lymph nodes and in the mammary gland (an enteromammaric system and an enterolymphatic system). Some of the IgA produced in the lamina propria finds its way into the systemic circulation after release from the cell, but most of it passes through or between the epithelial cells to be excreted.

During this active process, two molecules of the dimer IgA are bound to another protein, the transport piece, which perhaps among other functions makes the IgA molecule more resistant to enzymatic attack. The transport piece, or secretory piece, which is such an important part of the molecule in the secretions, is produced by secretory epithelial cells. Large amounts of IgA are excreted onto mucous epithelial surfaces. There it serves as the first line of immunologic defense against invasion of microorganisms, and it is particularly important in preventing gastrointestinal infections and infections of the secretory glands. IgA does not fix complement well by the classical pathway nor does it cross the placental barrier. Whether it utilizes the alternative pathway is still not certain, although it has been shown that aggregates of IgA in high concentration activate the alternative pathway. In ruminants and other animals, in which placental transfer of antibody does not occur, it may be important in providing the newborn with an immunological defense since, like the lactoglobulin antibodies of IgG type, it is absorbed across the newborn's gut as an intact molecule. IgA may act as a blocking antibody in vivo.

IgE

IgE represents an important class of antibody that includes the reagins. Reagins have a high affinity for human skin, leukocytes, and other cells, and they are the cause of many allergic disorders, including hay fever, asthma, and other types of atopy. IgE binds avidly to tissue mast cells and blood basophils by its Fc region. Subsequent exposure of the attached reagin to antigen results in the release of histamine and other mediators from the sensitized cell. IgE may represent an important line of defense in both the upper and lower respiratory tract, and it may represent an important defense mechanism against parasites.

IgD

This immunoglobulin is found in the serum in minute quantities, and no biological function has yet been ascribed to it. However, its presence usually is associated with IgM-containing cells, and this suggests that it may be involved in antigen recognition or that it has a precursor relationship to IgM.

GENETIC CONTROL OF IMMUNOGLOBULIN SYNTHESIS

Three autosomally inherited, nonlinked clusters of genes appear to determine immunoglobulin structure and antibody specificity. The first cluster codes for light chains, apparently with one constant region gene for the kappa type of light chain and at least four alleles for the constant region of the lambda type. The second cluster regulates various classes of heavy chains with approximately ten genes that determine the constant region. The third cluster, which codes for the variable (V) region, contains a much larger number of genes, and while the exact number is still disputed, it is probably on the order of 100 to 1000. Some evidence indicates that the V region has two and possibly three constellations, which code for different portions of the V region. As mentioned earlier, T cells may also use the same set of variable region genes as do B cells, as they have a set of constant region genes which are either entirely different or are no' part of the molecular complex.

How the products of these clearly nonlinked genes code for one polypeptide chain is still a matter of dispute. It is possible that linkage may occur at the DNA level, or at the level of m-RNA (Fig. 6–3). It has been clearly demonstrated that variable regions of heavy chains having identical amino acid sequences may be linked to constant regions of heavy chains possessing different amino acid sequences. Thus, it is almost certain that the constant and variable regions of each heavy chain are coded by different structural genes. Study of pairs of myeloma proteins from patients with two separate myeloma proteins has also shown that different constant regions may link to the same variable region. Since the carboxyl terminus of the variable portion of the immunoglobulin chain has several relatively constant amino acid resi-

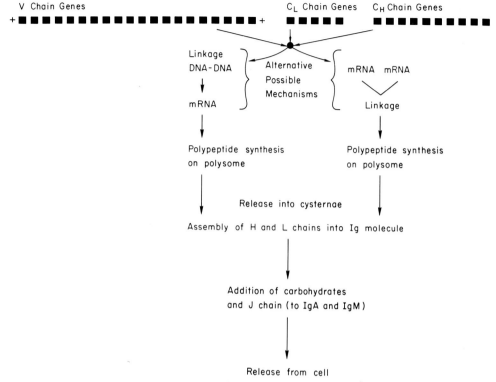

V Chain Genes

CL Chain Genes CH Chain Genes

Linkage
DNA-DNA

Alternative
Possible
Mechanisms

mRNA mRNA

mRNA

Linkage

Polypeptide synthesis
on polysome

Polypeptide synthesis
on polysome

Release into cysternae

Assembly of H and L chains into Ig molecule

Addition of carbohydrates
and J chain (to IgA and IgM)

Release from cell

Figure 6–3. Mechanism of antibody synthesis and release.

dues near the junction of the variable and constant regions, it has been suggested that the carboxyl end of the variable region may be involved in fusion with the constant region. Joining of the variable and constant regions most probably occurs with the aid of genetic-determined enzymes that link DNA or m-RNA, but the mechanism has not yet been elucidated.

The genome of each lymphocyte contains multiple genes for the V region, the C_L region, and the C_H region, but any given lymphocyte synthesizes only one specific kind of antibody molecule. Thus, only one member of each family of genes is expressed, while the others appear to be repressed. There is considerable evidence that, at least in some cells, there is switching of the phenotypic expression of one class of antibody to another, which involves derepression of a constant region gene with simultaneous repression of another constant region gene. The mechanisms involved in activation of repression of genes in mammalian cells is still enigmatic and no clear explanation of reciprocal activation and derepression of linked genes has been forthcoming, even though this is a subject of intensive investigation in molecular biology.

It is also noteworthy that immune response to certain antigens is genetically determined and that this responsiveness is somehow linked to the HLA or major histocompatibility system. This problem, which has been extensively investigated in relation to the major histocompatibility region of the mouse, will be discussed further in Chapter 21.

BIOSYNTHESIS AND SECRETION

Both light chains and heavy chains appear to be synthesized as intact polypeptides, the H chains being synthesized on 300s polysomes containing 11 to 18 ribosomes whereas L chains are synthesized on 200s polysomes containing 4 to 5 ribosomes. Both H chains and L chains, after completion of synthesis, are released into the cisternae of the rough endoplasmic reticulum, where they are assembled by covalent and noncovalent interactions. After the H and L chains have been assembled, carbohydrates are added, and the J chain, which is involved in polymer formation and perhaps polymer size determination, is attached to IgM and IgA shortly before secretion. The mechanism of secretion is not known, although it has been shown to be energy dependent.

ANTIBODY-COMBINING REGIONS

The antibody-combining region of immunoglobulin molecules is located in the variable portion of the Fab fragment. Antigens bind in or adjacent to the cleft between the heavy and light chains. In general, a high degree of specificity is found in antibody populations induced by specific immunization, and antibody may be able to discriminate between two proteins that differ from one another by as little as a single amino acid, between single functional groups on compounds, and between stereoisomers. The population of individual immunoglobulin molecules reacting with a specific antigen may be extremely diverse since as many as several thousand biochemically different immunoglobulin molecules, which bind to a defined antigenic determinant, may be found in a single animal. Conversely, some antigens may stimulate a very restricted response with remarkably homogeneous antibody. It has also been shown that when dissimilar antigens are capable of binding to one immunoglobulin molecule, both antigens will induce the synthesis of that immunoglobulin. The avidity of binding to the immunoglobulin is an important consideration in determining the degree of reactivity. With low energy interactions, the approximate frequency of cross-reactivity of antigens is in the range of 5 per cent. Higher energy interactions occur much less frequently (perhaps 10 times less). It is apparent that the ability of immunoglobulin to bind antigens with low affinity is quite frequent, whereas high affinity binding is relatively infrequent. Thus, while there is a large number of potential antigens, a great degree of cross-reactivity occurs between these antigens and specific immunoglobulin molecules, which increases with decreased avidity of the binding.

The antibody-combining site itself is relatively small, in the range of 30 Å $\times$ 14 Å $\times$ 6 Å. However, there may be multiple contact points with which antibodies can interact with antigens, occurring over an extensive region of the variable portion of the immunoglobulin molecule. Other experiments have presented clear evidence that binding sites of different specificities occur throughout the variable region and that the combining region is in fact a mosaic of binding sites for different determinants or even one determinant on a given antigen.

In the above discussion, it is apparent that antibody specificity is a population phenomenon. When antigen levels are high early in the immune response, there will be effective stimulation of cells producing both high and low affinity antibodies. Later, however, as antigen levels fall, only cells with high affinity receptors will be stimulated, and these cells will produce high affinity antibodies.

Affinity is the measure of binding of an antigen at a single binding site. It depends upon the complementarity of the functional groups and the degree of stabilizing noncovalent interactions involving hydrophobic and ionic contributions, as well as hydrogen bonding. For any given immunoglobulin molecule and antigen, this process appears to be genetically determined rather than directed by antigen. Measurement of affinity, however, involves examination of a population of different immunoglobulins rather than a single one. Avidity of antibody molecules for an antigen may involve more than one combining site.

7

Complement

To the majority of clinicians, complement represents an entirely new and poorly understood subject. For this reason, acquisition of new knowledge of complement is sometimes actively or, more often, passively avoided. This aversion is somewhat understandable since the field has advanced rapidly during the past 15 years, the system is complex, the terminology has changed several times, and many of the reactions within the system and interactions with other systems are still not completely understood. However, many scientific studies in recent years have served to stabilize both the field and its terminology and to bring agreement among its leaders about the major events so that explanations can now be simplified. As an aid for the reader, current terminology used in discussing the complement system is summarized in Table 7–1.

The term complement refers to a complex system of serum proteins which, interacting in a cascade or cascades, serves primarily to amplify the effects of an interaction between specific antigen and its corresponding antibody. There are two recognized pathways of complement activation, respectively known as the classical pathway and the alternative pathway (also called properdin pathway and formerly called C3 bypass mechanism, alternate pathway, or C3 shunt). These will be discussed separately and their interactions at C3 emphasized.

THE CLASSICAL PATHWAY OF COMPLEMENT

Activation of the classical pathway of complement usually requires an antigen–antibody reaction. However, only IgM and three of the four subclasses of IgG among the several immunoglobulins are known to activate the classical pathway. Most of the reactions have been studied in the fluid phase or at the site of antibody–antigen union on erythrocyte membranes. The physical and chemical nature of the reactions has been studied in detail, but this information will be presented only briefly. The single components are present in the serum in inactive precursor forms.

TABLE 7–1. TERMINOLOGY AND ABBREVIATIONS USED IN THE COMPLEMENT SYSTEM

TERM	SYMBOL OR ABBREVIATION	COMMENT
Complement	C	General term, usually precedes a designated component
Classical components	C1–C9	Nine separate components are in the classical pathway
Antibody	A	Refers to antibody capable of activating complement
Erythrocyte	E	Has antigenic sites (S), which will combine with specific A
Subcomponents of C1	q, r, s	Used as postscripts to C1
Properdin	P	Alternative pathway component
Properdin convertase	PC	Existence controversial
Factor B	B	Alternative pathway component. Same as C3 proactivator (C3PA) and glycine-rich beta glycoprotein (GBG) in older literature
Factor D	D	Alternative pathway component. Same as C3 proactivator convertase (C3PAse)
Initiating factor	IF	Closely related to nephritogenic factor. Involved in initiation of the alternative pathway activity
C3b inactivator	C3bINA or KAF	Latter abbreviation derives from the German spelling of the old name: Konglutinogen activating factor
Activated factor	$\overline{C42}$ *(example)*	Activated factors are often designated by placing a bar over the component(s) symbol
Degradation fragment	C3a *(example)*	Enzymatic cleavage of a molecule gives two or more fragments, usually designated as postscripts by small letters
Antigenic specificity	C3(B) *(example)*	The antigens of C3 are sometimes expressed as a large letter in parentheses following the component symbol. One must be careful not to confuse factor B, C3b, and C3(B), which represent entirely different things
Inactive fragment	C3bi *(example)*	Postscript i represents inactive state of a previously active molecule

SEQUENCE OF REACTIONS

The union of specific antibody with its corresponding antigen produces or reveals a site in the Fc portion of the heavy chain that combines with C1q to fix the trimolecular complex of C1 (C1qrs) in the presence of calcium ion and activate the proenzyme subunit (C1r), which in turn activates C1s to form an activated esterase. A single molecule of IgM can initiate complement activation, whereas at least two molecules of IgG are needed for activation, and the molecules of IgG must not be too far apart on the cell surface.

The critical distance for red blood cells is approximately 7000 Å. The immune complex and activated C1 (C$\overline{1}$) then interacts with C4 and C2 in the presence of Mg++ to split C4 and C2 each into two fragments. Splitting of C4 activates two sites, one that binds to the membrane and the other that binds to C2 to form a loose complex. One activated C1 molecule can assemble as many as 200 C$\overline{4b}$ molecules around it. The activated C$\overline{42}$ complex acts as an enzyme, called C3 convertase. The C$\overline{42}$ convertase can activate numerous C3 molecules, many of which become attached at different sites on surrounding areas of the cell membrane, and some bind with C3 convertase (C$\overline{42}$) to form the triple complex C$\overline{423b}$. The fixed C3b reacts with C5, C6, and C7, either in sequence or possibly wth C5, C6, and C7 as a trimolecular complex. C5 is split into two fragments, C5a and C5b, and C5b is bound to a site on the membrane that is distinctly different from that binding the C$\overline{423b}$ complex. C8 reacts next, and then C9. With the activation of C9, lesions that resemble small holes are produced in susceptible membranes. These functional holes appear to be due to insertion of terminal complement components into and through the membrane. A complement-damaged site on the cell membrane is often designated by the symbol S*. When lysis of human erythrocytes is produced in the presence of an excess of human complement, the erythrocytes show a maximum of 90,000 lesions approximately 100 Å in diameter per cell. Although the exact nature of the ultrastructural lesion remains somewhat obscure, the lesion permits loss of intracellular constituents, entrance of extracellular ions, and cellular swelling until the cell disintegrates.

The sequence of reactions of the classical pathway is shown diagramatically in Figure 7–1. On the red cell membrane, there appear to be four sites that are involved in the reactions. The first is at the antigenic site where antibody and C1 react, the second site binds C$\overline{42}$, the third site binds C3b (sometimes also bound at site of C$\overline{42}$ to form C$\overline{423b}$), and the fourth is the site for C56789 assembly and ultimate insertion of the terminal components into the membrane (Fig. 7–2).

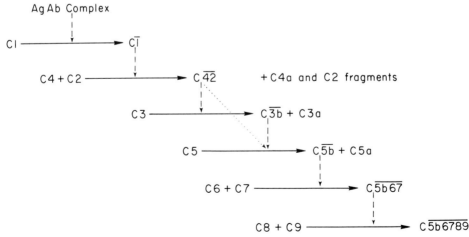

Figure 7–1. Schematic diagram of molecular sequences during activation of the classical pathway of complement.

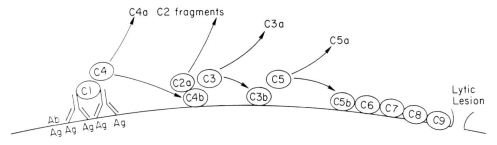

Figure 7–2. Diagrammatic representation of the reaction sites of the classical complement pathway on the red cell membrane.

PROPERTIES OF CLASSICAL PATHWAY COMPONENTS

The proteins of the classical pathway have now all been purified and partially characterized. Selected properties are shown in Table 7–2.

THE ALTERNATIVE PATHWAY

In 1954, Pillemer and his coworkers described properdin and some of its biological effects, but the findings were not well accepted by the scientific

TABLE 7–2. CHARACTERISTICS OF THE PROTEINS OF THE CLASSICAL PATHWAY OF COMPLEMENT

COMPONENT	APPROXIMATE SERUM CONCENTRATION (MCG/ML)	ELECTROPHORETIC MOBILITY	NUMBER OF CHAINS	MOLECULAR WEIGHT	SITE OF SYNTHESIS	SEDIMENTATION COEFFICIENT	LABILITY TO: HEAT	NH$_3$
C1q	180	γ_2	18	400,000	Gut epithelium, macrophages?, lymphocytes?	11.1	+	0
C1r	100	β	2	180,000	Gut epithelium, macrophages?, lymphocytes?	7.5	++	0
C1s	30	α_2	1	86,000	Gut epithelium, macrophages?, lymphocytes?	4.5	0	0
C4	450	β_{1e}	3	206,000	Macrophage	10.0	0	++
C2	25	β_1	–	117,000	Macrophage	4.5	++	0
C3	1400	β_{1c}	2	180,000	Liver	9.5	0	+
C5	80	β_{1f}	2	180,000	Liver?, spleen, macrophage	8.7	0	+
C6	75	β_2	1	95,000	Liver	5.5	+	0
C7	55	β_2	1	110,000	?	6.0	0	0
C8	80	γ_1	3	163,000	Many tissues	8.0	+	0
C9	2	α_2	–	79,000	Liver	4.5	0	0

TABLE 7-3. SELECTED PROPERTIES OF ALTERNATIVE
PATHWAY COMPONENTS

COMPONENT	APPROXIMATE SERUM CONCENTRATION (MCG/ML)	ELECTRO-PHORETIC MOBILITY	MOLECULAR WEIGHT	SEDIMENTATION COEFFICIENT	LABILITY TO: HEAT	NH$_3$
Properdin	20	γ	184,000	5.2	0	0
Factor B	200	β	80,000	6.2	+	0
Factor D	Trace	α_2	25,000	4	0	0
IF	Trace	β	150,000	?	?	?

community or apparently even well understood by the investigators. Tragically, despondency over the lack of interest and the negative reaction by his peers in part led to Pillemer's suicide. However, several more recent observations soon awakened new interest in properdin and the alternative pathway of complement activation. It was discovered that gram-negative bacterial endotoxin could activate the terminal sequence of complement components beginning at C3, without the apparent help of antibody. Cobra venom, which was first thought to be an inactivator of complement, was found to contain a factor that could deplete serum of C3 by activating C3 and the distal components, but not C1, C4, or C2, rendering the serum hemolytically and opsonically inactive. Also, serum totally deficient in C2 or C1 activity was fully active in opsonization of certain bacteria. These observations led to the elucidation of an alternative mechanism for activating the complement system at the level of C3. This is known as the alternative (or properdin) pathway, and it involves factor D, factor B, properdin (P), initiating factor (IF), and perhaps properdin convertase (PC), as well as C3 (or C3b). Selected properties of the alternative pathway components are shown in Table 7-3.

ACTIVATION OF THE ALTERNATIVE PATHWAY

While much has been learned about the alternative pathway in recent years and even precise biochemical schemes have been presented defining its component interactions, much remains to be learned and new interactions and functions are constantly being described.

A variety of substances has been shown to initiate activation of the alternative pathway, including zymosan (cell walls of yeast), lipopolysaccharides of gram-negative bacteria (endotoxin), cobra venom factor, inulin, a nephritogenic factor from serum of patients with hypocomplementemic nephritis, and aggregates of IgA and IgE. Pathways for activation are shown schematically in Figure 7-3. This represents a current view of the complex process, and it is unlikely to be completely correct. For example, the role of properdin itself may be multifactorial. It is not necessary for activation of the alternative pathway, but probably can be involved in this process as a convertase.

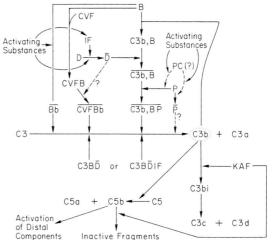

Figure 7–3. Schematic representation of the alternative pathway of complement.

Under certain circumstances, its primary role appears to involve an interaction to stabilize the C3bB convertase complex. It is uncertain whether activation is necessary for that function.

Exactly where and how initiation of activation of the alternative pathway is accomplished by many of the activating substances is also still a matter of discussion and dispute. Most probably, multiple mechanisms are involved. For example, trypsin can convert D to $\overline{D}$ and trypsin; plasmin or pronase can replace $\overline{D}$ in the activation of B. The role of antibody in initiation of the reaction is also unknown, but may be of considerable importance.

Despite our relative ignorance of the alternative pathway, it seems to be a primordial mechanism that may have even preceded the development of the classical pathway in evolution.

ADDITIONAL MECHANISMS FOR COMPLEMENT ACTIVATION

As study of the complement system progresses, evidence seems to be accumulating which indicates that this system plays major roles contributing to survival advantage far beyond its role as an important biological amplifier of certain antigen-antibody interactions. Obviously, the consequences of complement action can initiate numerous protective as well as destructive events. It seems to be involved directly and without antibody in destruction of certain abnormal cells. Complement can also be activated directly by cell wall components (like lipopolysaccharides of the bacterial cell surfaces) by acute phase reactants (e.g., C-reactive protein), by interactions of polyanions and polycations, and by a number of other chemicals.

With the complexity of the complement system, it is not surprising that a number of substances may activate complement at various levels. As examples, protein A from *Staphylococcus aureus* can induce marked depletion of hemolytic complement activity both in vivo and in vitro by activation of the classical pathway. Polyinosinic acid can activate complement by interaction with C1q; heparin and protamine in appropriate concentrations may bind and inactivate C1 without depletion of distal components. DNA and lysozyme may deplete the classical pathway. The reactions produced by polyanions and polycations may be markedly increased by the presence of C-reactive protein (CRP) which will itself react with C1q. CRP is an interesting acute phase protein, the concentration of which becomes markedly elevated—as much as 1000-fold—during an acute inflammatory process. It may bind C1q to activate the classical pathway. It also binds to many membranes and may participate in phagocytic mechanisms, but its precise role in host defense remains to be determined.

Certain viruses, such as the Maloney leukemia virus, may react with fresh serum to result in the consumption of classical pathway components. An important biological observation is that plasmin and streptolysin S, through activation of plasmin, activate C1s, and kallikrein has also been shown to activate C1s. These may be important reactions in inflammatory processes. Other pathways of direct activation of C3, exclusive of the classical and properdin pathways, include cleavage of C3 by plasmin, certain tissue proteases, and thrombin. Trypsin may also cleave C5. Lastly, altered membranes may activate the complement sequence, but the mechanisms remain incompletely studied.

REGULATORS OF COMPLEMENT REACTIONS

The potent biological consequences of complement system activation demand that activation be regulated. This is accomplished with the aid of several inhibitors and by a short biological half-life of some of the components and their derivative peptides. C1 inhibitor is a natural substrate for C1 esterase and interacts stoichiometrically with the activated enzyme, interfering with the reaction of C4 and C3. Deficiency of this inhibitor leads to hereditary angioedema. KAF (C3b INA) is an important regulator of complement activation, which cleaves biologically active C3b into two inactive molecular fragments, C3c and C3d. It may also inactivate C5b by cleavage. Breakdown of C3b by KAF is impaired by properdin. C3a is inactivated by an enzyme that has carboxypeptidase B–like activity, which acts by splitting the C terminal arginine residue from the polypeptide chain. A C6 inactivator has been described, but little is known of its mechanism of action or chemistry except that it inactivates cellbound C6. Another inactivating factor, apparently with effect on C7, is as yet poorly characterized.

BIOLOGICAL EFFECTS OF COMPLEMENT ACTIVATION

The biological consequences of complement activation may perhaps be appreciated best by examining the effects of the various activation steps (Table 7–4).

TABLE 7–4. BIOLOGICAL EFFECTS OF COMPLEMENT FRAGMENTS ADDITIONAL TO SEQUENTIAL ACTIVATION OF THE SYSTEM

MEDIATOR	EFFECT
C4a	Release of serotonin
C2b	Kinin-like activity
C4b	Immune adherence
C3a	Anaphylatoxin, vascular effect Chemotaxis Leukocyte mobilization
C3b	Opsonization Immune adherence; release of platelet Factor 3
C5a	Same effects as C3a
C5b	Opsonin for Candida (?) C5b may attach to platelets, active distal components, and cause platelet lysis as an innocent bystander
C$\overline{567}$	Chemotaxis
C$\overline{8}$	Initiates lytic process. Inserted into membrane
C$\overline{9}$	Completes lytic process

The smaller split product of C4, (C4a), is said to lead to the release of serotonin, and a fragment derived from C2, (C2b), has kinin-like activity. The latter is distinct from bradykinin and has been shown to produce permeability effects on small blood vessels without involving histamine release. The other product of C4, (C4b), derived by enzymatic action of C$\overline{1}$, may participate in immune adherence by attaching to membrane receptors on the cells in question.

C3 is the pivotal molecule in the complement sequence. Activation by either the alternative or classical pathway results in the release of two extremely important mediators. The smaller, C3a, has anaphylatoxic, chemotactic, and leukocyte-mobilizing activities. Its MW is approximately 7000 D. Principally through the anaphylatoxic activity, which causes release of mediators from mast cells, it may result in widening of capillary vessels, exudation of fluid, increased stickiness and adherence of cells to endothelial vascular membranes, and the deposition of inflammatory cells. Once phagocytic cells have reached the inflammatory focus, a concentration gradient of C3a may result in directed movement (chemotaxis) toward the cell wall of a microbe which has initiated the activation of the complement sequence. The larger C3 fragment (C3b) has much greater biological importance, since it becomes bound to foreign cells and microbes, acts to stimulate the alternative pathway amplification loop, and has potent opsonic properties. In addition, it may participate in the phenomenon of immune adherence. Neutrophils and macrophages both have receptors for C3b, which initiate phagocytosis. Immune adherence of microorganisms or cells to platelets may cause the release of platelet factor 3.

Activation of C5 is caused by enzymatic cleavage to release C5a, which has basically the same biological effects as C3a; however, their effects on mast cells are not cross-reacting. Apparently, they attach by different receptors or possibly attach to different subsets of cells. C5a is also a potent chemotaxin, perhaps the most potent of the chemotactic reactors. The trimolecular complex of activated C5, 6, and 7 (C567) apparently has additional chemotactic activity. Finally, partial degradation of the cell membrane is caused by assembly of several molecules of activated C8 at the surface, and activated C9 acts to complete the lytic process. C5b, which is released by fluid phase activation, may attach to adjacent platelets where it can initiate activation of the distal complement components and lyse the platelets as innocent bystanders. Another important consideration of the complement system is that it interacts with both the clotting system and kinin systems. These interactions and potential relationships are shown in Figure 7–4. It is not surprising that complement, which has such potent biological effects, may be both beneficial and harmful.

Through these powerful activities, complement plays a vital role in immunologic and nonimmunologic defense against bacteria of both high grade

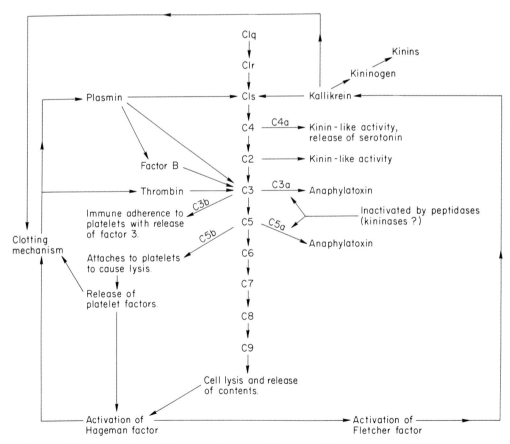

Figure 7–4. Interactions of the complement, clotting, and kinin systems. Inhibitory interactions are not shown.

and lower grade pathogenicity, fungi, viruses, protozoa, and possibly even helminth invaders. The complement system is also involved in elimination of effete and foreign cells. It plays important roles in initiating and controlling inflammatory reactions, coagulation of the blood, and circulation of blood through its potent influences on vascular reactivity. Indeed, the complement system stands at the very center of the effector processes for specific immunologic reactions with respect to defenses and tissue injury, and near the center of nonspecific mechanisms of resistance to infection and intoxication.

8

Mechanisms of Immunologic Injury

From the very earliest studies of immunity carried out by Jenner, it was apparent that immune reactions may be associated with both bodily defense and tissue damage. Jenner marveled at the observation that heightened resistance to smallpox and vaccinia viruses was regularly associated with the early development of increased inflammation. With the description of serum sickness by von Pirquet and Schick early in this century, it became apparent that immune responses to foreign proteins frequently led to disease and tissue destruction. However, many of the mechanisms involved in tissue injury produced by immune reactions have been elucidated only in recent years. There has been great effort to relate these mechanisms to the pathogenesis of human diseases, and progress has resulted largely from the incisive application of developing immunological technology and interpretation of experimental models. The clinical relevance of these models will become apparent.

Seldom does an immunological reaction stand as an isolated event in vivo. Instead, one reaction leads to others, eventuating in a complex and dynamic interaction of effector mechanisms and inhibitory controls. In this chapter, we shall attempt to describe as independent processes the primary mechanisms of immunologic reactions that may result in injury. Sometimes, these may be related to a specific disease, but more often, integration of events consequent to several immune processes is necessary to explain most diseases. The clinical features of this latter group with their interacting immunologic processes will be interpreted in later chapters.

IMMUNOLOGIC INJURY INITIATED BY ANTIGEN-ANTIBODY REACTIONS

REAGIN DEPENDENT ANAPHYLACTIC REACTIONS

IgE (reagin) is strongly cytophilic for mast cells and basophils, attaching to the cell membranes via the Fc portion of the heavy chains. When specific

90

antigen forms a complex with the cellbound IgE antibody, a series of reactions occur, which rapidly result in the release of granule bound histamine from the cells (the only source of stored histamine in the body). Histamine has numerous biologic effects, including constriction of smooth muscle (especially in the lung, gut, blood vessels, and uterus), increase of vascular permeability, and increase in gastric acid secretion (Fig. 8–1). The effect of histamine on the microvasculature is especially important since the vascular constriction results in an increase in capillary dilatation, separation of the junctions between endothelial cells, an increase in the adhesiveness of the endothelium, local acidosis, and hypoxia. Soon, there is extravasation of plasma proteins into the extravascular spaces and diapedesis of leukocytes from the capillaries. The clinical consequences of this set of reactions, when generalized and intense, include headache, flushing of the skin, sequestration of fluid extravascularly, asthma, diarrhea (occasionally), vomiting, and hypovolemic shock. Secondary effects may come from activation of Hageman factor which, in turn, activates the clotting mechanism and leads to release of kinins. This condition is known as anaphylactic shock, and it may result in death of the patient if treatment is not given promptly. More localized processes dependent on this immunologic mechanism may result in allergic rhinitis, angioneurotic edema, asthma, or urticaria.

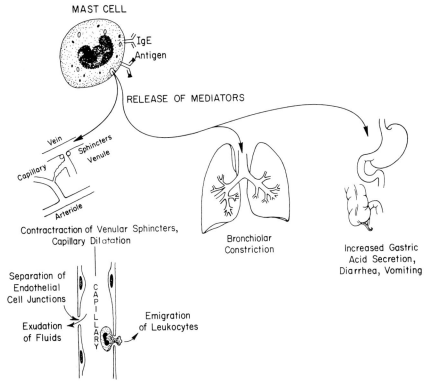

Figure 8–1. Effects of generalized histamine release from mast cells, caused by IgE-antigen reaction.

Histamine is not the only mediator of this response. Slow reacting substance-A (SRS-A), the prostaglandins, the kinins (notably bradykinin), and perhaps others may play variable but important roles. SRS-A has an effect similar to that of histamine in that it contracts smooth muscle of the bronchi, increases vascular permeability, and contributes to edema formation. It has a more prolonged effect than histamine (thus, its name) and unlike histamine is synthesized and released during anaphylaxis rather than being released from a preformed store.

The prostaglandins (PG) have received much attention as possible mediators in recent years. They probably play a role in IgE-mediated reactions, but that role is not yet well defined. Their effects are variable, depending upon the type of PG, but they include changes of permeability of vessels, contraction of smooth muscle, and potentiation of other vasoactive mediators.

Bradykinin, a simple nonapeptide, and other kinins are formed during anaphylaxis via the release of kallikrein and other proteases from cells that split kininogens to form kinins. Bradykinin causes contraction of most types of smooth muscle, increases vascular permeability, and causes sweating.

HOMOCYTOTROPIC IgG ANAPHYLACTIC REACTIONS

Some forms of IgG have been found to have the ability to bind to mast cells and basophils, although not as avidly as IgE. This activity has been attributed primarily to antibodies of the IgG4 subclass, although not all IgG4 binds to mast cells. Antigen interaction with this cellbound IgG antibody also results in the release of histamine, with the general consequences as described above.

ANAPHYLATOXINS

The formation of C3a and C5a during complement activation initiated by antigen-antibody reactions has already been discussed. These are called anaphylatoxins because one of their biologic activities is to cause the release of histamine from mast cells. Interestingly, C3a and C5a act either on different receptors on mast cells or on different populations of cells. These receptors are also different from those for IgE or IgG4. Since the effect on mast cells is similar to IgE-Ag, the end result of the release of large amounts of mediators may be anaphylaxis, and localized release can result in inflammatory lesions resembling those of atopy.

CYTOLYTIC REACTIONS INITIATED BY ANTIGEN–ANTIBODY REACTIONS

Fixation of antibody to specific antigens on the surfaces of isolated cells usually does not cause much discernible change in the cell. Certainly, the cells are not lysed. However, when IgM or IgG antibodies react with cell surface antigens and activate complement during the process, profound changes may follow that often include lysis and death of that cell. The IgM type of antibody is usually more efficient in this reaction than is IgG. Hemolytic transfusion reactions represent an example of such a reaction, and cytolytic processes involving cells affected by these immunologic reactions are especially important in cancer and transplantation. Reactions involving drug sensitivity, where haptens have become attached to the surfaces of normal cells, may also be cytolytic in nature. The mechanisms of cell injury involving complement-mediated cytolysis, as set in motion by IgM or IgG antibodies, have been described in the preceding chapter.

Cells of different types vary markedly in their susceptibility to immune cytolysis because of differences in the amount and kinds of antigens on the cell surface, topographical relationships of the antigens to complement-binding sites, variations in chemical structure of the cell surface, the amount and kind of complement and antibody that is fixed, and the capacity of the cell to repair damaged areas. Not only may a target cell be lysed in vivo by this immunologic reaction, but platelets with immune adherence receptors may undergo bystander lysis if C5-9 activation occurs near the C3 sites to which they are attached. Thus, an extremely complex set of events may be triggered by complement-mediated immune cytolysis.

The pathology of cytolytic reactions is probably expressed in its most dramatic form by intravascular hemolytic reactions (Fig. 8–2, also see

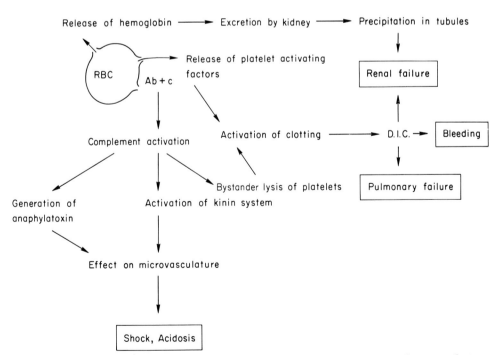

Figure 8–2. Immunologic injury associated with immune intravascular hemolytic transfusion reactions.

Chapter 17). The main clinical manifestations are consequent in large part to activation of complement rather than to hemolysis per se. In fact, lysis of large amounts of red blood cells by accidental dialysis of patient's blood against water instead of the usual dialysis fluid has resulted in few signs or symptoms except hemoglobinemia, hemoglobinuria, and jaundice.

OPSONIZATION OF CELLS WITH PHAGOCYTIC DESTRUCTION

Even when cells are not lysed by the effects of antibody and complement, they may be destroyed. If C3b has been deposited on their surface, they are vulnerable to phagocytosis by neutrophils and macrophages, and it appears that at least certain macrophages can ingest cells coated only with C3d. In some instances, antibody alone may be opsonic in vitro, but this opportunity occurs rarely in vivo. Removal and destruction of opsonized cells may occur with peripheral tissues or by removal from the blood by the fixed RES of the liver and spleen. Examples of such removal are represented by some of the diseases that involve autoimmune hemolysis, where full opsonization may not have occurred. Whether increased phagocytic destruction occurs largely as a function of liver or spleen depends upon the amount of antibody that has coated the red blood cells. Relatively weak opsonization results in removal of cells by spleen, whereas quantitatively greater opsonization results in removal by liver. The mechanisms of phagocytosis have been discussed in Chapters 4 and 5.

STIMULATION OF CELLS BY ANTIBODY

In a few instances, reaction of antibody with cellular antigens has a stimulating effect, but whether this represents a reaction to partial damage is unclear. Increased amounts of lysosomal enzymes may be excreted by the affected cells. One example of this stimulating effect of cell specific antibody in human disease is long-acting thyroid stimulator (LATS), an antibody which reacts with thyroid parenchymal cells to cause hyperthyroidism. Similarly, antibody reacting with surface antigens on certain cells can stimulate them to proliferate or undergo differentiation.

MECHANISMS OF INJURY CAUSED BY ANTIGEN–ANTIBODY COMPLEXES

During the immune process, when antibody is made against circulating or cell-free antigens, changing ratios of antigen and antibody appear, a result of increasing synthesis of antibody and increasing removal of antigen. Antigen–antibody complexes formed in moderate antigen excess often remain soluble, are locally toxic to tissues, and have a strong capacity to activate complement. Indeed, antigen-antibody complexes localized to vessels and tissues represent one of the most common and most damaging mechanisms of immunologic injury. When antigen–antibody complexes form at equivalence or in the region of mild antibody excess, the complex tends to become hydrophobic and precipitate. Such complexes are rapidly removed from the circulation by the phagocytic cells of the reticuloendothelial system. For this reason, precipitated complexes are less toxic than soluble antigen–antibody complexes, but they may cause damage when precipitated, particularly on basement membranes (Fig. 8–3). Recently, it has been found that the receptors on cells for the Fc portion of IgG or the C3b component of complement may serve to bind Ag-Ab–complement complexes to the cell surface, where the complex can produce damage to the cell (or platelet) even though it is an innocent bystander. Several types of clinically distinct processes can be caused by antigen–antibody complexes.

The Arthus Reaction.   The classical Arthus reaction is a vascular lesion that develops when IgG antibody and antigen combine at or in a vessel wall when one has been present in the intravascular compartment and the other distributed in the extravascular spaces. Subcutaneous injection of antigen in a previously immunized individual causes a direct Arthus type of reaction, but the reversed situation, where antibody is in the tissue and the antigen is intravascular, can produce the same lesion. The Arthus lesion is dependent upon the presence of neutrophils, but complement requirements are less well defined, since the reaction may be of normal intensity in C4-deficient guinea pigs and occurs in an attenuated form in animals depleted of C3-9 by cobra venom factor. Neutrophils contain a variety of enzymes that may dam-

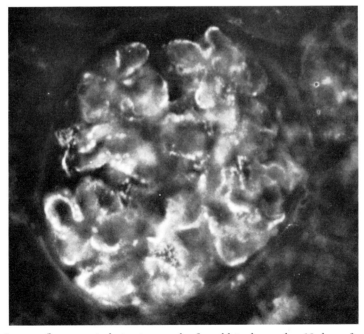

Figure 8–3.   Immunofluorescent photomicrograph of a rabbit glomerulus 10 days after the injection of bovine serum albumin, showing fine granular deposits of rabbit IgG. (From Fish, A. J., et al., Am. J. Pathol., 49:997–1022, 1966.)

age tissues when released. These include cathepsins, proteases, lipases, lysozyme, nucleases, phosphatases, peptidases, and others. Together, these products of cellular damage markedly amplify and expand inflammatory lesions initiated by other mediators, and they are important in nearly all immune processes that result in tissue damage. The assumed mechanism of damage is show in Figure 8–4.

Serum Sickness. When von Pirquet and Schick discovered serum sickness in 1905, they proved that immunity can be deleterious to man, as well as man's great benefactor. Clincal manifestations of serum sickness include fever, skin rash, eosinophilia, leukocytosis, arthralgias, arthritis, diffuse vasculitis, kidney disease, and even cardiac disease. Serum sickness reactions usually develop when a large single dose of foreign protein, such as horse serum, is given intravenously or intramuscularly. The clinical illness is highly variable and ranges from a relatively mild arthritis and fever to a progressive, fatal vasculitis with distinctive renal and cardiac disease.

The mechanism of injury in human serum sickness is almost certainly

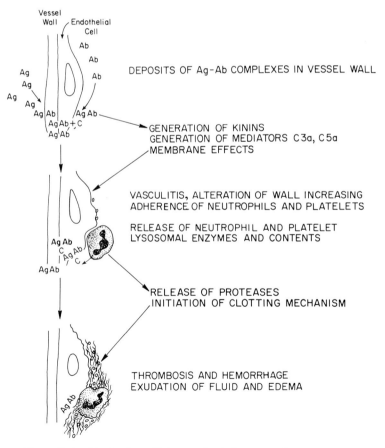

Figure 8–4.   Mechanism of injury in the Arthus type of reaction.

the same as in the well studied model of one-shot serum sickness in rabbits and can be attributed to the widespread renal and vascular deposition of soluble antigen–antibody complexes formed in antigen excess near the equivalence zone. Tissue damage is caused by activation of serum complement at the sites of deposition of these complexes, with consequent establishment of a widespread inflammatory vasculitis. Fortunately, the immunological injury in serum sickness is usually short-lived, and the renal lesions, vascular damage, arthritis, and carditis subside spontaneously as the antigen–antibody complexes are metabolized and disappear from the blood vessels. The acute disease does not subside completely until the damaging antigen–antibody complexes have been removed by phagocytic processes. In occasional instances, the process may be more persistent, and diffuse allergic vasculitis, similar to periarteritis nodosa, may occur. This illness, which may last for months and occasionally for years, is attributed to persistence of antigen or to sensitization to a new antigen from body constituents.

Massive Complement Activation by Antigen–Antibody Complexes or Endotoxin. Combination of large amounts of antigen with complement fixing antibody in the circulation or direct intravascular activation of complement by endotoxin or other substances results in a series of immunologic events that may produce shock, disseminated intravascular coagulation (DIC), and even death. The pathologic process is complement-mediated and therefore in some details may be similar to the events seen in anaphylactic shock or immune intravascular hemolysis. However, major differences from these, attributed to the fact that antigen–antibody complexes contributed in greater degree to the development of vasculitis and mediators released from neutrophils, play a more prominent role in the inflammatory reaction. In addition, both the vasculitis and bystander lysis of platelets contribute greatly to the development of DIC.

Mechanisms of Renal Injury. When conditions are ideal for production of soluble antigen–antibody complexes in the circulating blood for a prolonged period, large irregular ("lumpy-bumpy") accumulations of antigen and host antibody occur on the epithelial side of the glomerular basement membranes, and glomerulonephritis develops. The chronic nephritis of experimental animals produced in this manner has pathologic and clinical characteristics strikingly similar to those observed in the glomerulonephritis of systemic lupus erythematosus, certain types of chronic progressive glomerulonephritis, and one form of nephrotic syndrome of man.

In studies leading to the development and interpretation of this modification of the serum sickness model, Dixon and his associates found that rabbits injected repeatedly with bovine serum proteins could be divided into three groups: a few formed no demonstrable antibodies, some formed large amounts of antibody, and some were relatively poor antibody producers. Animals that formed no antibodies did not develop vascular or glomerular lesions. The rabbits that were especially vigorous producers of antibody developed lesions of acute serum sickness, which abated after free antibody appeared in the circulation. It proved difficult to give such animals amounts of antigen large enough to maintain a condition in which they had circulating soluble antigen–antibody complexes, and little or no tissue damage was observed. In the group of animals that were rather poor or only moderate producers of antibody, repeated injections of antigen over a prolonged period provided prolonged exposure to soluble antigen–antibody complexes that led to the development of chronic proliferative and inflammatory glomerulonephritis. The conditions obtained in those animals producing low amounts of antibody were ideal for achieving deposits of antigen–antibody complexes in renal glomeruli, which were capable of activating serum complement and initiating immunologic injury. Immunofluorescent and electron microscopic study of this model has demonstrated the presence of these damaging immune complexes on the epithelial side of the glomerular membrane in a "lumpy-bumpy" distribution adjacent to and between the foot processes of the epithelial cells (Fig. 8–5).

Both in serum sickness and in the Dixon model of chronic glomerulonephritis, the hallmark of indirect immune damage from deposition of antigen-antibody–complement complexes has been the interrupted or irregular deposition of these complexes in vessel walls, together with complement components. Similar complexes may be deposited along the basement membranes in the skin. This deposition, which can readily be demonstrated by immunofluorescent microscopy, is sometimes important in the pathogenesis of diseases like lupus erythematosus, where inflammation of the skin may be attributed to the deposition of the complexes in an extravascular site.

The so-called nephrotoxic nephritis is a classical model of immunologic injury, first studied by Masugi in 1933. In the original experiments, rabbits

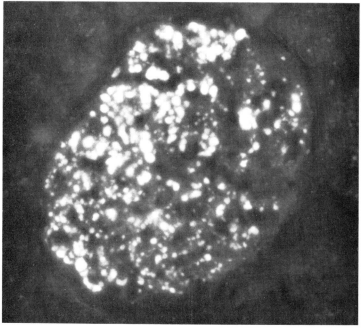

Figure 8–5.   Immunofluorescent photomicrograph of a rabbit glomerulus 2.5 weeks after the onset of nephritis in the Dixon model, showing large nodular deposits of rabbit C3. (From Fish, A. J., et al., Am. J. Pathol., 49:997–1022, 1966.)

were immunized with rat kidneys, and antiserum obtained two to three weeks later was found to be nephrotoxic when injected into rats. With very large doses of nephrotoxic serum, a rapidly developing nephrotic syndrome may be observed; but with smaller doses, a more gradually developing acute or chronic glomerulonephritis is seen. Nephrotoxic nephritis has been found to be produced by an immune assault of antibody against the glomerular basement membranes. When analyzed with modern immunochemical and ultrastructural techniques, one can demonstrate that the foreign immunoglobulin and complement are attached in a homogeneous linear fashion along the luminal side of the host glomerular basement membrane (Fig. 8–6). This experimental model reflects the mechanism of injury in Goodpasture's disease and in some other forms of chronic nephritis.

A number of modifications of the classical Masugi model have been developed. In one rather ingenious model, introduced by Kay, nephrotoxic antibody is raised in the duck against rabbit glomerular membranes. Upon injection back into the rabbit, some of this antibody attaches in linear distribution along the rabbit glomerular membranes. Considerable glomerular deposition may occur, but only minimal glomerular inflammation is induced because duck globulin activates rabbit complement poorly, even after it has reacted with the rabbit glomerular basement membrane. Two weeks later, when the rabbit produces antibodies against the duck gamma globulin, a violent glomerulonephritis may develop consequent to an immunologic as-

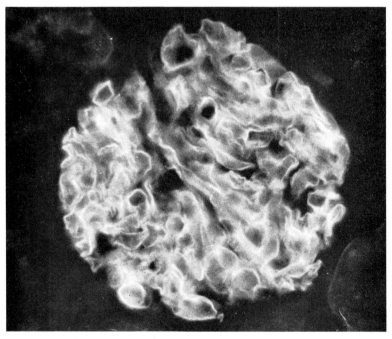

Figure 8–6. Immunofluorescent photomicrograph of a rat glomerulus 24 hours after the administration of rabbit antirat glomerular basement membrane (GBM) antiserum. The features of Masugi nephritis include ultralinear deposition of the administered rabbit IgG along the GBM. (Courtesy of Dr. A. J. Fish.)

sault directed toward the duck gamma globulin, which is still adherent to the rabbit's glomerular basement membranes. This immunologic reaction now involves rabbit antibodies to the duck protein and is capable of activating the complement system of the rabbit, which is essential for inciting an inflammatory exudate. The glomerulonephritis and kidney damage actually result primarily because of injury by host leukocytes in the exudate. The essential features of this model are illustrated in Figure 8–7.

Steblay developed a model of glomerulonephritis in sheep, which has contributed greatly to our understanding of certain renal diseases of man. In these experiments, sheep were injected with isolated glomerular basement membranes prepared from either human or monkey kidneys. The sheep recognized these membranes as being foreign and produced antibodies against them, which were capable of cross-reacting with the sheep's own glomerular basement membranes and of activating complement. Here again, activation of the complement system leads to inflammation, which produces severe glomerulonephritis and kidney damage. In the Steblay model, a direct immunologic assault on the host's own membranes has been produced by an immunologic response to a similar antigen of exogenous origin (Fig. 8–8). More recently, it has been found that identical lesions and comparable renal injury can be produced even when the host's own isolated membranes are injected with Freund's adjuvant. Thus, the host's glomerular basement membranes, modified perhaps only slightly, can initiate a directed immunologic assault on its own tissues capable of bringing about progressive and

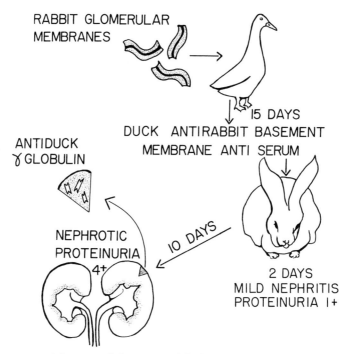

RABBIT GLOMERULAR MEMBRANES

15 DAYS

DUCK ANTIRABBIT BASEMENT MEMBRANE ANTI SERUM

ANTIDUCK γ GLOBULIN

NEPHROTIC PROTEINURIA 4+

10 DAYS

2 DAYS MILD NEPHRITIS PROTEINURIA 1+

Figure 8–7. Essential features of the Kay model (duck nephrotoxic serum model). (Adapted from Good, R. A., et al., Fed. Proc., 28:191–205, 1969.)

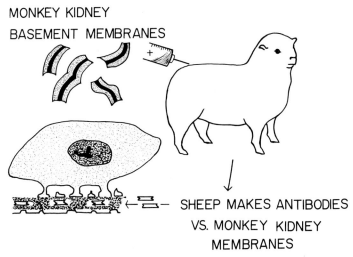

MONKEY KIDNEY
BASEMENT MEMBRANES

SHEEP MAKES ANTIBODIES
VS. MONKEY KIDNEY
MEMBRANES

Figure 8–8. Features of the Steblay model. (Adapted from Good, R. A., et al., Fed. Proc., 28:191–205, 1969.)

fatal chronic glomerulonephritis. The deposition of immunoglobulin and complement in a linear fashion on the basement membranes is typical of all of the models in which immunologic injury is directed specifically toward the membranous component of the kidney.

In the Heyman model of experimental chronic glomerulonephritis, kidney mixed with Freund's adjuvant was repeatedly injected in rats until glomerulonephritis ensued. After a long incubation period, most of the rats developed a form of nephritis that could be attributed to the formation of antibody against antigens present in renal tubular cells. However, like serum sickness, the Dixon model, and lupus of man, this autoimmune disease is also associated with deposition of complexes of antibody, renal tubular antigen, and complement in the glomeruli. Here is an example of a nephritis in which the glomeruli are being assaulted as innocent bystanders, as a consequence of antibody production against another part of the kidney. Study of this model clearly indicates that autoimmunity, just like immunity to antigens foreign to the host, may result in an indirect as well as a specifically directed immunologic assault.

IMMUNOLOGIC INJURY PRODUCED BY CELL-MEDIATED IMMUNE MECHANISMS

In contrast to antibody-mediated (or humoral) immunity, cell-mediated immunity (CMI) requires the presence of intact effector cells for its biological expression. This group of adaptive processes has been referred to as delayed hypersensitivity, transplantation immunity, cellular hypersensitivity, and thymus dependent immunity. The effector mechanisms require the participation of T lymphocytes, and macrophages are almost invariably involved, at least in vivo.

Injury can occur via three mechanisms, all of which may participate simultaneously in a single clinical lesion.

DIRECT CYTOTOXICITY OF T LYMPHOCYTES

Recognition of a cell surface antigen by the corresponding antigen receptor on a T lymphocyte (see Chapter 3) brings the T lymphocyte into close contact with a target cell. This initial contact triggers the lymphocyte to become an aggressor cell, which develops broader areas of contact, causing irregularity and some disorganization of the adjacent target cell membrane. Killing of the target cell by the effector T lymphocyte may then occur, apparently by the introduction of as yet undefined toxic products from the lymphocyte into the target cell at the points of contact (Fig. 8–9). The reaction is highly specific, and adjacent cells do not appear to be damaged. T lymphocytes not bearing specific receptors for antigens of the target cell do not participate in the process. A comparatively high antigenic density on the target cell is usually required to initiate this process. This type of cell-mediated damage appears to play a major role in allograft rejection.

CYTOTOXICITY BY T LYMPHOCYTE–ACTIVATED MACROPHAGES

Antigen specific T lymphocytes may participate in the killing of target cells by a mechanism other than direct cytotoxicity. When antigen combines

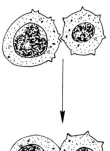

Combination of antigen receptors with site on membrane of target cell.

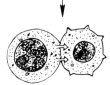

Intimate contact of membrane with destruction of target cell membrane.

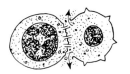

Lysis and death of target cell

Figure 8–9. Direct cytotoxicity of T lymphocytes.

with its specific receptor on T cells, it acts as a stimulus for the cell to become transformed (activated) and to undergo division. This response forms the basis for many laboratory tests used to investigate CMI, both clinically and in the laboratory. During the process, several mediators, often called lymphokines, are released (see Chapter 3). The lymphokines have several important biological effects which serve to amplify the specific response, the end result being analogous to the biologic amplification of specific antibody by complement. It has been estimated that this sort of amplification can increase the participation of cells in an inflammatory reaction several thousandfold. A current concept of this set of reactions is shown in Figure 8–10.

Activation of macrophages by lymphokines produced by antigen-stimulated T cells is a particularly important function, since the macrophages in this state act not only to destroy cells carrying the specific antigen,

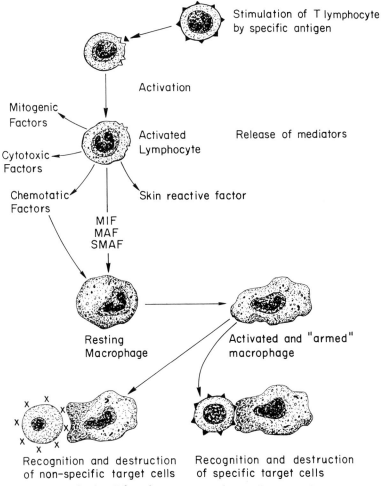

Figure 8–10. T lymphocyte–macrophage effector mechanisms.

but they may also react with cells or organisms carrying antigenic markers that have not induced specific immunity. Thus, while the release of mediators from sensitized lymphocytes is antigen specific, the mediators and cells they activate act nonspecifically. There is currently some debate concerning the specificity of specific macrophage arming factor (SMAF). Some investigators feel that this substance is the specific receptor released by the activated lymphocyte, which in turn attaches to the macrophage membrane, thus "arming" it with antigen specific receptor sites. Target cells with relatively weak antigenic expression, as well as soluble and other cell-associated antigens, are capable of triggering this response. T cell activation of macrophages appears to be important in immunity to tumors.

MITOGEN INDUCTION OF CELL-MEDIATED CYTOTOXICITY

A third mechanism has been shown to produce cytotoxicity of target cells by lymphocytes, but the effect is nonspecific and probably has little consequence in vivo. When nonspecific mitogens, such as phytohemagglutinin (PHA) or concanavallin A (Con-A), are used to induce mitosis of T lymphocytes, the transformed cells are capable of nonspecific lysis of target cells (Fig. 8–11). The target cells must be in contact with the transformed lymphocytes for lysis to occur. Some investigators have suggested that transformation aids in recognition of foreign antigens on cell surfaces, but others feel the effect is entirely nonspecific. Perhaps of more clinical significance, lymphocytes nonreactive to the antigen in question may be stimulated by the release of mitogenic factors from antigen-activated lymphocytes (see Fig. 8–10), and these lymphocytes may damage target cells in a nonspecific way.

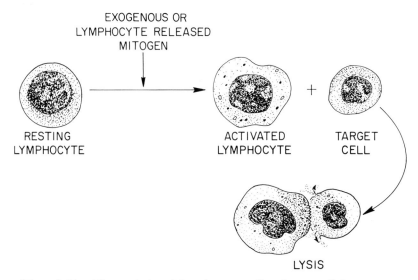

Figure 8–11. Mitogen-induced, lymphocyte-mediated target cell destruction.

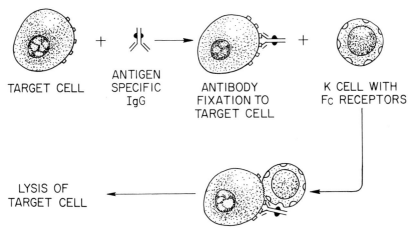

Figure 8–12.   Mechanism of antibody dependent cell-mediated cytotoxicity.

ANTIBODY DEPENDENT CELL-MEDIATED CYTOTOXICITY (ADCMC OR ADCC)

Another mechanism for direct cytolysis of target cells exists, which requires participation of both humoral and cellular components. Antibodies of certain types, which do not activate complement (or do so poorly), can combine with specific antigens on the cell surface of target cells to cause binding of a third population of lymphocytes (K cells) to the Fc portion of the molecule (see Chapter 3). This, in turn, activates the K cell to lyse the target cell (Fig. 8–12). The antibody, therefore, provides specificity to direct K cell activity, which in turn amplifies the immune response, as occurs with complement activation. K cells themselves do not possess specificity and have neither B cell or T cell markers. The best marker for the third population of circulating lymphocytes, at least some of which are K lymphocytes, is a highly avid receptor for the Fc portion of IgG. It is this capacity for avid attachment of the K cell to antibody that serves to provide the K cell with the capacity to attack and destroy foreign cells, or cells of the body against which an immune response has been directed.

Since macrophages and neutrophils also have Fc receptors, they may also participate in certain ADCC reactions.

9

Immunosuppression and Specific Negative Adaptation of the Immune Response

The prevention or reversal of established immune responses has become increasingly important in many clinical conditions, including transplantation, neoplasia, autoimmunity, infections, and allergic reactions. Immunologic unresponsiveness may be produced in a variety of ways, such as nonspecific damage or alteration of lymphoid tissues, induction of tolerance in the presence of specific antigen, and lack of response because of the presence of specific antibody. While the precise biochemical mechanisms for most types of unresponsiveness remain only partially understood, a working knowledge of negative adaptation is necessary for an effective therapeutic approach to many diseases.

ALTERATION OF IMMUNE COMPETENT CELLS BY NONSPECIFIC MEANS

A diminished immunologic response is an expected sequel of the destruction of a sufficient number of lymphoid cells or of a functional impairment of the immune competent cells by therapeutic manipulation. All of these have real or potential clinical usefulness.

MECHANICAL REMOVAL OF LYMPHOID CELLS

Neonatal excision of the primary lymphoid organs (thymus and bursa of Fabricius or its equivalent) will cause permanent immunologic crippling in many species of animals. Excision of these lymphoid structures, however, does not regularly produce any gross immunologic deficiency in other animals, although minor abnormalities may be detected when sensitive tests are used.

The effect of thymectomy in adult man on the induction or maintenance of negative adaptation has not been sufficiently evaluated, but from animal experiments, it would not be expected to cause significant immunodepression for several years. In adult animals, T cell immunodeficiency results from excision of the thymus after prolonged periods. The influence of thymectomy on functions of the shorter-lived lymphoid populations that may be involved in regulatory functions (e.g., suppressor functions) has not yet been adequately studied. Surgical excision of secondary lymphoid organs (the spleen and lymph nodes) has little apparent effect on the immunologic responsiveness of adult humans, although splenectomy during the first year of life renders children more susceptible to the development of fulminant bacterial infections, especially from pneumococci, and absence of the spleen may be a hazard even to an adult. This is because the spleen plays important roles, both in production of specific opsonins and in removal of nonopsonized or incompletely opsonized bacteria from the circulation. Splenectomy is regularly performed in many centers where clinical transplantation is being done, and there is some evidence that removal of the spleen improves homograft survival. However, many feel that this effect results from the ability to administer larger doses of azathioprine.

Chronic drainage of lymphocytes from thoracic duct fistulae has been utilized to produce a significant depletion of the long-lived, fully differentiated T_2 lymphocytes. Concomitant with a decrease in circulating small lymphocytes, there is an effect on the immune response, and graft survival can be prolonged by this technique. However, these fistulae are difficult to maintain for long periods, which limits their usefulness. In persons with intestinal lymphangiectasia, who have a chronic, persistent loss of lymphocytes into the intestinal tract, exceedingly prolonged survival of skin homografts has been demonstrated.

X-IRRADIATION

Many cells of the lymphoid system are particularly sensitive to the effects of irradiation. X-irradiation treatment was among the earliest types of therapy known to suppress the immune process, and it has been used extensively to modify the immune response of animals and humans to a wide variety of antigens. It acts by both destruction of lymphocytes and destruction of stem cells and is more effective in suppressing humoral immunity than cell-mediated immunity. Recovery after radiation damage can be modified by thymectomy in adult animals and by the administration of antilymphocyte globulin. Radiation has been valuable as an experimental tool, but the method has limited clinical usefulness because the damage is not selective for lymphoid cells. Lethal doses of total body irradiation have been used as a means for suppressing host immune response, and for destroying leukemic cells prior to bone marrow transplantation.

PHARMACOLOGIC SUPPRESSION OF IMMUNITY

The use of chemotherapeutic agents to modify adaptive immune responses has been widely utilized for transplantation and for treatment of a variety of "immunologic diseases" during the past few years. Their usefulness and their even greater potential have become increasingly apparent. Our review of the mechanism of action of these agents will be brief, partly because the pharmacologic pathways involved are often incompletely defined and partly because of the complexity of action in vivo where even the simplest biochemical lesion may result in far-reaching complex consequences because of its influence on cellular interactions.

The immunosuppressive properties of benzene, toluene, and the salicylates were discovered during the early part of the twentieth century, but therapeutic immunosuppression in man was not possible until the adrenal steroid hormones were discovered in the 1950s.

Adrenocortical Steroids. The adrenocortical steroids may affect the immune response at several sites (Table 9–1). Cortisone and its analogs can inhibit the cellular proliferation of many types of tissues, including lymphoid tissues, and in high concentrations may be lympholytic for cells at certain stages of differentiation in both B and T cell systems. Steroids bind to cytoplasmic receptors and are then transported to intranuclear receptors, causing initial synthesis of RNA and protein. In certain lymphocytes, this is soon followed by inhibition of uptake of small molecules, a fall in polymerase ac-

TABLE 9–1. SCHEMA FOR PROBABLE SITES OF ACTION OF COMMON IMMUNOSUPPRESSIVE AGENTS

	SITE OF ACTION	DRUG
Afferent arc	Development of nonspecific inflammatory lesion	Adrenal steroids Purine antagonists Alkylating agents
	Antigen uptake	
	Processing of antigen and transfer to lymphocyte	Adrenal steroids? Purine antagonists?
	Differentiation and proliferation of immune competent cell	Adrenal steroids Purine antagonists Alkylating agents
Efferent arc	Production of antibody	Adrenal steroids Purine antagonists Folic acid antagonists Alkylating agents
	and/or	
	Action of complement and development of specific inflammatory lesions	Adrenal steroids
	and/or	
	Cell-mediated immunological recognition and damage	Adrenal steroids Purine antagonists Alkylating agents
	and/or	
	Development of immunological memory	Purine antagonists

tivity, and inhibition of DNA, RNA, and protein synthesis. Within two hours, extensive death and lysis of small lymphocytes may occur. However, graft versus host activity of the remaining cells appears to be unimpaired. Adrenal steroids also alter cell membranes, have antiinflammatory properties, and can induce the formation of a variety of adaptive enzymes, some of which may have immunosuppressive properties.

An impressive number of reports have confirmed the fact that cortisone and its derivatives may regularly reduce the ability of an animal to synthesize circulating antibodies to an antigenic stimulus, but it is not often appreciated that the corticosteroids can enhance antibody production, depending on the time of administration and the dosage used. The maximum effect for suppression can be obtained when treatment is begun approximately 12 hours before administration of antigen.

The effect of adrenocortical steroids on cell-mediated immunity is pronounced, and steroids prolong the survival of normal tissue allografts in many experimental animals. Permanent immunologic tolerance has been achieved in a few. Steroids have been used extensively to suppress tumor immunity and are given frequently to increase the survival of tumor allografts and xenografts. Metastases from tumors may sometimes be strikingly increased by the administration of steroids. In addition to suppressing the inductive phases of immunity, the effector mechanism may be affected since the adrenocortical steroids have anticomplement properties in very high concentrations, and certain of the steroids, in high doses, may cause a direct or indirect pharmacologic inhibition of the development of vascular responses.

One of the most important mechanisms to explain the influence of adrenal steroids on immune responses is their suppressive effects on the inflammatory processes per se. Migration of both neutrophils and monocytes into inflammatory lesions is inhibited by adrenal steroids. A recently defined action that may explain the antiinflammatory activity is that the steroids suppress production of prostaglandin synthetase. It is, however, important to realize that a major, highly differentiated population of lymphocytes, in both thymus and peripheral lymphoid tissue, is highly resistant to adrenal steroids. Further, the fully differentiated antibody-producing cells, plasma cells, are resistant to the influences of the adrenal steroids.

Purine Antagonists. Azathioprine and 6-mercaptopurine (6-MP) are the purine antagonists that have been studied most extensively as immunosuppressants. These agents affect DNA synthesis primarily, but it is probable that they influence adaptive immunity in other ways. Depending on the dosage and time of administration, 6-MP may have a variety of effects on antibody synthesis (Table 9–2). If 6-MP is given in relatively small doses prior to the time of antigen administration, it has little effect, but, if larger doses are given for a shorter period of time and stopped several days before the administration of an antigen, a greater than normal immune response may be encountered. If treatment with these compounds is started at or shortly before the time of antigen administration and continued for several days, it may completely abolish delayed hypersensitivity responses, significantly in-

TABLE 9–2. TEMPORAL RELATIONSHIP OF ADMINISTRATION OF 6-MERCAPTOPURINE AND MOST IMMUNOSUPPRESSIVE AGENTS TO DEVELOPMENT OF IMMUNE RESPONSE

WEEKS					EFFECT
−2	−1	0	+1	+2	
⟵⟶					Enhanced response.
	⟵⟶				Slight or no effect.
		⟵⟶			Greatest immunosuppressive effect. Primary response predominantly affected.
			⟵⟶		Variable, depending on dose and agent. May get enhanced response in low doses.
		⟵⟶⟶⟶			Both primary and secondary responses affected.
	Administration of antigen				

fluence the development of inflammatory lesions, abolish the primary antibody response, promote specific induction of tolerance, suppress the secondary response, and promote allograft survival.

The synthesis of IgG is inhibited more readily by 6-MP than is the synthesis of IgM. Both 6-MP and azathioprine may profoundly prolong allograft survival and depress delayed hypersensitivity, but azathioprine has been used more extensively for clinical immunosuppression during transplantation of allogeneic organs than has 6-MP, since it appears to be slightly less toxic and may be slightly more effective. Still another reason for the use of azathioprine to prolong allograft survival is that it has a more selective effect on T cell-mediated immune responses than on antibody production. Administration of large doses of the drug causes depletion of lymphocytes in T dependent regions of lymph nodes and spleen, whereas the germinal centers and medullary cords are relatively unaffected.

The analogs of the pyrimidine bases have been studied extensively by cancer chemotherapists because of their antitumor properties. They are clearly immunosuppressive by virtue of their inhibition of RNA and DNA synthesis, but the degree of toxicity and the low therapeutic index associated with their administration have precluded their clinical use as immunosuppressants.

Folic Acid Antagonists.   Methotrexate and aminopterin are folic acid antagonists whose mechanisms of action are relatively well understood. Administration of these drugs inhibits dihydrofolate reductase, thereby blocking the conversion of folic to tetrahydrofolic acid, which is an essential step in many cellular biochemical processes, including the synthesis of DNA, RNA, and purine-containing coenzymes. They are potent mitotic inhibitors. Although the inhibition of dihydrofolic reductase has been well documented, the folic antagonists evidently have other less well characterized immunosuppressive effects.

The potential immunosuppressant properties of the folic acid antagonists were recognized not long after their introduction for treatment of leukemia. Toxicity has limited their usefulness in man, but recently, inhibition of toxicity without significant impairment of immunosuppressive effectiveness has been obtained experimentally by the administration of these agents with folinic acid (citrovorum factor) given on alternate days. Both cellular and humoral immunity are significantly affected. The folic acid antagonists are most effective as immunosuppressants when administration is begun shortly after antigen administration and continued for several days, including the period of maximum mitotic activity after the administration of antigens. With these agents, as with purine antagonists, effective immunosuppression has been associated with facilitation of development of specific immunlogic negativity. Several workers have shown that the concomitant administration of cell extracts and a folic acid antagonist can produce a significant prolongation of homograft survival.

Long-lasting immunologic tolerance has been produced in mice, especially across relatively weak histocompatibility barriers, by suppressing immune responses with these metabolic antagonists while challenging with injected cells or tissue grafts. In both experimental and clinical situations, treatment with amethopterin (methotrexate) has been used to prevent development of graft versus host reactions following bone marrow transplantation.

Alkylating Agents.   Alkylating agents, such as nitrogen mustard, have been known to be immunosuppressive since the 1920s. They have a profound effect on dividing cells, being both carcinogenic and metagenic, which suggests that one mode of action is to alter deoxyribonucleic acid. In addition, they directly inhibit synthesis of ribonucleic acid and proteins. They not only influence the proliferation and differentiation of cells in adaptive immune processes, but they also suppress the inflammatory response and thus block the afferent arc of the immune process (Table 9–1). Because of their cytotoxicity to all proliferating cells, they may cause extensive damage to the bone marrow and intestinal epithelial cells, as do most of the agents which have been under discussion.

Cyclophosphamide has been the alkylating agent most used for the suppression of immune responses. The intact molecule is inactive, but active metabolites appear rapidly with oxidation. There is a major species difference in the effects of this agent, and it has been best studied in the guinea pig. Antibody production may be significantly decreased by cyclophosphamide, especially if the drug is given just before and just after antigen administration. Widespread destruction of the lymphoid cells, particularly small lymphocytes, may be produced. In single dose treatments in animals, cyclophosphamide has been found to be especially damaging to B lymphocytes, particularly those in germinal centers. Administered in this way, the agent has selective depressing influences on antibody production. However, when given repeatedly, cyclophosphamide strongly suppresses both B cell and T cell functions, as well as inflammation. The development of inflammatory lesions may be significantly depressed, in part because bone marrow depression makes fewer neutrophils available for deposition at an inflammatory focus. Cyclophosphamide can profoundly suppress allograft rejection, particularly across weak histocompatibiltiy barriers or when it is used in combination with other agents. However, the drug is most useful in diseases of immune injury caused by antibody, since its effect on B cell function is greater than its effect on T cells.

Antibiotics. A number of antibiotics have been found to alter immunologic reactivity, but only a few are of importance. These include mitomycin, puromycin, actinomycins C and D, azaserine, and chloramphenicol. Puromycin has a well-defined effect on protein synthesis and acts by inhibition of amino acid transfer from soluble ribonucleic acid to ribosomal protein—the translation process. The usefulness of this agent has been limited to in vitro studies since the toxicity in vivo is prohibitive. Mitomycin C depolymerizes and cross-links DNA, and inhibits its replication. In higher concentrations, it may also directly affect RNA and protein synthesis. As with puromycin, toxicity of the drug prevents clinical utilization. The actinomycins C and D inhibit DNA-directed RNA synthesis. Experiments using actinomycin D, which acts specifically by inhibiting transcription of the DNA information in RNA production, have suggested that repressed messenger RNA may be responsible for immunologic memory. Recently, even very small doses of actinomycin D, which interfere to some degree with hematopoiesis, have been shown to be effective in preventing development of the lethal lupus-like renal disease and autoimmunity in (NZB/NZW)F_1 hybrid mice. The basis of this action is not clear as yet, but trials of this drug, perhaps with other therapy, should be tested in human lupus, where treatment with adrenal steroids with or without azathioprine often leaves much to be desired, though exerting a beneficial effect on the disease. Actinomycin C, which is a mixture of several of the actinomycins, was once used empirically in clinical transplantation programs for reversal of rejection episodes, but its value has not been proven. In high doses, chloramphenicol inhibits protein synthesis, thus having a rather nonspecific effect on antibody production. Azaserine is a poor immunosuppressant when used alone, but when used as an adjunct with purine antagonists, significant extension of allograft survival has been obtained.

Miscellaneous Drugs. A wide variety of other drugs has been shown to have some degree of immunosuppressive activity. Among these are: inhibitors of protein, DNA, and RNA synthesis, such as the plant alkaloids, including colchicine and the vinca alkaloids; inhibitors of proteolysis, such as epsilon-aminocaproic acid; asparaginase; inhibitors of inflammation, such as the salicylates or promazine derivatives; and others.

SUPPRESSION OF THE IMMUNE RESPONSE WITH
BIOLOGICAL MATERIALS

Antilymphocyte Globulin (ALG).   Antilymphocyte serum was first used by Metchnikoff around the turn of the century, but the important implications of its effect on adaptive immunity were not recognized until the last decade. Heterologous antilymphocyte globulin is one of the most effective immunosuppressive agents currently known, but the reported effects of its administration in man have been inconsistent because of the varying conditions under which ALG has been produced, purified, and administered.

Antibodies of the IgG class are the active components of crude antilymphocyte serum. The plasma membranes of the lymphoid cells contain the primary antigens that stimulate the synthesis of antilymphocyte antibodies, but other cellular components have been reported to stimulate the production of highly effective antisera. Antilymphocyte globulin has both specific and nonspecific properties, and many cross-reactions with similar but nonidentical antigenic structures occur on the plasma membranes of other types of cells. Some of the immunosuppressive activity of antilymphocyte globulin can be removed by repeated absorptions with nonlymphoid tissues, suggesting that these cross-reacting antigens contribute in a quantitative way to immune damage. Since the lymphocyte is the cell that has the greatest affinity for all reacting antibodies, it is the cell most affected.

The immunosuppressive properties of ALG are related to its specific combination with antigens of the lymphocyte plasma membrane. Just how it affects the cell, once this union occurs, remains a subject of considerable controversy. Studies in vitro with lymphocyte cultures have shown that antilymphocyte globulin alone has a mitogenic effect. If complement is present in the system, the lymphoid cells may be destroyed, depending on the affinity and concentration of antibody in the reacting system and on the ability of homologous complement to be bound and activated by the heterologous antibody. A difference in the relative inability of homologous complement to be activated by heterologous globulin could explain differences in in vivo immunosuppressive effectiveness of various kinds of antilymphocyte globulin and may also be related to the development of lymphopenia in individuals receiving antilymphocyte globulin. One of the most important biological effects of ALG is to coat lymphocytes with opsonic antibody, which causes their removal and destruction by phagocytic cells of the RES, especially Küppfer cells of the liver. Several investigators have hypothesized that coating the surfaces of the lymphocytes with antilymphocyte globulin masks specific binding sites, thus making them unavailable for reaction with the cellular antigens of allografts that would otherwise be rapidly destroyed by cytotoxic killer cells. The affinity of the specific antibody for the lymphocyte membrane probably also plays a decisive role in the effectiveness of this biological.

In experimental animals, great prolongation of allograft survival can be obtained when antilymphocyte globulin is used as the only immunosuppressive agent, but high doses are required. Antilymphocyte globulin has been prepared in rabbits, rats, horses, goats, sheep, cows, and dogs. The effectiveness of the antisera seems to be related both to the animal in which it is raised, and to the species of animal donating the lymphocytes used for immunization and in which it is tested. The mouse and guinea pig are the most receptive species while lesser effectiveness is seen in dog and man. Thymectomy potentiates the effect of antilymphocyte globulin, particularly in the mouse, but not the adult dog. The effect of combining antilymphocyte globulin therapy and thymectomy to induce permanent or long-lasting tolerance of allografts has not been studied in man.

It has been shown that antilymphocyte globulin possesses selective properties related to the type and source of lymphocytes used for immunization. Specifically, antisera raised against thymic lymphocytes, lymph node lymphocytes, or lymphocytes from gut-associated lymphoid tissues have selective effects. Antithymic lymphocyte globulin influences primarily the small recirculating T lymphocytes. Administration is associated with a moderate to marked depletion of the lymphocytes in the thymus dependent areas (TDA) or lymph nodes (i.e., the deep cortical or paracortical regions) and the perivascular lymphoid accumulation of the spleen. Administration of ALG raised against gut-associated lymphoid tissues, on the other hand, disrupts the architecture of the germinal centers and diminishes the numbers of large lymphocytes and plasma cells, but produces a much lesser effect on the population of small lymphocytes located in the TDA of lymph nodes and spleen. Antisera raised against lymph node cells cause damage to both types of lymphocytes. This differential effect of the various types of antilymphocyte globulin is not complete, either morphologically or functionally, although a partial separation of the functions of the thymic and gut dependent(B) types of lymphoid systems can be achieved by this method. It is possible by appropriate adsorption to develop antisera which are highly specific for each type of lymphocyte. Antisera against macrophages has also been shown to be an effective immunosuppressant in the laboratory, presumably by inactivating antigen-processing cells.

In humans, antilymphocyte globulin has not been used as the sole immunosuppressive agent for clinical allografting procedures. However, its administration in combination with a standard regimen of azathioprine and prednisone has significantly decreased the number and severity of rejection episodes and has increased survival rates, as reported by a majority of the centers where it has been used. In some centers, specially prepared aggregate-free ALG has been given intravenously in large doses, apparently without difficulty. However, other centers have avoided the intravenous route because of the potential for uncontrolled complement activation by Ig aggregates. One of the major problems with the clinical use of ALG relates to difficulties in assessing its potency. Currently, no universally accepted method exists for such evaluation, but inhibition of T cell rosetting (see Chapter 3) and prolongation of skin allografts in primates seem to correlate reasonably well with evidence of potency in man. It seems likely that improvement and standardization of this potent biological material will lead to its universal acceptance as an immunosuppressive agent for clinical transplantation. Additional experience in humans is needed to provide information concerning the optimal dosage and route of administration.

Antibody against Antibody. Recently, anti-Ig antibody has been shown to have immunosuppressive activity, probably by means of interfering with complement-activating activity or receptor sites on B lymphocytes or K cells. Antiidiotypic antibody promises to be a means for more effective immunosuppression for organ transplants in the future (see Chapter 15).

Alpha$_2$ Glycoprotein. In 1963, an alpha$_2$ glycoprotein fraction, which had immunosuppressive activity when administered intravenously to mice, was obtained from normal serum. This fraction is often called immunoregulatory alpha globulin (IRA). The possibility of being able to extract a naturally occurring protein that had an immunosuppressive activity from human serum was of considerable interest, particularly since it was reported to have little or no toxicity. This initial alpha$_2$ glycoprotein fraction was found to contain a ribonuclease which was thought to explain some, but not all, of the immunosuppressive activity. Later studies have shown that most if not all of the activity resides in a polypeptide associated with a larger α_2 glycoprotein. Some early investigators confirmed, while others were unable to confirm, the original work on the preparation of the immunosuppressive alpha$_2$ globulin, but there now seems to be little doubt of its existence. One group has prepared an alpha$_2$ globulin fraction from normal human plasma, which inhibits lymphocyte transformation and protein synthesis in the presence of phytohemagglutinin or specific antigens. Recent studies show that immunosuppressive action of IRA may be due to activation of suppressor T lymphocytes by the globulin. The clinical importance of these findings remains to be proved, but alpha$_2$ glycoprotein seems of great potential usefulness in immunosuppressive therapy. This immunosuppressive agent may have clinical relevance in a variety of diseases, since IRA is elevated in trauma, severe infections, and malignancies.

NEGATIVE ADAPTATION REQUIRING THE PRESENCE OF SPECIFIC ANTIGEN

In contrast to a diminished immunologic response to an antigen obtained by nonspecific damage or direct action on the cells of the lymphoid system, specifically acquired immunologic tolerance is a refractory state that develops only in the presence of specific antigen. Acquired tolerance is easily produced in immature animals before maturation of the lymphoid system and can also be produced in adults, although it is more difficult to achieve under most circumstances. Since there are many types of immunologic responses, the detection of tolerance sometimes depends upon the type of test used to detect it. Cellular immunity, humoral immunity, or both may be affected. It is only fair to say at the beginning of this discussion that the biochemical and cellular mechanisms of tolerance, although much discussed and studied since tolerance was discovered in 1952 by Medawar and his colleagues, remain poorly understood. Indeed, it seems very likely that there are several forms of tolerance.

Neonatal Exposure to Antigen

Owens' observation (1945) that dizygotic twin cattle often have two types of blood cells—their own and that of their genetically disparate twin—suggested a theoretic basis for acquired tolerance. Numerous investigators since that time have demonstrated that a variety of antigens administered in the neonatal period can produce a specific negative immunologic adaptation in some experimental animals (e.g., mice and rats), but in many species it is necessary to administer the antigen long before birth. If living cells capable of replication are used to induce the tolerance so that antigen persists throughout the life of the recipient, long-lasting or even permanent tolerance can be achieved. If a single injection of a soluble antigen is used to induce tolerance, repeated injections of antigen are required for as long as tolerance is to be maintained.

All of these observations argue that for tolerance to be lasting, antigen must be present. However, many attempts to demonstrate antigen during periods of persisting tolerance have been unsuccessful. This type of tolerance is central rather than peripheral and involves mechanisms that repress antigen reactions of cells that make them unresponsive. Either T cells, B cells, or both may be involved, and unresponsiveness of either B or T cells for a specific antigen results in a tolerant state, even when the corresponding T or B cell is capable of response to antigen. There is evidence that some forms of central immunologic tolerance involve exhaustive differentiation or elimination of a clone of cells reactive to the specific antigen, or both. This mechanism is clearly not the most important one for exogenous antigens, but it is thought to be largely responsible for the unresponsiveness to most self antigens. It is clear that some antigens are much more effective in producing tolerance than others. Smaller antigens, soluble antigens, and antigens with repeating subunits on a backbone are among the best with which to produce a tolerant state. Recent experimentations link forms of immunologic tolerance and immunologic unresponsiveness to the activity of so-called suppressor cells. T lymphocytes, adherent lymphocytes, and even monocytes and macrophages have been implicated as suppressor cells in certain tolerance phenomena.

Antigen Overloading (High Dose [Zone] Tolerance)

Immunologic paralysis with large doses of antigen was first demonstrated in 1942 when Felton reported that a specific loss of reactivity to pneumococcal polysaccharides could be induced in adult mice by the administration of large amounts of this antigen (Felton's paralysis). Since then, many types of antigens have been used to produce tolerance in the adult animal by the mechanism of antigen overloading. This type of paralysis requires the persistence of antigen and is more easily produced by antigens that are relatively resistant to degradation. Immunologic paralysis is specific, and it has been demonstrated that antibody is not formed during the period of paralysis. This type of tolerance can be terminated by the administration of antigens of similar but not identical specificities, particularly those differing only in haptenic groups.

A parabiotic union of genetically dissimilar animals often terminates with a toxic state in one or both partners. However, if the genetic disparity between the partners is not great, tolerance may be obtained. This type of tolerance seems entirely similar to that produced by Felton's immunologic paralysis, being dependent on the persistence of specific antigens. Similarly, repeated injection of whole cells and even of subcellular fractions in mice has led to the development of specific negative adaptation, even during adult life. Induction of this form of negative adaptation is easy when the histocompatibility barrier is relatively slight, but most difficult when histocompatibility differences are great.

The type of antigen has a profound influence upon whether or not immunologic paralysis can be induced. Antigens that possess a strong similarity to the naturally occurring constituents of the host are poorly antigenic, and paralysis can be induced with relative ease; on the other hand, antigens that are markedly different from the host constituents elicit a strongly positive immunologic response, and tolerance to these stronger antigens usually is difficult to produce.

LOW DOSE (ZONE) TOLERANCE

In contrast to the above techniques for producing paralysis with large doses of a specific antigen, it has been shown that very small doses of antigen may produce a specific immunologic negativity if the doses of antigen are correctly spaced. Some antigens, such as flagellin, produce tolerance at very low and very high doses, but are potent immunogens at moderate doses. In some instances, the effect can be potentiated by immunosuppressive drugs. Furthermore, the negative adaptation may affect only the cellular or humoral type of immune response (sometimes referred to as a split tolerance). This is an unusual type of tolerance, and its mechanism is not understood, but it demonstrates that tolerance, like immunity, may exist that involves one or another of the two functional lymphoid systems. Studies of mechanisms have shown that low dose tolerance tends to make T cell populations tolerant. With higher dose tolerance, both T and B cell populations appear to be involved in the specific negative adaptation.

OTHER METHODS

Another type of tolerance that can be induced by the administration of antigen is often referred to as the Sulzberger-Chase phenomenon. The oral administration of haptens may result in a specific decrease in the reactivity of the same hapten conjugated to a protein carrier when used for immunization. Of possible significance is the observation that the intraportal administration of many antigens may result in production of a specific immunologic negativity.

Suppressor T cells may significantly reduce immune responses, and undoubtedly are of major consequence in vivo. Just how the suppressor T cells accomplish this important task of regulation is still poorly understood. However, the response is antigen specific in some instances, and transfer experiments show that B cells normally responsive to antigens are suppressed. The molecular basis of this form of specific immunologic suppression has recently been analyzed. A powerful specific suppression of immunity is exercised by a molecule of some 45- to 55,000 D that is elaborated or released from stimulated T cells. This molecule seems to contain: (1) the V region present in Ig; (2) a component of the cell surface that contains antigens, which react with anti-Ia antibody; and (3) components of the antigen or hapten toward which the immunosuppression is directed. Thus, it could well be an antigen–antibody complex with the antigenic receptors of the T lymphocytes. In other instances, suppressive influences are exercised by cells that seem to react more generally to suppress T cell responses or B cell responses, or both. The molecular nature of the nonspecific suppressive influence exercised by T lymphocytes remains unknown, but a soluble substance called soluble immune response suppressant (SIRS) is liberated into supernatants of T cell stimulated by concanavallin A and apparently works through macrophages. Definition of the nature of this molecule could be a most important contribution to immunology.

RECOVERY FROM TOLERANCE

Recovery from tolerance may occur at a variable rate, depending on the type of antigen used to produce the tolerant state and upon the age of the animal at the time tolerance was induced. In young animals, recovery may be relatively rapid, whereas in aged animals the process is often considerably delayed. The rate of recovery from tolerance in thymectomized animals is exceedingly prolonged, suggesting that the recruitment of immunologically competent but uncommitted cells is necessary for recovery. Tolerance cannot be terminated by the transfer of normal lymph node cells, further indicating that recovery of immunologic tolerance or paralysis occurs through recruitment of new cells via the primary lymphoid organs. An apparent tolerant state has been transferred from animals in which tolerance was initially induced to syngeneic nontolerant partners by placing the two in parabiotic union. Further, lymphoid cells from animals with an immunologic paralysis to a given antigen, when transferred to an irradiated syngeneic host, may sometimes transfer the specific tolerance. On the other hand, cells from an immunized animal, when transferred to a syngeneic but tolerant host, sometimes confer the ability to produce specific antibody. This form of transfer has been called adoptive immunity.

Very dramatic immunologic tolerance has been produced by introduction of hematopoietic tissue lacking postthymic lymphocytes into fatally irradiated mice and rats. Fetal liver, neonatal spleen cells, spleen cells from 15 to 20 day old neonatally thymectomized donors, bone marrow freed of all lymphocytes by in vitro treatment with specific antilymphocyte globulin and bone marrow from germ-free donors have been used to reconstruct the hematopoietic tissues following fatal irradiation. Such reconstruction does not result in graft versus host reactions, and the lymphoid cells of the chimera produced are tolerant of both donor strain and recipient cells and tissues. They are, however, capable of responding with full vigor to third party cells or allografts. Such models of cellular engineering may eventually provide the basis for production of the long-desired tolerant state to facilitate organ transplantation, without need for the continuous or prolonged immunosuppression that still makes organ transplantation a hazardous undertaking.

ANTIGENIC COMPETITION

When two or more antigenic substances are administered, the response to each individual antigen may be less than the expected response if the antigen were administered by itself. Occasionally, an enhancing or adjuvant effect may be produced, but in general, the greater the number of antigens administered, the poorer will be the response to each. Living allogeneic cells can act competitively with bacterial antigens and soluble antigens. Antigenic competition could be caused by a relative lack of availability of the building blocks essential for the synthesis of specific antibody, but more recent evidence suggests that other mechanisms are more fundamental.

When competition occurs on the same molecule, it is called intramolecular competition, a process exemplified by the Fc and Fab determinants on heterologous IgG. When the intact molecule is given, Fc causes a more vigorous response, but equal responses occur when Fc and Fab are given separately. Once antibody is synthesized to Fc following administration of IgG as an antigen, a better response to Fab may occur, indicating that there is competition of B cells for antigen presented by T cells. B cells with receptors for the antigens on Fc apparently are more successful in competing for the antigen than are B cells with receptors for the antigens on Fab, perhaps because of greater affinity for the former.

Intermolecular competition occurs when antigenic molecules of different specificities compete. When they are administered sequentially, it is reasonably clear that the mechanism of reduced response to the second antigen is related to the elaboration of nonspecific inhibitors of the immune response, especially by suppressor T cells. Competition when antigens are given as mixtures is somewhat more difficult to explain, but the process involves competition at the level of helper T cell interaction. Perhaps suppression of some responses by suppressor T cells or inhibitory substances released by responding cells may be important as well. The clinical significance of competition in mixtures of antigens is especially important when mixed vaccines are given. The vaccine of diphtheria, pertussis, and tetanus is a good example. Diphtheria and tetanus antigens compete with each other. However, by adjusting the ratio of the two antigens, a vigorous response to both antigens can be obtained.

NEGATIVE ADAPTATION SPECIFIC ANTIBODY

SUPPRESSION OF HUMORAL IMMUNITY BY COMPLEXES OF ANTIGEN WITH ANTIBODY

The effect of the administration of antigen–antibody complexes to an animal is quite variable, sometimes resulting in a suppression of antibody synthesis and sometimes leading to an increase in responsiveness. The neutralization of tetanus or diphtheria toxoid (or toxin) with the corresponding antitoxin, for example, may completely abolish the immunogenicity of the antigen. This difference undoubtedly results from the method of presentation to macrophages or antigen-reactive lymphocytes.

SUPPRESSION OF ANTIBODY RESPONSE BY THE PASSIVE ADMINISTRATION OF ANTIBODY INDEPENDENT OF ANTIGEN

Prevention of hemolytic disease of the newborn caused by Rh_0 (D) incompatibility has been one of the most important contributions of immunology to clinical practice (see Chapter 17). During delivery, fetal blood of Rh positive infants usually enters the maternal circulation and may cause immunization of an Rh negative mother. Infants of subsequent pregnancies may be affected by the transplacental passage of immune IgG causing damage to Rh positive cells of the infant. Immunization of the mother at the time of the initial delivery can be presented by the passive administration of relatively small amounts of anti $Rh_0(D)$ IgG antibody. The specific unresponsiveness is not permanent, and subsequent challenges by pregnancy (or transfusions) of the $Rh_0(D)$ antigen may cause sensitization.

The mechanism for prevention of the immune response has not been completely elucidated. The antigen-bearing cells are more rapidly removed from the circulation than they normally would be, and degradation of the antigen by macrophages may be so complete as to render it nonimmunogenic. However, the passive administration of anti-Rh antibody as long as 48 hours after introduction of the antigen during delivery can completely prevent immunization. By this time, antigen-reactive cells would already have been stimulated by antigen. It, therefore, seems more likely that the antibody has a selective effect in repressing antibody synthesis by cells primed by the specific antigen. Whether this entails antigen–antibody interaction or reaction at the level of RNA or DNA is unknown. A likely possibility is inactivation through RNA–antigen-antibody complexes. The possibility that the mechanism involves selective activation of suppressor cell populations should be considered and tested.

The same mechanism has been used to prolong graft survival across weak and intermediate strength histocompatibility barriers in animals, and it has potential usefulness in clinical transplantation. Thus far, however, specific suppression of immune responses by antibody, although permitting dramatic acceptance of renal allografts in a hemiallogeneic rat model, has not been proved of value in allografts involving other histoincompatibilites in rats, other animals, or man.

ENHANCEMENT AND BLOCKING FACTORS

The effector mechanisms of cell-mediated immune responses can clearly be inhibited by certain kinds of antibody, generally of the IgG class, which do not activate complement sufficiently to cause damage to the cell, sometimes because of low antigenic density. This effect is called enhancement since it was first observed in tumor grafts and caused an increased (enhanced) rate of growth of tumors. However, the process is a general one and extends to most clinical considerations of immunity and disease processes. A simple explanation for enhancement has never been entirely satisfactory, and it seems likely that several mechanisms are involved. Included among the influences that could attribute to enhancement, besides those mentioned below, is a stimulating influence of antibody on proliferation of tumor cells and modulation of antigen on tumor cell surfaces. One clear mechanism of enhancement is peripheral (Fig. 9–1), but antibody may have a more central

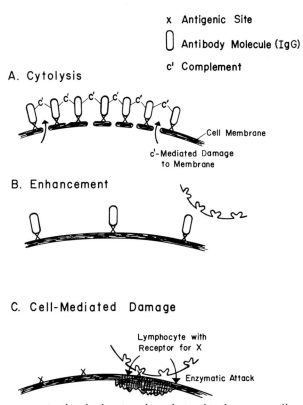

Figure 9–1. Diagrammatic sketch showing the relationship between cell-mediated cytolysis, antibody-mediated cytolysis, and enhancement. Note how antibody may help the cell to survive.

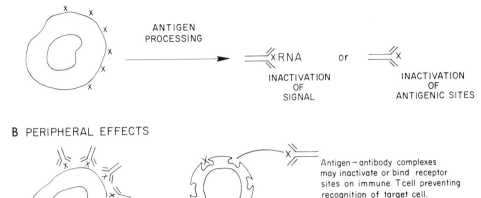

A CENTRAL EFFECT

ANTIGEN
PROCESSING

RNA   or

INACTIVATION   INACTIVATION
OF   OF
SIGNAL   ANTIGENIC SITES

B PERIPHERAL EFFECTS

Antigen – antibody complexes
may inactivate or bind receptor
sites on immune T cell preventing
recognition of target cell.

Inactivation of antigen on receptor sites.

Masking of receptor sites on target cell
by blocking antibody prevents recognition
by antigen receptor sites on immune T cells.

Filling of receptor sites by free antigen
prevents recognition of receptor sites
on target cell.

Figure 9–2.   Possible mechanisms of enhancement and blocking factors.

effect, as discussed in the preceding section. In addition, blocking of effector cells appears to occur as a consequence of free antigen and antigen–antibody complexes (Fig. 9–2). Enhancement is exceedingly important in clinical medicine and appears to be a primary mechanism for immunologic adaptation of allogeneic grafts in their new hosts. As might be expected, enhancement is easier to produce when antigenic differences between donor and recipient are not great.

10

Immunopotentiation

Clinical observations made by physicians practicing in the last part of the nineteenth century led to initial studies on immunopotentiation as an attempt to control cancer in man. Several patients with inoperable or incompletely removed malignant neoplasms were noted to have regression of tumor following an attack of erysipelas. W. B. Coley studied these reports after making a similar observation, and deliberately produced erysipelas in a small number of patients. However, the lack of control of the infections led him to seek safer methods. Heat-killing a culture of *Streptococcus* destroyed its activity, but this could be partially restored by adding toxins from *Bacillus prodigiosus (Serratia marcescens)*. The mixture came to be known as Coley's toxin. Scattered clinical trials yielded variable results, with some preparations clearly inactive, and the toxin did not find general popularity. However, subsequent analysis of well-documented, long-term regression of established malignancies has shown that many of these patients received Coley's toxin. The successful treatment of cancer with immunoadjuvants is now well demonstrated, both experimentally and clinically, and these studies will be discussed in more detail in Chapter 14.

Early studies on antibody production also led to the realization that certain combinations of antigens could increase the antibody response. Furthermore, it was discovered that guinea pigs infected with tuberculosis produced more antibody to certain antigens than did noninfected animals. This phenomenon was applied to develop mixed cell vaccines, and the phenomenon of enhancing antibody response became known as adjuvant action. Perhaps the best known and most potent of the older adjuvants is Freund's complete adjuvant, which is extensively used to enhance antibody production in animals, but is not safe for man. Nonbacterial adjuvants were also developed, but, in general, they have not been as potent as adjuvants containing bacterial products.

Metchnikoff (1901) was one of the first investigators to show that infection with some organisms could increase resistance to infection by others. Numerous recent studies have shown that such resistance is usually conferred by the group known as the facultative intracellular bacterial pathogens. Notable among these are Listeria, BCG, and Toxoplasma. This bio-

TABLE 10–1. POTENTIATING EFFECTS OF SELECTED AGENTS
ON IMMUNE SYSTEM

INCREASES MACROPHAGE ACTIVITY	INCREASES B CELL RESPONSES (Continued)
C. parvum	Mycobacterium
B. pertussis	Silica
Pyran	Beryllium
BCG, mycobacteria	Cationic detergents
Levamisole (slightly)	Saponin
Polyribonucleotides	Retinol
Glucan	BCG, Freund's adjuvant
	Tilorone
IMPROVES T CELL RESPONSES	
Levamisole	INCREASES COMPLEMENT ACTIVITY
BCG, Freund's complete adjuvant	Levamisole
B. pertussis	
	INDUCES INTERFERON PRODUCTION
INCREASES B CELL RESPONSES	Pyran
Pyran	Endotoxin
Glucan	Polysaccharides
C. parvum	Tilorone
B. pertussis	
Endotoxins	INCREASES GRANULOCYTE FUNCTION
Bordetella	None known

logical response has been used clinically in only the crudest sense. Before the introduction of antibiotics, many patients with chronic infections were treated with a variety of vaccines and bacterial extracts, including those from *Staphylococcus*, *Salmonella*, and *Pseudomonas*. Some patients showed clear benefit, but many did not. Since fever was usually produced by bacterial vaccines, the therapeutic value of fever alone was evaluated. Hyperthermic chambers were constructed and used for the treatment of certain infectious diseases, especially the venereal diseases, again with quite variable results. The dramatic effect of the antibiotics on infectious disease in the 1940s virtually abolished clinical interest in nonspecific means for the treatment of infection.

Within the last two decades, several truths have become evident, among which are the realization that antibiotics have limited usefulness, and that cancer chemotherapeutic agents are potent but often ineffective and rarely curative. Such drugs are regularly toxic, and diminished immune responses caused by the drugs are associated both with progression of cancer and infection. Together, these problems have once again forced a reevaluation of and search for agents that have the property of immunopotentiation. Although still in its infancy, the field has made great progress in recent years. Table 10–1 provides a partial listing of immunopotentiating agents and their effects upon various components of the immune system. The more important of these will be discussed individually.

CORYNEBACTERIUM PARVUM

C. parvum belongs to a group of organisms referred to as the anaerobic coryneforms, which include the *Corynebacteria* and closely related

Propionibacteria. Many of the species within this group have similar effects on the immune system, although they may vary considerably in their effectiveness, with some species and strains being quite ineffective. *C. parvum* and *C. granulosum* are currently used the most in laboratory and clinical investigations. Because of the similarity of action among this group, only *C. parvum* will be discussed.

In 1958, it was found that administration of *Corynebacterium parvum* causes reversible hyperplasia of the reticuloendothelial system and increases phagocytic activity. Further investigation showed that its administration would inhibit the growth of certain neoplasms. Because of this, *C. parvum* is one of the better studied immunopotentiators, and the effects of the administration of the killed organism, gleaned from several studies, are shown in Table 10–2.

Activation of mononuclear phagocytes is undoubtedly the most important of the biological effects. Macrophages activated by *C. parvum* develop an increase in lysosomal enzymes (especially acid phosphatase), increased adherence to glass, an increase in intracytoplasmic vacuoles, and increased bactericidal capacity. Activated macrophages are cytotoxic for tumor cells in vitro and are distinct from either "armed" or "immune" macrophages. Animals injected with *C. parvum* develop an increased weight of the liver, spleen, and lung, with an accelerated clearance of particles from the blood upon subsequent challenge. The mediator of macrophage activation appears to be identical to a chemotactic factor that has been recovered from cultures or culture filtrates of the bacteria. This substance attracts macrophages, but not neutrophils, and acts independently of serum factors.

TABLE 10–2. EFFECTS OF *Corynebacterium parvum* ADMINISTRATION ON IMMUNE RESPONSES

Macrophages
   Direct chemotaxin for mononuclear phagocytes (MP), but not neutrophils
   Increases acid phosphatase activity of MPs
   Increases particle uptake by RES
   Increases clearance of intravenously injected bacteria
   Activates macrophages (T cell presence sometimes necessary)
   Increases resistance to infection by intracellular pathogens
   Causes MP-mediated regression of tumors, especially when injected directly in tumor

T Cells
   Decreases thymic weight
   Decreases T cells in lymph nodes and spleen
   Decreases delayed hypersensitivity response to intradermal tests
   Prolongs skin grafts
   Decreases response of T lymphocytes to PHA
   Decreases graft versus host reaction

B Cells
   Increases antibody response to most antigens, especially to T independent antigens
   Causes B cell proliferation

Complement
   Decreases both classical and alternative complement activity via activation

Bone Marrow
   Stimulates bone marrow macrophage and neutrophil colony production

Because of the increased activity of macrophages, treatment with *C. parvum* increases resistance to infection caused by intracellular pathogens, including some viruses and malaria. Increased macrophage activity seems to be responsible for an increased resistance to malignant cells, with inhibition of tumor growth in treated animals. The degree of inhibition depends upon the type of tumor, the tumor load, and the route and timing of injection of *C. parvum* in relation to the inoculation of the tumor. Different preparations of *C. parvum* have been shown to differ considerably in biological potency. Tumor regression is best accomplished when the material is injected directly into the tumor mass, in which case it sometimes causes a regression of both the injected tumor and noninjected tumors. The effect of *C. parvum* on tumor growth may be potentiated by concurrent irradiation or administration of cyclophosphamide. However, the most dramatic regressions in tumor-bearing animals were found when *C. parvum* was given 12 days after a single dose of cyclophosphamide.

The protective effect of *C. parvum* against tumors or intracellular infections clearly seems to be related to activation of macrophages, since *C. parvum* exerts a depressive effect on T cells. The systemic administration of *C. parvum* results in a decrease in delayed hypersensitivity responsiveness, including the responsiveness to intradermal skin tests (such as PPD or mumps antigen), prolongation of skin grafts, decreased response of T lymphocytes to phytomitogens, and decreased graft versus host reactions. This inhibition is not a direct effect of the immunopotentiation, but rather is mediated by a negative feedback of the activated macrophages on T cells. On the other hand, *C. parvum* will expand the B cell population, and its administration is associated with an increased and prolonged antibody response to most antigens, particularly T cell independent antigens. The response to T cell dependent antigens is interesting: it may be increased, decreased, or remain the same when *C. parvum* has also been given.

The beneficial effects of chemotherapy on cancer in man have been improved by the additional administration of *C. parvum*. Patients receiving *C. parvum* seem to tolerate chemotherapy better than when no *C. parvum* has been given, perhaps through stimulation of the bone marrow, and this may have contributed to the improvement in therapeutic response. It is of interest that the tumor inhibitory effects of *C. parvum* seems to be no greater in animals previously immunized to *C. parvum* than in nonimmunized controls, an observation which supports the concept that the antitumor activity results from nonspecific stimulation of the immune system and not a specific response to cross-reacting antigens.

BCG AND MYCOBACTERIAL PRODUCTS

BCG is an abbreviation for bacillus Calmette-Guérin, an attenuated strain of *Mycobacterium bovis*, developed from a virulent culture by Calmette and Guérin in 1908 at the Pasteur Institute. All subsequent BCG vaccines have derived from this parent strain, but there may be considerable differences in biological potency because of variations in culture technique and genetic drift of the cultures. Apparently, the best results of immunopotentiation have been obtained by investigators using subcultures recently obtained from the Pasteur Institute.

BCG has long been used as a vaccine for the prevention of pulmonary tuberculosis in humans, and has been especially effective in areas where tuberculosis incidence is high. Since the administration of the attenuated vaccine was found to activate macrophage activity, Old and Benaceraf tried BCG treatment as an adjunct for the therapy of malignant neoplasms in 1958. In experimental systems, BCG treatment has been shown capable of preventing and effectively treating many malignant neoplasms. The effect of administration of reasonably large doses of BCG to patients with minimal residual malignant neoplasms has been impressive in some studies. Significant prolongation of the interval before appearance of metastasis and improvement in survival have been reported. The best results have been obtained when material was injected directly into the tumor. In some systems, intratumoral injection has provided clear evidence of systemic immunity to the tumor. The beneficial effect of BCG seems to be mediated primarily through activation of macrophages (Table 10–3). Active infection with BCG will stimulate the release of a lymphocyte-activating factor from macrophages, which, in turn, secondarily activates other macrophages, thereby amplifying the response. BCG augments helper T cell function, enhances antibody production, and enhances development of delayed allergies and cell-mediated immunity. Presumably, because of the macrophage activation, there is increased resistance to virus infections and infections by intracellular bacterial pathogens and fungi.

Since BCG is a living organism, it may cause disease in susceptible individuals, particularly those with significant immunodepression. Disseminated infection as well as infections at specific sites, such as the site of injection, regional lymph nodes, or the eye may occur. Widely disseminated BCGosis has been observed in children with severe combined immunodeficiency or T cell immunodeficiency. Hepatotoxicity may be an important feature of BCGosis, but the symptoms usually disappear with antituberculosis chemotherapy.

Because of the potentially adverse effects of the living vaccine, various extracts derived from BCG have been evaluated for their biological activity. One of these, a methyl extraction residue (MER) seems to have shown prom-

TABLE 10–3. EFFECTS OF BCG ON IMMUNE RESPONSE

Activates macrophages

Stimulates the release of lymphocyte-activating factors from macrophages

Augments helper T cell function
Causes blast transformation of lymphocytes
Enhances antibody production

Inhibits tumor growth, especially when given intralesionally

Increases resistance to virus infection

Increases resistance to intracellular pathogens

ise, especially when given in combination with radiation therapy or chemotherapy. Both MER and BCG increase T cell activity to augment cell-mediated immune responses. Cell walls prepared from BCG when used together with oil droplets also have a similar potentiating effect on the immune response.

Other forms of mycobacteria have a marked effect on the immune response. In particular, extracts from *Mycobacterium smegmatis* and *M. kanasasii* have significant antitumor effects. A water soluble preparation (WSA) from *M. smegmatis* has been obtained from lysosomal digestion of purified mycobacterial cell walls. This preparation is primarily an adjuvant for antibody formation. Another preparation from *M. smegmatis,* known as interphase material, has been shown to have an antitumor effect and to activate macrophages.

Freund's complete adjuvant is a widely used immunopotentiator which consists of the killed mycobacteria suspended in a water-oil emulsion with mineral oil and Arlacel A. When antigen is mixed with Freund's complete adjuvant and injected subcutaneously or intradermally, a remarkable potentiation of antibody production can be achieved, especially with protein antigens. However, it does not potentiate immune responses to thymus independent antigens. The major effect is a long-lasting and persistent level of cell-mediated immunity to protein antigens. It is the mineral oil acting together with the mycobacteria that is the critical component conferring a long-lasting influence on immune response. Immunization with Freund's incomplete adjuvant (lacking mycobacteria) will stimulate antibody formation, but only a transient form of delayed hypersensitivity response is observed. Another interesting feature is that incomplete Freund's adjuvant stimulates predominately a gamma-1 type of antibody, whereas the complete Freund's adjuvant incites the stimulation of gamma-2 type of antibody (IgG2). When Freund's complete adjuvant is injected with extracts or suspensions of tissues, autoimmune phenomena and disease may result. Various extracts have been made from *M. tuberculosis* to substitute for the intact organism in Freund's complete adjuvant. One of these, wax D, was found to be quite active. Its principal component is a peptidoglycolipid.

Several water-soluble adjuvants have been developed, and it has been shown that monomeric peptidoglycans are active adjuvants. As a result of this information, several synthetic analogs have been prepared by workers in Japan and at the Pasteur Institute in Paris. These investigators independently showed that the adjuvanticity of bacteria, such as BCG, tubercle bacilli, *Nocardia,* and many other organisms, resides entirely in the relatively simple chemicals in the cell wall skeleton. These are the muramyldipeptides, such as N-acetylmuramyl-L-alanyl-D-isoglutamine. They can be purified, are completely defined chemically, and are simple, relatively nontoxic substances that can be synthesized. It seems quite certain that much of the immunopotentiation of the future will be carried out with defined molecules of this class. Cruder but chemically defined cell wall skeletons act to stimulate both antibody and cell-mediated immunities. Although these cell wall skeletons cannot be synthesized, they have great advantages of relative simplicity, chemical definition and consequent uniformity, and freedom from many side reactions that complicate preparation of crude organisms like BCG.

Other exciting data indicate that enhancement of the T cell-based cell-mediated immunities may be attributed to another relatively simple chemical known as cord factor because of its influence on the manner of growth of acid-fast organisms. This substance is a potent enhancer of the development of cell-mediated immunities and, like the simple muramyldipeptides for antibody production, may become a standard immunopotentiator of cell-mediated immunities.

BORDETELLA PERTUSSIS

Whole killed pertussis vaccine contains a number of substances that have a significant effect on the immune system (Table 10–4). One property of significant interest is the ability of pertussis vaccine to induce anaphylactic sensitivity to an antigen in experimental animals. Not only does it increase the production of homocytotropic antibody, but it also sensitizes for the development of passive anaphylaxis and increases sensitivity to histamines and other mediators of the anaphylactic reaction.

Another prominent feature associated with the administration of pertussis vaccine is the induction of a striking peripheral lymphocytosis. The mechanism for the lymphocytosis appears to be release of the mobile small lymphocyte population from the peripheral lymphoid organs into the blood, and failure of these lymphocytes to recirculate for a time to the lymphoid organs. These lymphocytes, which are predominately T lymphocytes, lose their ability to "home" to the postcapillary venule, therefore becoming unable to exit from the circulation. The relationship of this peripheral lymphocytosis to its known potent effect as an adjuvant is unknown.

Some of the adjuvant effect of pertussis vaccine undoubtedly occurs because of endotoxin contained in the vaccine. However, a more potent effect seems to be mediated by direct stimulation of macrophage activity. *B. pertussis* vaccine accelerates clearance of antigen from the circulation and enhances both primary and secondary responses. The adjuvant effect on an-

TABLE 10–4. IMMUNOMODULATION BY *Bordetella pertussis*

Provokes striking peripheral lymphocytosis secondary to delivery of small lymphocytes from lymphoid organs to blood

Stimulates macrophage activity

Increases susceptibility to anaphylaxis
Increases sensitivity to histamine and other mediators
Increases antibody synthesis (adjuvant effect)

Stimulates both B cells and T cells

Primary adjuvant effect appears to be via expansion of antigen sensitive cells

tibody formation occurs only after uptake of the antigen by macrophages. Thus, the effect seems to be primarily upon the multiplication of antigen-sensitive cells. Pertussis vaccine can increase the rate of cell division, and stimulates both B cells and T cells. The vaccine given alone can result in an anamnestic response.

ACTION OF ENDOTOXIN

Endotoxins have long been known to stimulate antibody production, especially in mixed bacterial vaccines, such as tetanus toxoid and typhoid bacilli. The early work with endotoxins also demonstrated an early but transient (days) increase in resistance to infection following the systemic administration. In experimental animals rendered refractory by prior administration of endotoxin, this increased resistance to infection could no longer be demonstrated. Interestingly, animals rendered refractory to endotoxin by repeated administration also became unable to show an adjuvant effect when endotoxin was administered.

Bacterial endotoxins are complex lipopolysaccharides of the cell walls of gram-negative bacteria, composed of three principal chemical regions, a specific (O) polysaccharide, a core polysaccharide, and lipid A. The polysaccharides are antigenic, and the O polysaccharide provides the major antigenic specificity of the molecule. Lipid A is responsible for most of the other biological effects of the endotoxin, including the principal toxicity, mitogenic effects, and the adjuvant effects (Table 10–5). While lipid A may act on a variety of cells, one important effect is its mitogenic stimulation of B cells, especially in the mouse. It is a potent adjuvant for the formation of antibody, probably as a consequence both of this direct mitogenic stimulation and because of inhibition of the negative feedback influence on B cells. The effect of lipopolysaccharide on macrophages appears to be primarily indirect, through stimulated B cells, which synthesize and release MIF and macrophage activating factor (MAF). However, endotoxin will activate macrophages directly in vitro. Because of the enhanced B cell activity, endotoxin often results in a premature inhibition of T cell responses specific for an inducing antigen. Its relationship to T cell activity is interesting, in that T cells may be necessary for an adjuvant effect of endotoxin for many thymus dependent antigens.

Besides enhancing antibody production and activating macrophages to

TABLE 10–5. MECHANISMS OF ACTION OF ENDOTOXIN

Active portion causing adjuvant effect is lipid A

Direct stimulation of B cells

Macrophage activation secondary to effect on B cells

Inhibits negative feedback on B cells, thus increasing antibody production

May increase resistance to infection transiently

Adjuvant effect requires presence of T cells at least for many thymus dependent antigens

Induces formation of tumor necrosis factor (TNF)

the bodily defense against microorganisms, endotoxins have long been known to exert destructive or necrotizing influences on certain tumors. Recent studies have shown endotoxin to generate in the blood a fascinating substance called tumor necrosis factor (TNF). This glycopeptide of approximately 130,000 D is capable of producing in vitro necrosis of certain tumor cells, but not normal cells in tissue culture. Tumor necrosis factor appears more regularly and in higher concentrations when endotoxin has been given to animals pretreated with BCG. Purification and definition of TNF may yield antitumor agent of great specificity.

A variant form of immunopotentiation by endotoxin, which looks extremely attractive, was recently developed in Freiberg, where investigators found that when the outer coat of 2-keto-3-deoxyoctanoic acid is removed by acid hydrolysis from a rough strain of salmonella (S. minnesota), a sticky inner layer composed of lipid A is revealed. Many weak antigens, such as blood group substances, can be applied to these altered salmonella organisms. Upon injection of the organism with its outer coat of weak antigen, the immune system perceives the weak antigen as though it were the outer coat of a bacterium. In some instances, massive immunopotentiation can be accomplished. This new principle of immunopotentiation will surely have much to offer when cancer specific antigens, likely to be weak antigens, are defined, evaluated, and developed for the treatment of cancer.

OTHER MICROBIAL PRODUCTS

Glucan is a purified lipopolysaccharide derived from brewer's yeast. It is a potent stimulator of macrophage activity and has many of the properties of BCG, including the ability to increase clearance of injected particles, to enhance humoral immunity, to inhibit tumor growth, and to enhance sensitivity to endotoxin. Its effect on resistance to infection has not been fully evaluated.

A variety of infections, such as those caused by *Salmonella enteritidis* and *Listeria monocytogenes*, increases resistance to both tumor growth and bacterial infection, especially during the stage of active infection. Also, a variety of vaccines and bacterial products has been used to increase nonspecific resistance to infection, as mentioned earlier. Undoubtedly, as more advanced scientific methodology is applied to determine the precise chemicals involved and the specific effect on the immune system, chemical products of these organisms may also become available for potential manipulation of immunologic functions.

LEVAMISOLE

Imidazole is the parent moiety of both levamisole and its optic isomer, tetramisole. Both drugs are widely used as effective antihelminthic agents, and levamisole, the best studied in man, has remarkably few side-effects. The action of the drugs is similar and both will hereafter be referred to as levamisole.

TABLE 10–6. MECHANISMS OF ACTION OF LEVAMISOLE

Increases cyclic GMP and lowers cyclic AMP levels in T lymphocytes

Increases proliferative response of cultured lymphocytes to antigens (PPD, measles, *Candida*)

Augments proliferative response of lymphocytes to PHA and allogeneic cells in culture

Restores cell-mediated immune responses in immunodepressed patients

May augment antibody synthesis by accelerated priming of T cells

Decreases tumor incidence when given one day before IV challenge, but increases tumor incidence when given five days before challenge

Administration associated with long-term remission in leukemia and delayed recurrences in breast cancer with increased survival

Increases phagocytosis by macrophages and possibly by neutrophils

Increases resistance to infection with intracellular bacterial pathogens, helminths, many viruses, and *Candida*

Increases levels of hemolytic complement

The primary immunopotentiating effect of levamisole is mediated through an augmentation of the response of lymphocytes to the antigens that cause delayed hypersensitivity reactions (Table 10–6). Levamisole increases cyclic GMP levels and decreases cyclic AMP levels of T cells. Culture of T lymphocytes with levamisole in vitro, in the presence of antigens like PPD, measles, or *Candida* will increase the reactivity of those lymphocytes to the antigens. It will also augment the response to phytohemagglutinin and allogeneic cells in culture. In patients with a diminished delayed hypersensitivity response to several common antigens, the oral administration of levamisole will often cause restoration of these responses to normal. In some patients who have failed to respond to sensitization using DNCB, levamisole therapy has restored reactivity. Its effect on antibody production appears to be variable, but the synthesis of antibody may be increased by an acceleration of the priming of T cells. The drug may also have an effect on macrophages since it can increase phagocytosis by these cells and also possibly by neutrophils. A beneficial effect in infections has been shown with intracellular pathogens, including bacteria, viruses, and fungi. However, initial attempts of therapy for anergic patients with severe acute bacterial infections have not shown a beneficial effect in limited trials, and it is probable that the primary therapeutic value of the drug will be in restoring altered delayed hypersensitivity responses where these are diminished in cancer patients or in patients with chronic infection. Levamisole has prolonged remissions in leukemia and delayed recurrences in patients with breast cancer, both being associated with increased survival. The effect is reasonably prompt, and 150 mg given daily for three days will often restore depressed delayed hypersensitivity responses.

PYRAN

Pyran is a synthetic, negatively charged polyanion consisting of a maleic acid – divinyl ether copolymer. It has antiviral activity, partly because of its

TABLE 10-7. IMMUNOMODULATING EFFECTS OF PYRAN

Initial depression, then stimulation of phagocytosis by RES, maximal effect 5–7 days after administration

Increases antibody response

Induces synthesis of interferon

Administration diminishes complement activity

capacity to induce interferon. In mice, the drug is also effective in protection against lethal bacterial and fungal infections. When administered systemically, it causes splenomegaly and hepatomegaly, which is associated with an expansion of the reticuloendothelial systems and improved clearance of particulate matter (Table 10–7). Pyran treatment causes an initial depression of phagocytosis, which lasts for two to three days after the last injection of the drug. This returns to normal by six days, and by seven to nine days, there is marked stimulation of phagocytic activity. Part of the effect on antibody production may be through T cell macrophage interaction. Pyran is mitogenic for spleen cells in vitro, but mitogen-induced blastogenesis of spleen cells to PHA and lipopolysaccharide in vitro is inhibited following administration of pyran in vivo. The drug clearly has some antitumor activity, which seems to be macrophage-mediated.

TILORONE

Tilorone is another drug of potential interest. It induces the synthesis of interferon and enhances antibody formation. On the other hand, cell-

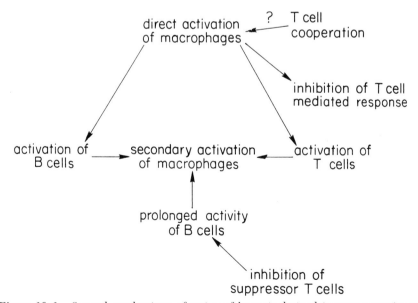

Figure 10–1. Several mechanisms of action of bacteria-derived immunopotentiators.

mediated responses are depressed, and the drug depresses tuberculin sensitivity, prolongs skin grafts, and inhibits graft versus host reactions. Its potential as a drug for preventing viral infections in immunosuppressed patients should be investigated further.

THE FUTURE USE OF IMMUNOPOTENTIATORS

From our present knowledge base, it would appear that the primary effect of these immunopotentiators will be on the macrophage (Fig. 10–1). However, many avenues remain unexplored. In particular, the effect of immunopotentiators on the complement system needs extensive study, and the use of immunomodulators to favor the production of either enhancing or cytotoxic antibody remains in its infancy.

It can be envisioned that it will soon be possible to regulate (modulate) much of the immune response at will. Certainly, it will be possible to improve resistance to infection and cancer, and to selectively depress some types of immune responses while enhancing others.

SECTION II
LABORATORY AND CLINICAL TESTS

Tests of immunologic function provide the tools for
investigating and understanding the complex immune
process. A working knowledge of the basic principles
underlying commonly used procedures is therefore necessary
for the well prepared clinician in almost any specialty.
Technical details of these tests will not be presented in the
following two chapters since good descriptions can be found
in the standard texts of immunology. Instead, we offer a brief
survey of the general concepts, usefulness, and applications
relevant to clinical practice or animal models of human
disease.

11

Tests for Cellular Function in Immunity

Increasing numbers of patients have been shown to have either primary or associated abnormalities of immunity related to cellular function. Since many of these diseases appear amenable to correction, it becomes especially important to document the specific defects, not only to gain further insight into the basic mechanism of the immune process, but also to formulate a rational approach to therapy.

For convenience, the tests will be divided into those performed in vivo and those performed primarily in vitro.

IN VIVO TESTS

DELAYED HYPERSENSITIVITY REACTIONS TO SKIN TEST ANTIGENS

Observation of the response to an intradermal injection of an antigen is a time-honored procedure of considerable value. The classic response is elicited by the introduction of a small amount of PPD. Transient early reactions may occur, but the ones of interest are those related to the delayed hypersensitivity process, which involves an infiltration of the subepithelial tissues with lymphocytes and mononuclear phagocytes. This lesion reaches a maximum of intensity between 24 and 48 hours and may persist for several days. Only the development of induration is important in interpretation of the test, and erythema should be disregarded.

Delayed hypersensitivity to skin test antigens can be used in two ways. First, and classically, it has been a valuable tool in the diagnosis of certain diseases or for demonstrating that an individual had a given disease (such as tuberculosis) in the past. Recently, skin testing for delayed hypersensitivity reactions has been used to investigate the immune competence of an individual. The common antigens used for such testing include tuberculin (or PPD), histoplasmin, coccidioidin, mumps antigen, candidal antigen, and

137

streptokinase-streptodornase (SKSD). Normal individuals usually respond to more than one of these antigens; persons with a lack of responsiveness are said to be anergic. Anergy may be transient, and its presence may be related to a complex set of factors, including diminution of T cell function and macrophage function, or vascular reactivity, or a combination of these. Since virtually everyone has been exposed in the past to one or more of the above antigens, a positive skin response should be elicited regularly in normal individuals.

DNCB SENSITIZATION

Dinitrochlorobenzene (DNCB) is an industrial chemical that usually causes intense sensitization when applied to the skin of normal individuals. The small molecule acts as a hapten, binding to normal protein of the skin, and elicits a T cell-mediated, delayed type of contact hypersensitivity. Since the compound does not normally appear in nature, few persons have preexisting sensitivity.

DNCB is used clinically to determine the ability of a patient to respond to a stimulus that normally causes T cell dependent immunization (contact sensitivity). A small sensitizing dose is applied to the skin of the arm, together with a smaller testing dose to rule out prior sensitization. Two weeks later, a small test dose is applied to a separate site on the arm. The sensitizing application should cause erythema but no induration, and the second application should cause both erythema and induration. A negative test indicates that the individual has diminished T cell function. DNCB testing has been especially useful in assessing immune competence in cancer patients and in patients prior to transplantation.

ALLOGRAFT REJECTION

Primary rejection of an allograft is a potent cell-mediated immunologic reaction that is mostly a measure of T cell function. It is sometimes used to test immunologic competency in patients, but the result also reflects histocompatibility differences (Chapter 15). Graft rejection of allogeneic skin is frequently used to test the potency of immunosuppressive regimens and to measure the biological activity of antilymphocyte globulin. For the test, a small full thickness or thick split thickness piece of skin is transferred from one individual and grafted to an appropriately prepared site on the recipient. The bed of the test site should be deep enough to have removed all epithelial elements. Often, the graft rejects in an irregular fashion over several days, and the end point is usually taken as that time when 50 per cent of the graft has lost viability, as evidenced by marked discoloration, loss of circulation, or desiccation. Allograft rejection has been useful in detecting decreased cellular competence in seriously burned patients and in patients with immunodeficiency diseases.

Graft versus Host (GVH) Reactions

While this reaction occurs clinically in humans, it is never used as a test. However, its widespread application in the laboratory as a measure of immunologic reactivity warrants its inclusion in this discussion. GVH reactions are caused by the injection of immunocompetent lymphocytes (T cells) into recipients who have a reduced or no reactivity against the injected cells. Thus, the response is one in which grafted cells reject the host. To avoid rejection of the injected cells, the recipient is usually given a lethal dose of a cytotoxic drug or irradiation, or the experiment is performed using parent strain cells injected into F_1 hybrids. The GVH response causes a number of clinical features, including enlargement of the spleen and lymph nodes, cutaneous lesions, and wasting (runting in immature animals). Splenic enlargement is the easiest and most accurate of these to measure, and measurement of splenic weight is often used to evaluate the degree of GVH response. The splenic weight assay has the advantage that only low doses of injected cells are required, and the results can be obtained in about nine to ten days in mice. Splenic enlargement occurs because the injected "foreign" T cells "home" to the spleen and lymph nodes after IV or IP injection, later expanding their population by division. Popliteal lymph node enlargement can also be used when the cells are injected into the footpad.

Lymph Node Biopsy

Histologic examination of lymph nodes provides a crude but often semiquantitative measure of T and B activity. Marked depletion of lymphocytes in the deep cortical or paracortical thymus dependent areas (TDA) usually reflects a systemic reduction in functional T cells, whereas marked depletion of cells within germinal centers, follicles, and medullary cords usually reflects a systemic reduction of B cells. On the other hand, evidence of accumulation by cells, and cell enlargement, cell division, or both in the TDA indicate that the cells of thymus dependent regions are responding to antigenic stimulation. Similarly, enlargement of the size of the outer cortex, increased numbers of germinal centers, enlargement of the lymphoid follicles, and accumulation of plasma cells in medullary and postfollicular regions reflect stimulation and terminal differentiation of the cells of the thymus independent or B lymphoid system. Figure 11–1A and B illustrates these two separate responses. In many instances, both T and B cell regions of the node will be expanded simultaneously as antigenic stimulation affects both lymphoid systems simultaneously. Accurate interpretation requires that the section be taken perpendicularly through the hilum.

Skin Window Techniques (Rebuck Test)

Epidermal abrasion to the point of causing punctate bleeding will result in the exudation of cells from the blood to the site of injury. The cellular

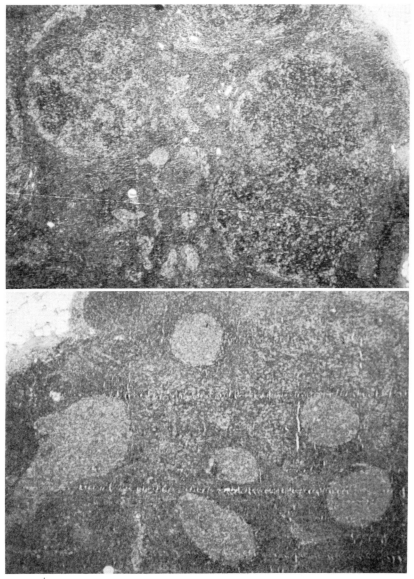

Figure 11–1. *A*, Lymph node showing stimulation of thymus dependent areas. *B*, Lymph node showing stimulation of B cell dependent areas.

composition of the exudate can then be studied by sequential application of coverslips to the abraded area, followed by microscopic examination. Qualitatively, neutrophils first appear in the exudate, followed by lymphoid cells, and then macrophages. The number of cells in the exudate can only be estimated crudely, and attempts to make quantitation more accurate by the use of chambers placed over the abraded area have been hindered by technical problems. The response to certain stimulating substances, placed on the abraded surface, has sometimes been used. The test has been most useful in man to determine the ability to develop a normal inflammatory response to mechanical injury.

Particle Clearance

Particulate material introduced by the intravenous route is usually rapidly removed from the circulation by the reticuloendothelial system (RES), thereby providing the basis for a series of tests to measure RES function. These tests have used various materials, including colloidal carbon, lipid emulsions, aggregated isotope-labeled albumin, bacteria, chromium phosphate, colloidal gold, fluorescent particles, and chromium phosphate. After an intravenous injection, these substances are rapidly cleared from the circulation in an exponential fashion (about 90 per cent by the liver for colloidal carbon). Serial sampling of the blood must be done to measure the rate of clearance, which is expressed by the constant K that represents the slope of the line when the logarithm of blood concentration is plotted against time. Most of these substances require opsonins for their removal so that individuals with reduced opsonic activity may have inaccurate assessments of RES activity, as measured by particle clearance.

In experimental animals, colloidal carbon and bacteria are the substances most commonly used. None is entirely suitable for use in patients, but lipid emulsions and labeled aggregated albumin appear to be the most frequently employed in recent experiments. At the present time, such tests are of limited clinical value.

Tests of B Cell Function

Evaluation of in vivo B cell function against a defined antigen is accomplished in a number of ways. The most common evaluation used clinically is simple quantitation of the amount of antibody present in the blood against an antigen to which the host has previously been stimulated. This is done in a variety of ways, including Schick testing with diphtheria toxin if the person has been immunized with diphtheria toxoid, in vitro flocculation or neutralization tests for diphtheria and tetanus toxins, neutralization tests for polio virus, streptolysin O titers, agglutination against *Salmonella* or other bacterial organisms, and quantitation of agglutinins against blood group substances. For better analysis of the currently existing state of B cell function, response to active immunization with a specific antigen may be used. If the patient has not been previously immunized or shows no titer against a given antigen, measurement of antibody formation to injections of tetanus toxoid, diphtheria toxoid, or killed polio vaccine is perhaps most frequently used. However, immunization with other killed virus vaccines like influenza; with bacterial vaccines such as brucella, typhoid, or pneumococcal polysaccharide; or with other antigens, such as keyhole limpet hemocyanin or $\phi\chi 174$, has value in evaluating the functional state of B cells in patients.

IN VITRO TESTS

In vitro testing has several obvious advantages, including the ability to test the function of purified cell populations. With this, however, must come the disadvantage of an artificial environment in which the cells must reside or function.

TESTS OF LYMPHOCYTE FUNCTION

Measurement of lymphocyte function has become increasingly important in clinical practice. Lymphocytes can be recovered from blood or efferent lymph channels such as the thoracic duct, or from tissues such as lymph nodes, spleen, or thymus. As might be expected they have different properties, depending upon the source. To obtain purified lymphocytes, it is necessary to use additional procedures, which include sedimentation, the use of centrifugation and gradients, erythrocyte attachment and lysis, and the employment of columns to remove adherent cells (macrophages and neutrophils).

T cells can be separated from B cells in a purified lymphocyte population by passing the mixture over a column coated with IgG or C3, which will retard the movement of B cells through the column. B cells can be separated from an initial mixture of T and B cells by adding sheep erythrocytes to cause rosette formation with T cells and centrifuging to remove the rosettes. Antigen-reactive lymphocytes can be extracted from a purified lymphocyte mixture or even whole lymph or blood by the use of antigen-coated columns. These cells can subsequently be eluted from the columns, using mild conditions. In addition, many other physicochemical techniques have been exploited for separation of various lymphocyte populations.

Purified lymphocytes can be labeled with a variety of radioisotopes and introduced in vivo to study tissue distribution, traffic patterns, and cellular relationships. They can also be used in vitro to study biosynthetic pathways and response to stimuli.

Tests for Measuring Lymphocyte Responsiveness to Mitogens. A variety of agents can stimulate lymphocyte activity, specifically or nonspecifically. These are variously called mitogens, activators, or stimulators. While activator is probably the preferable term, mitogen is more commonly used. The essential components of this group of tests are shown in Figure 11–2. When such tests were first derived, comparisons were made using morphologic examination of the lymphocytes for blast transformation, but the test now customarily utilizes incorporation of radioisotopic precursors as an index of responsiveness, and is often automated. Tritiated thymidine is used to determine the rate of synthesis of DNA, ^{3}H L-leucine is used to measure the rate of protein synthesis, and other isotopes may be used to measure different components of cellular activation. Still another method for evaluating the increase in DNA and RNA has recently employed vital staining with acridine orange, which stains DNA so that it fluoresces green while

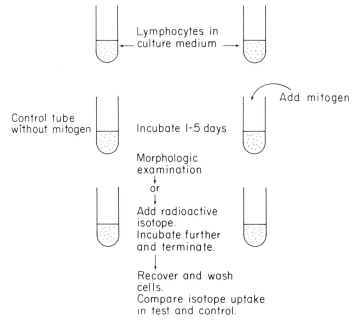

Figure 11–2. Essential components of tests that measure responsiveness of lymphocytes to mitogens.

RNA fluoresces red. Fully automated analysis of responses of the cells to mitogens has been possible employing this technique. By varying the conditions of these tests, it is possible to determine the reactivity of different, highly purified lymphocyte populations to various activators or mitogens, to compare the reactivity of lymphocytes from one individual with that of others, to detect inhibitors of the reaction, to measure the effect of drugs, and to study products of the activation.

Responsiveness of blood lymphocytes to one or more nonspecific mitogens is an often used clinical test. Phytohemagglutinin (PHA), which activates primarily T cells, is perhaps the most widely used mitogen for this purpose. In contrast, endotoxin selectively activates B cells of animals, but not man, and pokeweed mitogen (PWM) activates T cells and also B cells in the presence of a helper T cell population. Some substances, such as staphylococcal protein A attached to Sepharose, may act as a selective mitogen for human B cells.

Mixed lymphocyte cultures (MLC) are even more useful from a clinical standpoint. In this test, allogeneic cells, usually lymphocytes, are used as the activator. When lymphocytes are used as activators, they are treated with mitomycin C or irradiation to prevent a mitogenic response of the stimulating cells to the responder cells (one-way MLC). The one-way MLC is especially useful in selecting the best donor-recipient combination when several potential donors are available for organ transplantation. The donor cells causing no stimulation are well matched with those of the recipient, and when several potential donors are tested, cells causing the least stimulation are considered to come from the donor least likely to elicit a vigorous rejection reaction.

Specific antigens can be used as the activators to measure preexisting sensitization, as well as to measure the ability to respond to given antigens.

Cytotoxicity Tests. A variety of tests is available for measuring the ability of lymphocytes to kill target cells, and these are referred to as cell-mediated cytotoxicity (CMC) tests. One frequently used technique (Hellström) plates target cells in Petri dishes, then adds lymphocytes. After incubation, dead target cells are detected as plaques or enumerated by adding vital stains or other techniques. In a more widely applied test, target cells are labeled with ^{51}Cr, washed, and incubated with the lymphocyte suspension (Fig. 11–3). The cells are removed from suspension, and the supernate counted in a gamma counter. Dead cells release their bound chromium, and the amount of free chromium released into the supernate is proportional to the degree of cytotoxicity. Both types of tests may be used semiquantitatively, but must be carefully controlled. They are often used to determine the presence of blocking factors or potentiating factors in serum, and they have frequent clinical application.

Suppressor Cell Functions. Since it has now been shown that T lymphocytes not only proliferate in response to mitogens, antigens, and allogeneic cells, but also can regulate normal proliferative responses including synthesis and secretion of antibodies or immunoglobulins, direct analysis for these suppressor functions has recently been developed. The capacity of T cells, after stimulation with specific antigen or with the activator Con-A, to inhibit the response of other T cells to antigens, mitogens, or allogeneic cells can be measured. In addition, analyses of the capacity of stimulated T cells to inhibit the responses of B lymphocytes to synthesize and secrete im-

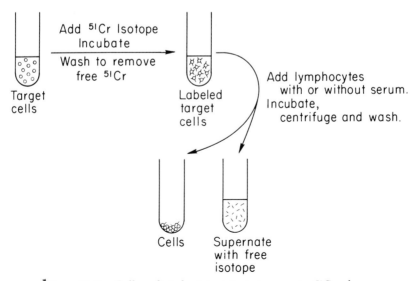

Figure 11–3. Cell-mediated cytotoxicity test measuring ^{51}Cr release.

munoglobulin molecules or specific antibody have also been perfected. Figure 11–4 illustrates the tests for analysis of suppressor function of T cells.

Helper Cell Function. It has also become possible to evaluate the function of T cells as helper cells in antibody production or in terminal differentiation to Ig-synthesizing and secreting cells. Ordinarily, these helper functions are evaluated with purified T and B cell populations. The purified T cells, stimulated with either a specific antigen or with an activator like Con-A, are evaluated for their capacity to assist the purified population of B cells in responding to antigen or the activator PWM. Figure 11–5 illustrates the analysis of helper function of T cells.

Helper T cells and suppressor T cells have been shown in mice to represent distinct populations of T cells with different antigenic surface markers (see Chapter 3).

Assays of B Cell Activity. Quantitation of the levels of each of the immunoglobulins by radial immunodiffusion is perhaps the simplest measure of B cell activity. The numbers of B lymphocytes in the circulation can be assessed by measuring the proportion and absolute number of circulating lymphocytes that have surface Ig. The number of peripheral blood lymphocytes that differentiate in culture to plasma cells can be assessed, using fluorescent microscopy to detect cells that contain IgM, IgG, IgA, or total Ig in their cytoplasm. Alternatively, quantitation of the amount of Ig that is synthesized and secreted by the peripheral blood lymphoid cells after six or seven days of stimulation in culture can be measured. These analyses have proved to be excellent means for evaluating responses of the B lymphocyte population, and for evaluating defects of B cell function.

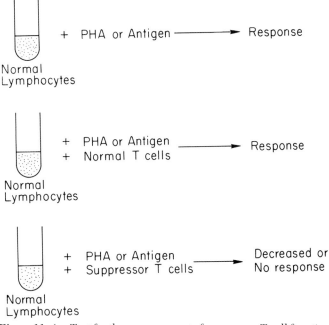

Figure 11–4. Test for the measurement of suppressor T cell function.

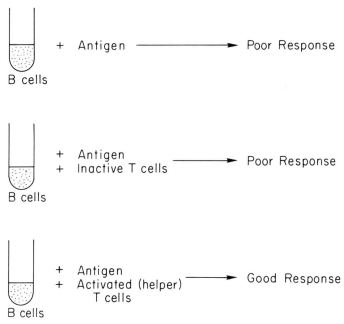

Figure 11–5. Tests for helper T cell function.

Assays for the Presence of Antibody-Producing Cells. The most widely used technique for detection of antibody-producing cells is localized hemolysis in gel, originally described by Jerne. Basic details of the test are shown in Figure 11–6. As originally described, the test detected only those cells capable of producing antibody (largely IgM), which would directly fix complement and lyse the red cells. However, by the use of appropriately absorbed antiglobulins to other immunoglobulin classes or substructures (e.g., anti-IgG, IgA, κ chain, or λ chain), it is possible to detect secretion of most types of antibody. Sheep cells and other erythrocytes have been used not only for direct assays, but also as carriers for numerous antigens, which can be chemically bound to their surface. The Jerne plaque technique has been particularly popular for measuring the development of antibody-producing cells in the spleens of mice during the induction of an immune response. However, cells from blood or any lymphoid organ may be used. The technique has the advantage of detecting small numbers of antibody-producing cells among large populations. Mishell and Dutton have applied a technique using peripheral blood lymphocytes to measure in vitro production of antibodies to sheep erythrocytes.

Measurement of Lymphokines. Using appropriate conditions for culture, lymphocytes will produce lymphokines that can be extracted from the culture filtrate. Appropriate test systems have been designed to detect which cells produce lymphokines under varying conditions, and to measure mitogenic properties, effects upon the vascular system, cytotoxicity, macrophage-activating activity, interferon activity, chemotactic activity, and other activities.

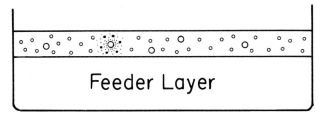

Figure 11–6. Detection of antibody-producing cells by the classical Jerne plaque technique. Lymphoid cells (large circles) are mixed in agar with sheep erythrocytes (small circles). Antibody (small dots) elaborated into the medium by antibody-producing cells sensitizes nearby erythrocytes (large black dots). After a period of incubation, the agar is overlaid with a solution containing lytic complement, which produces visible hemolysis of the sensitized cells.

The most widely used test is probably the migration inhibition test (Fig. 11–7). In this test, a mixture of lymphocytes and macrophages (most often obtained from blood or peritoneal exudate) is placed in the end of a capillary tube. The tip of the tube is then placed on a glass surface in a chamber and incubated. Normally, the macrophages will migrate from the end of the capillary tube and spread over the glass surface. However, in the presence of an antigen of the type that will induce delayed hypersensitivity, previously sensitized (immune) T lymphocytes will elaborate a substance that will inhibit macrophage migration (MIF — migration inhibition factor). This test seems to be a rather specific indicator of delayed hypersensitivity, and immune B cells in the presence of the appropriate antigen will not cause inhibition of migration. The LMIF (leukocyte migration inhibition factor) test is similar to the MIF test except that a purified population of neutrophils is employed as the indicator system.

TESTS OF MACROPHAGE FUNCTION

Macrophages can be obtained from a variety of sources, and they have well established differences in their functional properties, depending upon the source. Most of the studies on abnormalities of macrophage function have been performed in laboratory animals, since in man no convenient

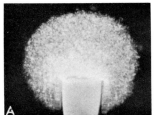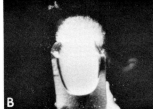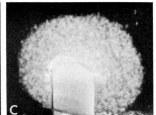

Figure 11–7. Inhibition of macrophage migration. *A* and *B*, a capillary tube containing cells from a peritoneal exudate of an animal with a delayed type of allergy to tuberculin. Tuberculin was added to the culture medium of tests *B* and *C*. *C* is a control with peritoneal cells from a nonsensitized animal.

source of cells is readily available that can be tested repeatedly. In laboratory animals, large numbers of peritoneal macrophages can be harvested from the peritoneal cavity several days after the injection of inducing agents such as glycogen, mineral oil, casein, thioglycolate broth, and so on. They can also be harvested from lungs (by lavage or after mincing) or from liver, spleen, or lymph nodes (after mincing).

Numerous biochemical and functional tests may be performed. Those which may be of value in clinical medicine are the response to chemotaxins and lymphokines, the ability to ingest and kill microorganisms, and the ability to kill target cells. The first two types of tests will be described for neutrophils and they are quite similar for macrophages. The population to be tested in man is generally isolated from the peripheral blood (monocytes). The cytotoxic tests are similar to those shown in Figure 11–3.

TESTS OF NEUTROPHIL FUNCTION

Neutrophils are relatively easy to harvest from peripheral blood, with 10 ml providing about 10^7 cells for study.

Tests of Phagocytosis and Intracellular Killing. Heparinized blood is mixed with dextran to promote sedimentation of erythrocytes. After sedimentation, the leukocyte-rich plasma is removed and centrifuged, and the white cell pellet is washed, counted, and resuspended to a concentration of about 10^7 cells per ml. A few contaminating erythrocytes and mononuclear cells will not interfere with accurate results. Bacteria (usually staphylococcus) are added to the cell suspension and incubated in the presence of normal pooled serum to provide an optimal amount of opsonins. Numbers of cells and bacteria must be carefully controlled, usually in a 1:1 ratio. After varying periods of incubation at 37°C by a technique to promote bacteria-neutrophil contact, samples are removed for quantitation of bacteria. Defects in phagocytosis can be distinguished from intracellular killing by adding antibiotics to the medium to kill extracellular bacteria after a short initial period of incubation. If staphylococci are used as the test organism, lysostaphin kills extracellular organisms and gives excellent and reproducible results. This basic test and its modifications have been used extensively to evaluate neutrophil function in a variety of diseases, and there has been a good correlation between poor neutrophil function and susceptibility to infection.

The NBT Test. When neutrophils phagocytize latex particles in the presence of a nitroblue tetrazolium, the formazan dye is reduced, forming dark granules within the neutrophils (NBT positive cells). This may be read directly or optically after extraction. Bacterial infection is usually associated with a spontaneous increase in the number of NBT positive cells. Stimulation of neutrophils with endotoxin causes a marked increase in NBT positive cells, and lack of a significant increase after endotoxin stimulation signifies cells that are unable to respond and have poor antibacterial function.

Chemotaxis. Directed migration of neutrophils by chemotactic substances can be measured in several ways. The most popular is with a Boyden chamber (Fig. 11–8). A cell suspension is placed in the upper chamber, which is separated from the lower chamber by a porous membrane (such as a

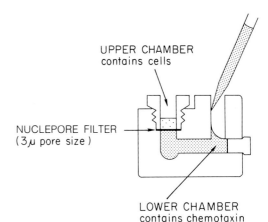

UPPER CHAMBER
contains cells

Figure 11–8. Diagram of a chemotaxis chamber.

NUCLEPORE FILTER
(3μ pore size)

LOWER CHAMBER
contains chemotaxin

Nuclepore membrane with 3-μ holes). In the lower chamber is placed a chemotactic stimulus. After incubation, the membrane is removed, and the numbers of cells migrating through the membrane and the numbers on the starting side are enumerated to provide a chemotactic index. A functional chemotactic index may be calculated by comparing the results of tests with patients to those from normals. Abnormal chemotaxis has been formed in a number of disease states, but its relevance to the etiology and pathogenesis of these conditions remains obscure.

12

Detection and Measurement of Antigen – Antibody Reactions

The methods for detection and quantitation of antigens by their reactions with antibody or the converse provide important tools for both the investigator and the clinican. Many types of reactions and tests have been described, but each depends upon the specific binding of antigen to antibody. These tests usually provide only semiquantitative answers since the affinity of this union may be variable, the antibody may be heterogeneous, and numerous cross-reactions may occur between antibody and antigens from unrelated sources. Table 12–1 shows the limits of sensitivities of many of these tests.

IN VIVO TESTS

REAGIN DEPENDENT ACUTE ALLERGIC REACTIONS

Allergens in dilute solution may be injected intradermally, or introduced into small epidermal lesions (prick test), into the conjunctival sac, intranasally, or even intrabronchially. Within a few minutes, individuals allergic to a specific allergen develop characteristic erythema and wheal lesions of the skin, acute conjunctivitis, rhinitis, or asthma, depending on the route of administration. Conjunctival and intranasal tests are rarely used at the present time. Prick tests seem to have replaced scratch tests as a screening procedure, and intradermal challenges are then used for more definitive diagnosis. Intrabronchial challenge may be helpful both in identifying specific allergens and in distinguishing allergic from nonallergic asthma in some patients, but must be used with caution.

150

TABLE 12-1. RELATIVE SENSITIVITY OF QUANTITATIVE TESTS MEASURING ANTIBODY NITROGEN OF HIGH AVIDITY ANTIBODY

	MG AB N/Ml OR TEST
Precipitin reactions	3–20
Immunoelectrophoresis	3–20
Double diffusion in agar gel	0.2–1.0
Complement fixation	0.01–0.1
Radial immunodiffusion	0.008–0.025
Bacterial agglutination	0.01
Hemolysis	0.001–0.03
Passive hemagglutination	0.005
Passive cutaneous anaphylaxis	0.003
Antitoxin neutralization	0.003
Antigen-combining globulin technique (Farr)	0.0001–0.001
Radioimmunoassay	0.0001–0.001
Bactericidal test	0.0001–0.001
Virus neutralization	0.00001–0.0001

ARTHUS REACTIONS

Skin reactions developing several hours after intradermal injection of an antigen, which reach a maximum in 7 to 8 hours and resolve in 24 to 36 hours, are the result of immune complex–complement dependent reactions. The lesions are usually soft, edematous, and pruritic. The test has some clinical value in determining previous sensitization to an antigen, but many more sophisticated tests for in vitro measurement are now available.

PASSIVE CUTANEOUS ANAPHYLAXIS (PCA)

Certain types of antibody (cytotropic) readily become fixed to cells of the skin after intradermal injection. IgE is the most avid of the cytotropic antibodies, but certain types of IgG also bind well enough to the surface of cells, especially mast cells, to cause the cells to respond to the union of antigen with the bound antibody. Antibody that binds only to skin of the same or closely related species is termed homocytotropic and antibody that binds to the skin of more distantly related species is termed heterocytotropic.

Prausnitz and Küstner first discovered that serum from an allergic individual could be tested for the presence of skin-fixing antibodies by passive transfer to another person (the PK test). After 24 hours to allow displacement of all but IgE antibody, a small amount of the antigen in question is injected adjacent to the initial site at which the serum or plasma was injected. A positive reaction is indicated by development of a typical wheal and flare response. This test is rarely used today because of the possible transfer of hepatitis. However, it launched investigations into other forms of PCA.

The most common clinical application involving PCA employs injection of a small amount of gamma globulin or serum intradermally into a guinea pig. Several hours later, the antigen is given intravenously, along with a dye such as Evans blue. Vascular damage caused by antigen reacting with skin-fixed antibody is indicated by leakage of the dye into the interstitial tissues at the injection site. This test, employing human serum, measures the presence of antibody in three of the four subclasses of IgG rather than IgE, since the latter does not fix to guinea pig skin.

IN VITRO TESTS

Extensive testing of antigen-antibody reactions can be done by in vitro methods, and literally thousands of assays have been described. These will be grouped for convenience of presentation. Although not specified in each case, each test or group of tests must be closely controlled with appropriate negative and positive samples to insure accuracy.

PRECIPITIN REACTIONS

The divalent structure of the antibody molecule permits the development of cross-linkages with soluble antigen and precipitation from solution as a macromolecular lattice complex when mixed in equivalent proportions (Fig. 12–1a). When there is an excess of antibody, all of the combining sites on the antigen molecule may be preempted to prevent lattice formation (Fig. 12–1b). When there is an excess of antigen, small complexes form, which become larger only with the addition of more antibody (Fig. 12–1c). These

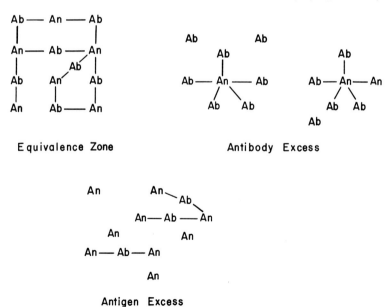

Figure 12–1. Diagrammatic representation of the reaction between divalent antibody and multivalent antigen.

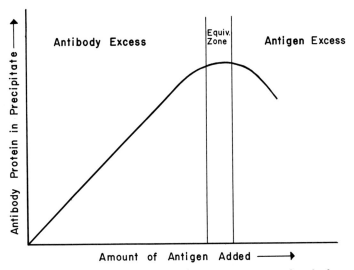

Figure 12–2.   Precipitin curve with a constant amount of antibody.

variable ratios account for the rapidity and completeness of the precipitation. A fairly good quantitative estimate of the amount of antigen or antibody in an unknown can therefore be made by determining the zone of equivalence (maximum amount of precipitation in the reaction mixture at or near antigen excess) for an unknown, and comparing it with that of a standard (Fig. 12–2). Although this basic reaction is the grandfather from which subsequent generations of tests have emerged, it is rarely used now.

Other types of precipitin reactions, however, have great value. The detection of the precipitation of antigen-antibody complexes at the fluid inter-

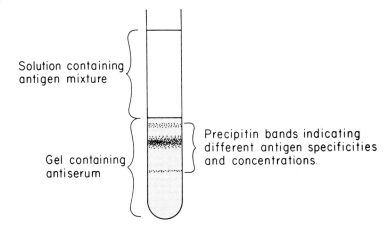

Figure 12–3.   Single diffusion reaction in agar gel. Antiserum is incorporated into the gel which is placed in the bottom of a capillary tube or test tube. The antigen containing solution is layered on top and diffusion is allowed to occur. After several hours, precipitin bands form in the gel which correspond to different antigen-antibody specificities.

face between a solution of antibody and a solution of antigen in capillary tubes has been used with great success in forensic medicine for rapid identification of small quantities of biological materials; for example, small stains on clothing can be identified as human semen or blood.

The precipitin reaction has been refined by allowing it to take place in agar gel or other semisolid media through which soluble molecules will diffuse. Differences in the concentration and rates of diffusion of different molecules within the gel determine the location and density of precipitin bands, allowing greater precision in the identification of multiple components in mixtures of antigens and antibodies (Fig. 12–3). In single diffusion tests in agar, the concentration of the antigen in solution can be estimated by the distance the precipitin band travels into the agar gel when the concentration of antibody in the gel is constant. A modification of this original test (Mancini quantitative radial immunodiffusion) is done by incorporating the antibody in a gel which is poured to form a thin uniform layer in a plate. Numerous uniform holes are cut into the agar, and the solution to be tested (which contains the antigen) is placed in the wells to fill them completely. By comparing the size of the rings (zones of precipitation) that form about the wells in these tests with appropriate standards, accurate measurements can be made of the concentration of antigens in unknown samples (Fig. 12–4). Radial immunodiffusion is routinely used for measurement of specific serum proteins such as IgG, IgM, C3, and so on, as well as many other biological antigens that occur in moderate concentrations in body fluids. Double dif-

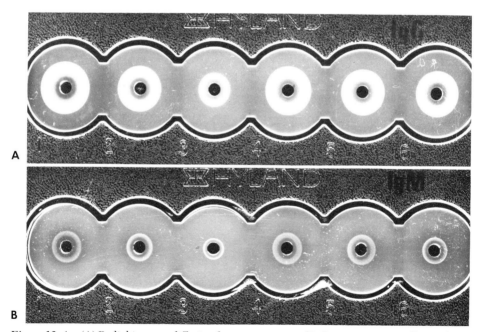

Figure 12–4. (A) Radial immunodiffusion for measurement of IgG using commercially available plates. Zone sizes are clearly demarcated.

(B) Radial immunodiffusion for measurement of IgM concentrations in serum. Note that considerable differences exist among the individuals tested.

Figure 12–5. Sketch of double diffusion reactions in agar gel. Antigens from three different sources are in wells Nos. 1, 2, and 3. Two antigens in well No. 1 are identified by the antiserum. One antigen in well No. 2 has reaction with the antiserum which is identical to one of the antigens in well No. 1. Another antigen shows no identity with the second antigen in well No. 1 (crossed lines). Well No. 3 has a single antigen which shows partial identity with the antigen from well No. 2, as evidenced by the spur.

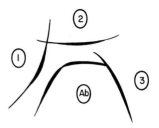

fusion tests in gels are used largely for qualitative analysis, but can be quantitative and can be done with minute amounts of reactants, using microscope slides with a layer of agar between the slide and a template. Use of these tests has led to the easy identification of identical and dissimilar antigens (Fig. 12–5). An increased sensitivity of the gel diffusion technique can be obtained by using antibody labeled with radioisotopes, such as ^{125}I or ^{131}I, and detecting precipitin bands with radiosensitive emulsions.

Immunoelectrophoresis is an even more powerful tool for the separation and identification of antigens within a mixture, although this method is not very sensitive for low concentrations of reactants (Fig. 12–6). This test, which combines the principles of gel diffusion and electrophoresis, is especially useful for the study of proteins. A method of immunoelectrophoresis has also been devised for semiquantitative measurement of antigen concentration. The antigens are placed in wells on one side of a layer of agar in which antibody has been incorporated. Application of an electrical field will cause unidirectional movement of the antigen into the agar proportional to its concentration, the extent of which can be measured by the leading edge of a precipitin band.

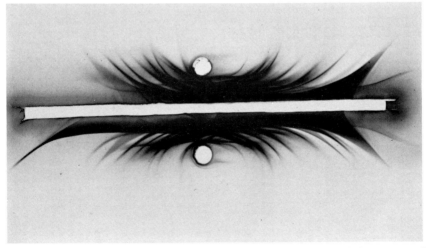

Figure 12–6. An immunoelectrophoresis of the serum from a patient with hypogammaglobulinemia (upper well) and from a normal patient (bottom well). The center trough contained rabbit antiserum against normal human serum proteins. (Courtesy of Dr. R. Hong.)

ANTIGEN-BINDING CAPACITY

Since not all antibody binding with antigen results in precipitation, complement fixation, or other readily detectable reaction, a method was devised by Farr that allows detection of all antibody which binds with soluble antigen. In this test, the antigen is labeled with a radioisotope and mixed with an unknown sample containing antibody. After a period of reaction, an equal volume of saturated ammonium sulfate is added to precipitate all of the immunoglobulin, including antigen-antibody complexes. The precipitated radioactivity therefore reflects the antigen-binding capacity. Of course, the antigen must be one which can be radiolabeled without interfering with antigenic binding sites and which does not precipitate with ammonium sulfate, thereby somewhat limiting the usefulness of this type of test. Within these limitations, the test is highly accurate and reproducible.

USE OF IMMUNOABSORBENTS

The principle of the above test has been applied to an even better advantage by linking the antigen to an insoluble support. The serum sample to be tested is then added and incubated. The amount of bound antibody can be measured in several ways, including the use of labeled antigen-specific antibody to saturate unbound sites (decreased uptake proportional to amount of antibody in original sample) and interaction with labeled antiimmunoglo-

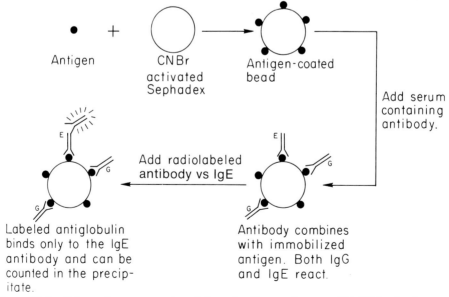

Figure 12–7.   Schematic representation of the radioallergosorbent test (RAST) for the detection of IgE antibody. Modifications of this test can be used for the detection of any antibody.

bulin antibody (amount of uptake directly proportional to amount of specific antibody in the original sample). The radioallergosorbent test (RAST) for the detection of IgE antibodies utilizes this principle (Fig. 12–7).

RADIOIMMUNOASSAYS

The technique of radioimmunoassay has literally revolutionized the field of endocrinology by making assays of hormones readily available. The test can also be used for many other substances, such as specific drugs (digoxin is an example) and small molecular weight compounds (such as vasoactive mediators). Its principal value is that material can be measured accurately in nanogram and picogram concentrations. Table 12–2 lists compounds for which radioimmunoassay has been developed for routine clinical analysis. This method, employing solid phase iron containing beads on which antigen or antibody can be coated, lends itself to complete automation, and this is revolutionizing much of clinical chemistry.

The test requires availability of a radiolabeled compound that will react specifically with a high dilution of an appropriate antiserum, usually raised in animals in response to the compound injected as a hapten-conjugate. In performance of the test, the material to be assayed is mixed with the diluted antiserum in the presence of a specific amount of radiolabeled compound. In certain instances, the sample and antiserum are mixed and incubated before addition of labeled antigen. After equilibrium between bound and unbound antigen is achieved, the bound radio-labeled compound is quickly separated from the unbound by a physical method or by precipitating the immunoglobulin with specific antisera (to the immunoglobulin) or by salts. The precipitated and/or nonprecipitated radioactivity can then be measured and compared to controls. The concentration of compound in the original sample will be inversely related to the amount of radiolabeled compound bound to the specific antibody. In some instances, the antibody is coated onto tubes or other solid supports. The degree of accuracy, of course, depends entirely upon the specificity of the antiserum used and adequate separation of bound and free antigen. Figure 12–8 illustrates the radioimmunoassay technique.

TABLE 12–2. PARTIAL LISTING OF SUBSTANCES FOR WHICH RADIOIMMUNOASSAY HAS BEEN DEVELOPED FOR ROUTINE CLINICAL ANALYSIS

Insulin	Chorionic gonadotropin
Gastrin	Thyroxin
Angiotensin I	Triiodothyronine
Angiotensin II	Thyrotropin
Growth hormone	Cortisol
Parathormone	Estradiol
Luteinizing hormone	Progesterone
Follicle-stimulating hormone	Testosterone
	Digoxin

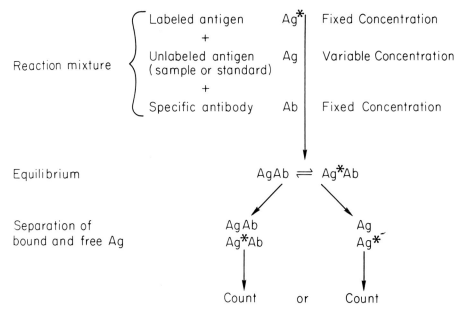

Figure 12–8. Principle of radioimmunoassay test.

AGGLUTINATION REACTIONS

Agglutination reactions are in every way similar to precipitin reactions except that the union of antibody occurs with antigens on suspended particles rather than on soluble molecules. These reactions are particularly useful for the detection of antibodies against microbial organisms, erythrocytes, and other suspended cells. The end points of these tests can be determined in several ways, but are usually reported as a titer, which represents the reciprocal of the last dilution of antiserum that gave a distinctly positive reaction. Either gross or microscopic examination of the particles can be made, and positive tests can be determined by the pattern obtained by settling or after light centrifugation, which increases the opportunity for particle contact. The length of incubation and the temperature at which the test is done will influence the observed titer, and considerably different results can be obtained by using different criteria for determining the end point. This should be kept in mind when comparisons are made of reported results from different laboratories or different personnel within the same laboratory. Even within a single series of tests done with the utmost of care by the same person, the accuracy of these tests is often no better than $\pm \log_2$. Nevertheless, agglutination reactions form a backbone of laboratory methods for blood banking and many diagnostic and investigative procedures.

The sensitivity of many antigen-antibody reactions can be increased considerably by coupling soluble antigens to suitable particulate carriers (passive agglutination tests). Several types of particles such as polystyrene can be used for this purpose, but tanned or formalin-treated erythrocytes are the most common carriers (Fig. 12–9). As with any sensitive test, adequate

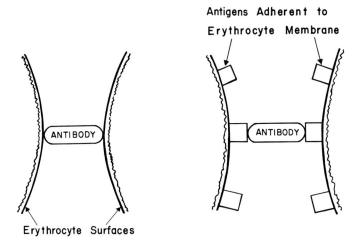

Figure 12-9.   Schematic diagram of simple hemagglutination and passive hemagglutination reactions.

controls must be run to demonstrate specificity and rule out false negative reactions. Microtechniques have been developed for these tests, and analysis may be performed on minute quantities of serum. Passive hemagglutination tests are used in the quantitation of antibody to a wide variety of protein and polysaccharide antigens. Mixed agglutination tests are used to detect similar antigenic determinants on two different types of cells.

Antibodies to certain erythrocyte antigens will not cause agglutination. These have sometimes been called incomplete antibodies, although they have the normal divalent structure of all immunoglobulins. Their presence on the erythrocyte membrane may be detected by the use of antisera against IgG, which will then cause agglutination (the antiglobulin test of Coombs, see Chapter 17). As presently practiced, Coombs' reagent also contains antibody against C3 and sometimes C4. The indirect Coombs' test checks for the presence of nonagglutinating antibodies in serum.

NEUTRALIZATION TESTS

Many viruses are neutralized by antibody, and the presence of antibody can be detected by the prevention of virus plaque formation in tissue cultures. Under favorable conditions, only a few antibody molecules are required for the effect. Specific antibody provides major protection in several infections caused by bacteria that elaborate exotoxins. The toxin-inactivating ability of antiserum can be assayed by observing the in vivo neutralization of the toxin in laboratory animals. The Shick test in man measures for the presence of antibody to neutralize diphtheria toxin injected subcutaneously in small amounts.

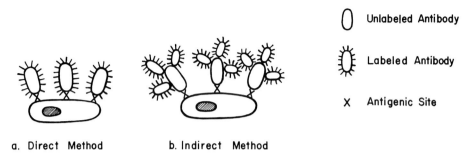

a. Direct Method   b. Indirect Method

Figure 12–10. Technique of fluorescent microscopy. In the indirect method, the labeled antibody is specific for the species of gamma globulin used to react with the antigen, X, and does not itself react with X.

FLUORESCENT AND ELECTRON MICROSCOPY

The localization of cellular antigens and antibodies within tissue sections by immunologic reactions was a difficult task before the application of fluorescent microscopic techniques for this purpose. Antibodies can be conjugated to dyes that fluoresce in ultraviolet light without appreciably altering their properties as a specific antibody. When applied to tissue sections, fluorescinated antibody is bound to specific antigenic sites, which can be visualized when viewed under ultraviolet light. The test is sensitive and must have proper controls to differentiate specific from nonspecific fluorescence. However, immunofluorescence is a powerful tool with many modern applications. Indirect methods for labeling may increase the sensitivity of the test (Fig. 12–10). Ferritin-tagged or peroxidase-tagged antibody has been used to detect localization of tissue antigens by electron microscopy.

COMPLEMENT REACTIONS

Several types of complement reactions can be used to detect antigen-antibody reactions indirectly, but since there are several classes and subclasses of antibody that do not activate the complement systems, these techniques are not always applicable. Since all of the complement components have been purified and antibody prepared against them, it is possible to quantitate the individual complement components both by radial immunodiffusion and by functional assays using hemolytic analysis.

Complement fixation tests, such as the Wassermann test, have been used for many years, but are seldom employed now. The technique depends upon detection or measurement of the removal of hemolytic complement activity by antigen-antibody interaction, using an indicator system of erythrocytes and specific antierythrocyte antibody, which fail to produce lysis in the absence of complement. In measuring hemolytic complement reactions, the point at which 50 per cent of the target red cells are lysed gives the most reproducible end point (CH_{50}).

Cytolytic or cytotoxic reactions are often convenient methods for detecting antibody interaction with susceptible cell membranes. These techniques have been particularly useful in tissue typing for transplantation procedures. In the microcytotoxicity test of Terasaki, antibody fixation to susceptible lymphoid cells is detected by adding rabbit complement and observing cell damage, which is detected by the addition of a vital dye (eosin). Very small quantities (microliters) of reactants are required.

The generation of biologically active fragments of complement such as C5a and C3a during complement activation can be measured by chemotactic assays or the effect on indicator cells (e.g., release of histamine from mast cells).

Opsonic tests have become increasingly useful in the analysis of mechanisms of resistance to infection. The alternative pathway of complement is primarily involved, and sera devoid of C2 or C6 and distal components may function normally in these assays. The serum is usually diluted, and concentrations of 1 to 5 per cent are customarily used. Killing of bacteria by normal neutrophils (or macrophages) is used as the indicator. Since certain substances, such as inulin, may directly activate the alternative pathway, they may be used to assess functional activity by activating the pathway and measuring the disappearance of the B antigen of C3 during incubation. The B antigen (C3B) disappears upon activation of C3 to C3a and C3b.

SECTION III
CLINICAL APPLICATIONS

The application of immunologic principles affects most, if not all, areas of clinical practice. In this section we provide perspectives for the daily use of these principles in patient management. Clinicians not familiar with immunologic terminology, or who do not have a working knowledge of the current fundamentals of immunology, are advised to review Section I before proceeding to the following chapters.

13

Infections

The impact of the partial control of infectious disease cannot readily be appreciated by clinicians now in practice. Before the time of Pasteur and Lister, little more than a century ago, infections stood prominently in the destiny of mankind. Because of infectious diseases, wars were won or lost, kingdoms rose and fell, and cities perished. It is a wonder that the American Revolution was won by the colonial forces since ten times more deaths occurred from contagious diseases than from British guns. Smallpox, typhus, and a malignant form of dysentery were the most important among the many diseases that took the lives of one of every five soldiers each year. By the time of the Civil War, almost a century later, conditions had improved somewhat, yet there were twice as many deaths from infectious diseases as from battle injuries (62 per 1000 per year) and virtually all wounds became infected. This deplorable condition resulted in a 59 per cent death rate for patients with amputations at the knee joint and an 83 per cent mortality for those with amputations at the hip. Data from the Crimean war in the mid-nineteenth century also serve to illustrate the significance of infection before the time of Lister's application of antiseptic principles; one fourth of the fighting forces died as a result of various types of infections, and the mortality from amputation for fracture of the femur was 92 per cent. The advances of medicine during this century have made remarkable differences in the control of infection. During World War I the ratio of "other deaths," including those from infection, to "battle deaths" fell to 1.08; during World War II, it was 0.35; and during the Viet Nam War, it was 0.22.

No one would question that modern medicine faces far fewer problems with infection at the present time. Nevertheless, we continue to pay a significant toll. Approximately 1 of every 20 patients admitted to acute care hospitals develops a nosocomial infection, accounting for approximately 2,000,000 hospital-acquired infections in the United States of America each year. About one half of these are infections in surgical wounds, which alone have been estimated to result in an economic loss to the nation of almost $10,000,000,000. Gram-negative septicemias account for between 50,000 and 80,000 deaths per year in the U.S.A., considerably greater than the number of patients dying from cancer of the colon and rectum or from automobile accidents. While of the viral diseases only hepatitis, influenza, and childhood viral pneumonia cause more than 1000 deaths per year in the United States,

165

morbidity and economic loss from viral infections are also impressive. Current data indicate that the common cold causes about 35 acute illnesses per 100 persons annually and that acute respiratory infections account for approximately one third of all visits to physicians. Data from the National Center for Health Statistics indicate that in 1973, influenza, colds, and upper respiratory infections accounted for 403 days of restricted activity per 100 persons in the nation, almost twice as much as for injuries. Thus, at any given time, an average of more than 1 per cent of the population is restricted by a viral infection of the respiratory tract.

Despite these persistent problems, progress has been made through immunization, the appropriate use of antibiotics, and better standards of hygiene, nutrition, and environmental control. Some of these advances come as mixed blessings, perhaps best illustrated by the changing pattern of important pathogens causing infection following serious thermal injury, which has occurred largely because of the pressure of antibiotic therapy (Fig. 13–1). We have now reached the realization that antibiotics have limited usefulness because of the emergence of the antibiotic-resistant microbial pathogens and the development of complications consequent to their administration. We must continuously examine methods to increase host resistance to infection by detecting abnormalities of immune resistance and correcting these abnormalities by appropriate therapy. This problem has recently been placed in dramatic focus by the gonococcus, so long held in check by the efficacy of penicillin. This organism now threatens to cause a worldwide epidemic since an antibiotic strain, apparently first appearing in the Philippine Islands, has spread rapidly to North America. It seems certain that this problem, like that with so many organisms, will have to be addressed in immunologic perspective.

The deposition and proliferation of microorganisms within tissues are obvious prerequisites for the development of any infection. Epithelial sur-

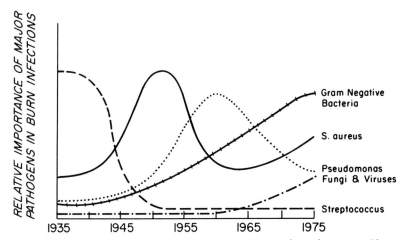

Figure 13–1. Changing patterns of infection in burns. (From Alexander, J. W., Chapter 6, *in* Artz, C. P., Moncrief, J. H., and Pruitt, B. A., Jr., (eds.), Burns: A Book for the Whole Team. Philadelphia, W. B. Saunders Company, in press.)

faces are continually bathed by a sea of both desirable and undesirable microorganisms, which can become pathogenic under the proper conditions. Although epithelial surfaces provide an amazingly effective barrier against the entrance of bacteria into the host, this barrier is by no means perfect, and viable microbes frequently reach the physiological interior, especially when the epithelial surfaces are damaged by injury or surgical intervention. Careful bacteriological studies have shown that the majority of clean surgical wounds and probably all traumatic wounds have one or more types of bacteria that can be detected by careful sampling at the time of closure. However, clinically apparent infections in normal persons develop infrequently, and only when the number of organisms within a given microenvironment exceeds the capabilities of the host to destroy them (Fig. 13–2). One of the most important lines of defense, in addition to the integrity of the external and internal surfaces of the body, is inhibition by organisms of very low pathogenicity, which compete with more pathogenic organisms for the ecological niche on the surface of the body or within the upper respiratory or gastrointestinal tracts.

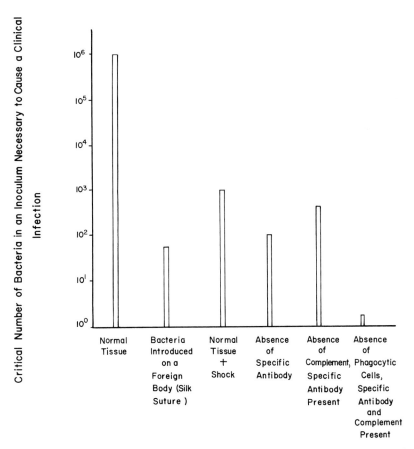

Figure 13–2. Chart of the relative importance of host defense mechanisms on the development of infections in selected conditions.

The range of pathogenicity among different species of microbes is vast. In some, such as *Yersinia pestis* (the plague bacillus), the introduction of a single organism in certain instances may result in a fulminant and fatal infection. On the other hand, there are many nonvirulent species that fail to cause clinical infection, even when large numbers (greater than 10^9) are injected. Despite the extreme range of variability in the characteristics of different strains and species of microbes, the majority that cause infection in man require an inoculum of considerable size to overcome the capabilities of normal host defense. In a healthy person, it has been shown that it is necessary to inject approximately 10^6 staphylococci intradermally, subcutaneously, or intramuscularly to produce a discernible infection. Only slight differences in the critical inoculum were found among the different species of staphylococci studied.

The variables which may influence the pathogenicity of an organism have not been documented completely, but many bacterial characteristics may be contributory. For example, the surfaces of certain bacteria such as *E. coli, Klebsiella,* or pneumococcus may inhibit phagocytosis in the absence of immune antibody, whereas other bacteria may be readily opsonized in sera containing no immunoglobulin at all. In one recent report, resistance to opsonization was found to be the most important determinant in the development of gram-negative bacteremia in nonleukopenic patients. The ability of an organism to produce a chronic infection depends primarily upon its ability to resist destruction within the digestive vacuoles of phagocytes.

GENERAL MECHANISMS OF RESISTANCE TO INFECTIONS

Entrance of bacteria and other microorganisms into healthy tissues incites a series of physiologic events similar but not identical for all species studied (Fig. 13–3). In fact, the initial events in the microcirculation are similar whether inflammation has resulted from bacterial invasion, traumatic injury, or the introduction of noxious materials. Attendant to injury with or without microbial colonization, there is an immediate vascular response which reaches its peak in five to ten minutes and which is accompanied by an increase in endothelial permeability. The chemical mediators of early inflammation produce constriction of the venular sphincters at the junction of venules with the veins (Fig. 13–4A). This produces increased venular and capillary pressures and increased permeability of the endothelium to plasma proteins, exudation of fluids into the tissues, and decreased rates of blood flow leading to stasis, hypoxia, and acidosis (Fig. 13–4B). As a result of the exudation of plasma proteins and fluids from the intravascular to the extravascular compartments, an increase in lymphatic flow occurs. The arterioles may be variably affected, and small arteriolar-venular shunts may become functional. In the established inflammatory lesion, total blood flow is usually significantly increased. Following the brief initial phase of increased permeability, or concurrent with it, is a more sustained phase characterized by ad-

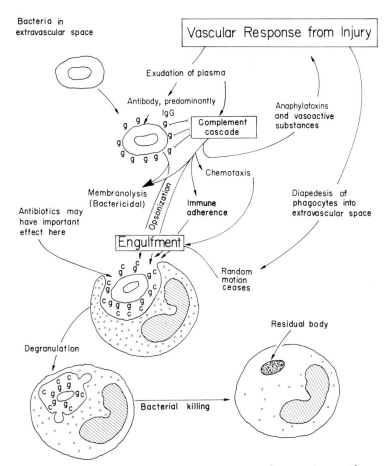

Figure 13–3. Diagram on inflammatory response at sites of injury. (From Altemeier, W. A., and Alexander, J. W., Chapter 17, *in* Sabiston, D. C., Jr., (ed.), Davis-Christopher Textbook of Surgery. 11th ed. Philadelphia, W. B. Saunders Company, 1977.)

herence of blood phagocytes to the endothelium of the venules and capillaries. These leukocytes marginate because of the decreased rate of flow and become "sticky" upon contact with the activated endothelium. They exit from the blood vessels by emigrating through the spaces at intercellular junctions (Fig. 13–4C).

Many investigators have studied the phenomenon of sticking and emigration of leukocytes since it was described in 1824, but numerous questions remain unanswered. The exact mechanism by which leukocytes adhere to the endothelial surface is unknown, although it apparently involves an enzymatic reaction. After their exit, phagocytic cells wander about randomly in the inflammatory lesion until chemotaxins affect their movement. For the most part, these chemotaxins are generated by activation of complement (C3a and C5a). When a leukocyte is positively attracted, its random motion ceases, and it progresses in a relatively straight line toward the attracting particle. The importance of chemotaxins has been disputed in the past, but it

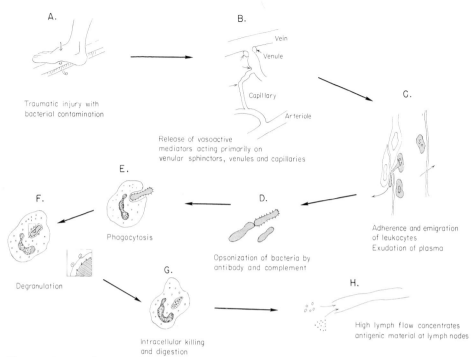

A.

Traumatic injury with
bacterial contamination

B.

Vein

Venule

Capillary

Arteriole

Release of vasoactive
mediators acting primarily on
venular sphinctors, venules and capillaries

C.

Adherence and emigration
of leukocytes
Exudation of plasma

D.

Opsonization of bacteria by
antibody and complement

E.

Phagocytosis

F.

Degranulation

G.

Intracellular killing
and digestion

H.

High lymph flow concentrates
antigenic material at lymph nodes

Figure 13–4. Schematic development of an inflammatory lesion following traumatic injury with bacterial contamination.

is now apparent that chemotaxis may play a major role in the removal of certain bacteria and foreign substances from an inflammatory site. The distance involved in the chemotactic influence is relatively short, usually less than 0.1 mm. The exact mechanism of chemotaxis is poorly understood from a biochemical standpoint, but the phenomenon is related to a chemical concentration gradient which affects the gel-sol state of the membrane.

A variety of both endogenous and exogenous chemical mediators of the vascular response has been described, which might play an important initial role in the development of an inflammatory lesion. Some of these serve only to release other more specific vasoactive substances. Different mediators may produce different manifestations, particularly concerning reactivity of the arterioles, but the venules seem to be affected by all. The exogenous mediators may act directly, but in most cases they seem to function primarily to release or activate endogenous mediators. The anaphylatoxins, C5a and C3a, also cause release of endogenous mediators.

Histamine is the most extensively studied of the endogenous chemical mediators. It is widely distributed throughout the body, being particularly located within the mast cells, which undergo degranulation in response to tissue injury. Histamine causes constriction of the venular sphincters with consequent dilatation and increased permeability of the venules and capillaries. The increased vascular permeability causes exudation of plasma proteins into the area, which may in turn play an important role in the delayed vascular response. Bradykinin, whose pharmacologic action is similiar to that of histamine, is probably the most important mediator of the early vascular response. Serotonin plays little if any role in the development of most inflammatory lesions, but prostaglandins may be important mediators of some types of inflammation.

Vascular permeability and adhesiveness are also closely related to activation of the clotting mechanism. Hageman factor is a plasma protein, which can be activated by negatively charged particles and by contact with glass. Activated Hageman factor activates the antecedent of plasma thromboplastin and thus can initiate the series of biochemical reactions which lead to clotting of blood. Activated Hageman factor also has been shown to act on kallikreinogen to produce plasma kallikrein, and the kallikrein serves as a catalyst for the release of the octapeptide bradykinin from a kininogen, which is an alpha$_2$ globulin. Activated Hageman factor evidently has an additional effect: it contributes to production of permeability other than by the release of plasma kinins, since the effects of Hageman factor and bradykinin as observed in the rabbit ear chamber have been considerably different. Bradykinin produces an immediate and transitory response in which leukocyte emigration is not a prominent feature, whereas Hageman factor produces a prolonged and delayed response in which sticking and emigration of leukocytes are prominent.

A number of other endogenous mediators have been described that may be of importance. Among these are partially characterized substances derived from tissue extracts, and a globulin permeability factor that migrates as a beta globulin on electrophoresis and has trypsin-like activity. Hydrolytic enzymes released by injured leukocytes may also play an important role, as it has been shown that the inflammatory response of the Arthus reaction can be reduced markedly in animals by inducing neutropenia.

It is clear that there is no one mediator of the vascular response in an inflammatory lesion and that each type of injury may invoke the release or activation of mediators that are somewhat characteristic for that injury. Nevertheless, the final result is essentially the same, with the production of a biphasic vascular response or a modification of it. This biphasic response is usually characterized by an early, transient, vascular permeability, and a delayed phase in which leukocyte sticking to the vascular endothelium is a prominent feature. All of these responses have an alteration of vascular endothelium as an underlying characteristic.

The extracellular interstitial fluids already contain some immunoglobulin, predominantly IgG, and complement components. If injury is present or inflammation occurs, more of the blood proteins will escape from damaged vessels. Bacterial products also may have a direct effect on vascular tissues, resulting in exudation of plasma proteins. When antibodies are present that combine with antigenic sites on the surfaces of the bacteria (as is usually the case because of prior exposure, cross-reaction, or maternal transfer), complement may be activated, generating chemotaxins and vasoactive products that cause further recruitment of opsonic plasma proteins and phagocytic cells.

In the absence of phagocytes, antibody and complement do little to most microorganisms except to cause agglutination, but some highly susceptible species are killed outright by a process similar to hemolysis when complement is activated on their surfaces. Lysozyme may potentiate the reaction and is sometimes required. Such complement-mediated bactericidal reactions may kill *Vibrio cholera, T. pallidum,* leptospira, hemophilus, gonococcus, meningococcus, *Pseudomonas,* salmonella, mycoplasma, and a few viruses. Gram-positive bacteria and mycobacteria are resistant, and organisms grown in vivo are usually more resistant than those grown in vitro.

Microbicidal lytic reactions appear to play a minor role in resistance to the majority of infections. Much more important is ingestion and killing of opsonized particles by phagocytic cells. Opsonization is the result of a critical series of steps which varies from species to species and even among different strains of the same species of microbes. Unfortunately, data concerning the exact requirements for effecting opsonization of different species of bacteria are still incomplete. It is known, however, that some are opsonized effectively by IgG antibody (IgG1 and IgG3) whereas IgM and IgA antibodies are not usually effective opsonins by themselves. This is not surprising since phagocytic cells have receptors for IgG1 and IgG3, but not IgM or IgA. IgG in excess may block these receptors and actually decrease phagocytosis. Phagocytic cells also have receptors for C3b which primarily causes binding, according to some studies, whereas IgG causes ingestion. However, for at least some bacteria, such as *E. coli* 075, antibody is not necessary for effective ingestion whereas C3b is required.

C3b is probably the most important and potent of the opsonic proteins. It can be generated by activation of either the classical complement pathway or the alternative pathway, and it has been demonstrated that either or both pathways may be involved in opsonization of many bacteria and other microbes. From a practical standpoint, the alternative pathway appears to be the more important since patients with homozygous deficiencies of C2 do not usually have an increased susceptibility to infection, and their sera opsonizes most bacteria normally. Other proteins may be opsonic for bacteria, but as yet, there is no clear evidence for their role in vivo. Neither is it clear why C3b is necessary for opsonization of some bacteria but not for others.

Once opsonization has occurred by deposition of IgG or C3b or both on the bacterial surface, ingestion by phagocytic cells may take place. Neutrophils are the primary line of phagocytic defense against bacterial infections in man. Once the neutrophil comes in contact with an opsonized microbe, the process of ingestion begins, and intracellular destruction usually follows in short order. These events are described in detail in Chapter 5. When the ingested microbe is resistant to intracellular digestion, it may outlive the neutrophil—only to be ingested again by other phagocytic cells, usually a macrophage. T cell immune mechanisms play a major role in antimicrobial immunity when macrophages becomes significantly involved, since they may cause further recruitment and activation of these cells (Chapters 3 and 4). In addition, immune T lymphocytes may directly kill some microbial species (see Chapter 8).

Finally, an adaptive immune response occurs with most infections, which results in the synthesis and release of specific antibody and the formation of immune T lymphocytes, thereby potentiating the existing antimicrobial defense.

BACTERIAL INFECTIONS

Even among the bacteria, considerable differences exist in the mechanisms of host resistance to infection. For the purposes of discussion, the bacteria can best be classified as extracellular pathogens, intracellular pathogens, and variant forms.

EXTRACELLULAR PATHOGENS

Most of the serious bacterial infections in man are caused by extracellular pathogens. These organisms produce disease primarily by the elaboration of toxic products that have an adverse effect on the host. For some organisms, such as *Clostridium tetani,* exotoxins cause the entire clinical disease, and growth of the organisms in the host has little other apparent effect. For others, endotoxins intrinsic to the structure of the bacterial cell wall are the primary cause of clinical disease, and much of the damage is mediated through an immunologic response involving the endotoxin. For most bacteria, however, a number of toxic products, both endotoxins and exotoxins, contribute to the development of disease, and these often act synergistically, especially in mixed infections.

Abnormalities of Host Defense Which Increase Susceptibility to Extracellular Bacterial Infections. The vast majority of extracellular bacterial infections occur in association with an abnormality of host defense. Some of these are generalized abnormalities, whereas others are localized to the microenvironment of the area of contamination and generally affect the development of a normal inflammatory response. An important observation has been made during prospective longitudinal studies of immune function in susceptible burn and transplant patients, as patients who did not develop systemic immune abnormalities remained free from systemic infection.

Any condition that results in a relative impairment of the delivery of phagocytic cells or opsonic proteins to the microenvironment where bacterial contamination has occurred will encourage the development of infection. These conditions include inhibition of mediators of the inflammatory response, diminution in blood flow to the affected area (such as may be caused by the use of vasopressors, by hypovolemic shock, or by vascular occlusive disease), the presence of devitalized tissues or foreign bodies, and collections of blood or tissue fluids. Vascular reactivity may be inhibited by the presence of uremia or by the administration of high doses of corticosteroids or other antiinflammatory drugs. Decreased delivery of phagocytes to an area of inflammation may also accompany a decrease in the total circulating pool of these cells, thereby decreasing the number of available phagocytic cells which might be carried to a lesion. In each of these conditions, the opportunity for bacteria-phagocyte interaction is diminished because the condition leads to their physical separation. The bacteria, therefore, are not phagocytized, remaining free to multiply, and what would ordinarily be a subinfectious inoculum may grow to become many times the critical number necessary to cause an infection.

The observation that the presence of a silk suture may decrease the size of the inoculum necessary to cause an infection by a factor of 10,000-fold illustrates this point well. This potentiation of infection occurs perhaps in part because bacteria entering the interstices of the multifilament material are protected from phagocytic cells since monofilament sutures are generally more resistant to bacterial contamination than multifilament sutures. Similarly, all types of foreign bodies potentiate infection to a variable degree by preventing phagocytic cells from reaching the microenvironment of the contaminating bacteria. Not only is it necessary to consider exogenous causes of diminished phagocytic deposition in areas of bacterial contamination, but anatomical variations are important as well. Surgeons have known from antiquity that lacerations of highly vascular areas, such as the face, become infected much less frequently than lacerations in less vascular areas, such as the pretibial region or abdominal panniculus in obese individuals.

Deficiencies of opsonic proteins have become increasingly recognized as a major factor in the pathogenesis of infection. The first clear clinical demonstration of an antibody deficiency which predisposed to infection came with the description of agammaglobulinemia in 1952, only a quarter of a century ago. Since then, many conditions with associated hypogammaglobulinemia or dysgammaglobulinemia have been shown to have an increased susceptibility to infection, especially by organisms such as pneumococcus, hemophilus, meningococcus, streptococcus and *Pseudomonas*. Not surprisingly, the presence and concentration of specific antibody in these conditions is the crucial element for antibacterial defense. Patients with normal levels of immunoglobulin may not have antibody against a specific pathogen and are susceptible to infection by that organism if it requires Ig for opsonization, as most do. Furthermore, specific antibody may be consumed during acute infection, rendering the subject even more susceptible to the pathogen. Depletion of opsonins by consumption of specific antibody or complement components or both during infection is known as consumptive opsoninopathy. Fatal consumptive opsoninopathy has usually been associated with some degree of malnutrition where decreased synthesis and release of opsonins may contribute to low concentrations in the blood.

Opsonic proteins of the complement system are as important as specific antibody in resistance to most extracellular bacterial infections, and it could be anticipated from in vitro studies that complement abnormalities would predispose to infection. In fact, it has been the inherited abnormalities of complement components that have aided greatly in our understanding of their biological role in infection. Individuals with homozygous deficiency of C2, although showing some increased susceptibility to infection, usually do not show greatly diminished resistance. Similarly, individuals with absence of Clr, Cls, C4, C6, or C7 are often only moderately susceptible. Patients with C5 deficiencies or abnormalities exhibit diminished resistance (abnormal chemotaxis) to certain infections, such as *Candida*, but not to others. By contrast, patients with homozygous C3 deficiencies usually are markedly susceptible to infection, emphasizing the critical role of C3 and the less general role of C5 in complement-mediated resistance. Patients with absent properdin, Factor B, or Factor D have not yet been reported. It follows logically that anything that will deplete C3 or diminish its activity will increase susceptibility to infection, and this has been shown both clinically and experimentally. The administration of cobra venom factor to animals to reduce C3 and distal components by activating them will strikingly reduce the LD_{50} of a bacterial challenge. Likewise, liquoid, mucin, and hemoglobin are examples of substances that inhibit complement, and they will increase infection when injected with bacteria.

In prospective sequential studies of patients highly susceptible to infection, reduced levels of C3 and properdin have been shown to be associated with the development of infection. Other studies on patients with severe or fatal infections have shown that the level of C3 and properdin correlate both with the opsonic capacity of the patients' serum and the clinical outcome. In this regard, measurement of C3 using radial immunodiffusion with an antiserum against the B antigenic determinant is necessary, since it measures only functionally intact C3. The B determinant disappears upon cleavage. Antisera to βlc/β1a also measures nonfunctional C3 products and may provide misleading results. When bacteria are incubated with serum, C3(B) may fall to very low levels in a short period of time as the result of complement activation, while C3 measured using antisera to βlc/βla actually increases in concentration. An insufficient number of patients have been studied to determine whether low levels of properdin, Factor B, or Factor D without reduction in C3 occur significantly often and result in increased susceptibility to infection. Extreme malnutrition appears to exert a major influence in reducing blood levels of most complement components.

Abnormalities of phagocytic cells may also potentiate infection. Both neutrophils and mononuclear phagocytes ingest and kill bacteria at sites of inflammation, but neutrophils are the primary line of defense against bacterial infections, partly because they can be mobilized rapidly, and their numbers in the circulation can be rapidly expanded by the host. When there is a functional impairment of their ability to ingest and kill bacteria, the critical number of organisms required for the development of an infection becomes considerably less. Abnormalities of phagocytic ingestion in the presence of adequate quantities of opsonins have been demonstrated, but occur rarely, and the mechanism is not understood. In one study, virus infections caused a reduction in the ability of neutrophils to ingest pneumococci. On the other hand, the process of ingestion of bacteria is often normal or increased in a wide variety of conditions in which the phagocytic cell is unable to kill the phagocytized microbe. Abnormalities of intracellular killing may have a genetic basis, as in patients with chronic granulomatous disease of childhood, or they may be acquired, as in patients with severe thermal injury as severe malnutrition.

Many patients with severe infections have been demonstrated to have abnormalities of neutrophil function if they are studied soon after the development of the infection, and some investigators have felt that infection causes these defects. However, in burn patients and other patients who have been studied prospectively, the development of infection has regularly been preceded by appearance of an abnormality of neutrophil function (Fig. 13–

5). Also, in experimental animals, induction of severe infection does not influence neutrophil function adversely, a finding which suggests further that these abnormalities are etiologically related to the development of clinical sepsis rather than a consequence of it.

Significant dysfunction of neutrophils was more commonly demonstrated in patients studied five to ten years ago than in patients studied currently. While the reasons for this may be multifactorial, it seems certain that the *major* influence for this change has been more aggressive nutritional support of seriously ill patients using methods of oral and parenteral hyperalimentation. Nutritional defects can also result in other abnormalities of immune defense, affecting antibody synthesis, complement activity, and T cell function. Although hyperalimentation has usually been given without thought as to its influence on the immune system and its functions, improved nutritional support has probably been the most significant advance in the control of infection in the last 30 years. Using this method, acquired defects associated with infection can often be readily reversed. This important subject will be discussed in greater detail in Chapter 20, but mention here can hardly be avoided.

Recently, a cyclical variation in the ability of neutrophils to ingest and kill bacteria has been demonstrated in normal individuals, patients with a variety of diseases, and a variety of laboratory animals. In normal humans, the periodicity of the cycle averages about 17 to 21 days, but it may be shorter in stressed patients. There is reason to believe that unexpected occurrence of infection in many patients may be related in part to the relative abnormality of neutrophil function during this cyclical variation. Abnormalities of neutrophil chemotaxis have been demonstrated repeatedly in vitro and seem to have a relationship to infection. However, it has still not been determined whether chemotactic dysfunction predisposes to infection or occurs as a consequence of infection.

Finally, most seriously ill patients with infection can be shown to have abnormalities of T cell function. However, infections caused by extracellular bacterial pathogens do not seem to be much influenced by T cell abnormalities, and there has been no great predisposition to these types of infections

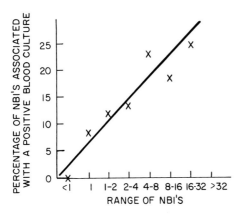

Figure 13–5. Relationships of poor neutrophil as evidenced by increased neutrophil bactericidal index (NBI), with recovery of positive blood cultures during the 48 hours following determination of the NBI. Note that the risk of having a positive blood culture was directly related to the value of the NBI. (From Alexander, J. W., and Meakins, J. L., Ann. Surg., *176*:273–287, 1972.)

in hereditary T cell disorders. However, recovery may be influenced when T cell helper function is necessary for synthesis of specific antibody by B cells.

Correction and Prevention of Immunological Defects Predisposing to Extracellular Bacterial Infections. Clearly, the most important and simplest means for correction of acquired immunologic defects is through nutritional support (Table 13–1) since, at the present time, it appears that most acquired defects of neutrophil function, opsonic activity, and antibody synthesis are related to undernutrition. Patients who experience stress or injury often have increased nutritional requirements, which are not met by customary therapy. As examples, patients with severe burn injury or peritonitis may require a caloric intake twice their basal needs to prevent a negative balance, and the metabolic requirements are increased by 20 to 100 per cent in most other septic states. Thus, to prevent weight loss and negative nitrogen balance in an average-sized (70 kg) adult with severe peritonitis or a large burn, it may be necessary to administer 7000 to 9000 kcal and over 200 gm protein equivalent per day. Since certain B vitamins, vitamin C, and trace metals, especially zinc, may affect the immune response, it is usually wise to administer them to patients with suspected marginal nutrition or stress.

At the present time, the following recommendations can be made for the use of nutritional therapy to prevent or supplement treatment of infections: In previously healthy, nutritionally normal individuals, intravenous hyperalimentation should be instituted if a patient is expected to be unable to take food orally for periods longer than five days. Correction of nutritional defects should be accomplished in patients with preexisting malnutrition before the time of planned therapeutic procedures, especially surgical operations. Pa-

TABLE 13–1. ADJUNCTIVE THERAPY FOR CORRECTION OF ACQUIRED IMMUNOLOGIC DEFECTS IN TREATMENT OF EXTRACELLULAR BACTERIAL INFECTIONS

ACQUIRED IMMUNOLOGIC DEFECT	METHOD FOR CORRECTION	COMMENT
Antibacterial function of neutrophils (intra-cellular killing)	Nutritional supplementation	Oral hyperalimentation probably more effective than intra-venous. Precise biochemical defect not defined
Severe neutropenia	Granulocyte transfusion	Probably not helpful if neutrophil count >1000/mm³
Defective chemotaxis	Nutritional supplementation (hyperalimentation)	Benefit not established
Low levels of specific antibody	Passive administration of IgG	Hyperimmune globulin most effective although rarely available
Low levels of complement opsonic proteins	Passive administration of plasma	Amount necessary not deter-mined. Plasma in CPD-stored blood retains opsonic activity for at least 21 days

tients with severe infections who do not respond promptly to therapy should have supplemental nutritional support by oral or intravenous hyperalimentation. Provision of adequate proteins or amino acids or both is probably more important than caloric intake. Hyperalimentation can be administered either by a continuous drip via a nasogastric tube or intravenously through a central venous catheter; the former method is preferable when it can be accomplished. When oral hyperalimentation is used, the continuous drip method is associated with less diarrhea than are divided intermittent feedings. The formulae used for hyperalimentation will obviously vary with the condition being treated, but should insure adequate caloric intake to meet both basal metabolic needs and requirements of the hypercatabolic state, and the formulae should provide adequate protein or amino acid composition, considering basal metabolic needs, increased metabolic rate, increased urinary loss, and loss from wounds or other sources.

For patients not previously vitamin deficient, supplementation with vitamins in the range of 2 to 3 times the minimum daily requirement should be sufficient. Pronounced excesses of vitamins should be avoided. Vitamin C should be administered in amounts approximating 500 mg per day. Iron therapy should not be given during acute bacterial infections since the infection may be aggravated. Although the requirements for trace metal supplementation have not been determined, it is apparent that they are necessary, especially zinc and copper, and should be added in small amounts to intravenous hyperalimentation regimens.

Serum opsonic defects occurring in the malnourished person can clearly be corrected in vitro by the addition of antibody (normal or hyperimmune gammaglobulin), normal plasma, or both. In certain instances, it has been possible to demonstrate that selected complement components could be added to restore opsonic activity, but in many instances a combination of C3, properdin, and Factor B is required. It thus seems probable that opsonic deficiencies can be corrected in vivo by the passive administration of gammaglobulin, plasma, or both. However, the exact requirements in terms of quantity necessary to correct certain defects have not been determined. In seriously burned children, the combination of oral hyperalimentation and the passive administration of blood or plasma in an amount of 200 ml per m² per day will prevent opsonic defects. However, it has not yet been determined whether the opsonic proteins administered passively or the hyperalimentation is more important. In a few patients with severe infections who have opsonic defects caused by complement component deficiencies, correction seems to have been achieved by the passive administration of plasma. In a larger number of patients, clear evidence that the passive administration of antibody will improve resistance to infection has been shown when there is an opsonic defect that represents a deficiency of antibody for the infecting organism.

Granulocyte transfusions have been advocated for adjunctive therapy in the treatment of patients with severe infection and concomitant leukopenia. However, large numbers of neutrophils are required, and they are rapidly destroyed following transfusion, partly because of their intrinsically short life span and also because antineutrophil antibodies are rapidly stimulated by alloimmunization. At present, it would appear that granulocyte trans-fusions are beneficial primarily in those patients with neutrophil counts less than 500 per mm^3 who have suppression of the bone marrow, which is likely to recover. When marrow suppression is caused by the infection, and not drug or radiation related, granulocyte transfusions are less effective. Perhaps when granulocytes, like red blood cells, can be given in larger numbers from well-matched donors, greater benefit will be obtained. Although still not de-termined with certainty, it is unlikely that transfusion of granulocytes will be of significant benefit to individuals with peripheral neutrophil counts greater than 1000 per mm^3.

Perhaps of more importance to a greater number of people will be at-tempts to increase the delivery of neutrophils to infective foci. This can be accomplished in part by the time-honored practice of applying heat to localized infections. Whether the use of peripheral vasodilators will be of benefit remains to be answered.

Another time-honored practice of proven benefit in the management of severely contaminated wounds is delayed primary closure. If a high level of bacterial contamination has occurred in a traumatic or surgical wound, or if complete debridement is not advisable or possible, the wound should be left open and a delayed primary closure performed four or five days later. Delayed primary closure at this time may be accomplished in the face of a relatively large bacterial contamination without the development of infec-tion. It has been shown experimentally that the number of organisms neces-sary to cause an infection in a surgical wound increases logarithmically dur-ing the first few postoperative days and by the fifth day may actually exceed the number necessary to cause an infection to uninjured tissues (Fig. 13–6). The reason for this increase in resistance to local infection is apparent if one remembers the progressive increase in reactive capillary vessels at the margins of a healing incision, which results in an increased potential for the deposition of phagocytic cells. If the wound is too large for a delayed primary closure, grafting with split-thickness skin can be done at the same time with excellent graft acceptance.

The use of immunopotentiators in the treatment and prevention of bac-terial infections has not been studied well enough to formulate current rec-ommendations. It is known, however, that in experimental animals, certain of the immunopotentiators can result in increased resistance to bacterial challenge, but they have not been used in man in any well controlled study. These agents are discussed in detail in Chapter 10.

Immunization for the Control of Extracellular Bacterial Infections. The introduction of antibiotics gave such impressive results initially that at-tempts to perfect effective vaccines were virtually abandoned for many years. Only recently has it become obvious that antibiotics have limited use-fulness and that their use often produces harm. With this realization has come a return of interest in methods to improve host resistance by biological means; immunization is the best studied and most familiar.

Active and passive immunization procedures for the prevention or treat-ment of extracellular bacterial infection have proven merit in only a few spe-cific instances. Immunoprophylaxis and immunotherapy of tetanus have had

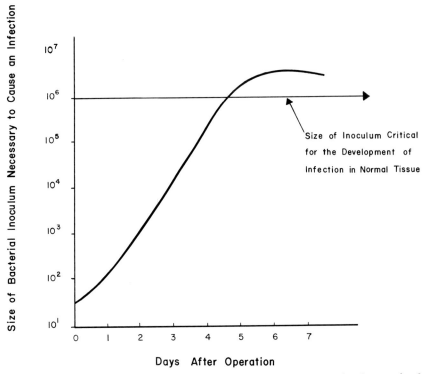

Figure 13–6.   Chart of the increasing resistance of a healing wound to bacterial infection.

outstanding success, virtually eliminating the disease in this country. The vaccine is composed of inactivated exotoxin (toxoid) and does not prevent growth of the organism. Persons who have had a full course of active immunization are protected against the development of clinical tetanus for many years; most are probably protected for a lifetime. In individuals who have been fully immunized, a booster injection of tetanus toxoid has regularly elicited protective levels of antibody when the booster has been given within a ten to twenty year period following initial immunization. The administration of antitoxin for prophylaxis is not indicated in such patients, except under most unusual circumstances. The use of homologous gammaglobulin (antitoxin) from immunized human donors had made passive immunization a safe and effective, albeit temporary, measure. Surprisingly, antitoxin against the exotoxin of *Clostridium welchii* has not been particularly effective.

Specific bacterial vaccines have sometimes been beneficial in selected situations in which there has been a failure of other treatment modalities. In our experience, the utilization of a polyvalent *Pseudomonas* vaccine has been outstandingly successful in the prevention of invasive *Pseudomonas* infections in patients with large thermal injuries. Vaccines for cholera, typhoid, pneumococcus, meningococcus, gonococcus and others are at least partially effective, and several are undergoing current development and evaluation.

Antibiotics and the Immune System.   Antibiotics have been extremely valuable in controlling most of the extracellular bacterial infections. However, they have proved to be a double-edged sword, and overuse has many deleterious effects. Of particular interest is the interrelationship of antibiotics with the immune system since almost any component of immune defense can be affected. Rifampin, chloramphenicol, and certain other less frequently used antibiotics affect protein synthesis significantly. It is not surprising, therefore, that they may depress T cell function, prolong graft survival, and inhibit delayed hypersensitivity reactions. Probably of far greater importance, other antibiotics may interfere with complement activity. Tetracyclines, sulfadiazine, and to a lesser extent cephalosporins, synthetic penicillins (especially oxacillin), aminoglycosides, erythromycin, and clindamycin in concentrations of 10 mcg per ml or more may interfere with the generation of complement-mediated chemotactic factors from serum. Presumably, since they inhibit complement, they may inhibit the opsonic activity of serum for antibiotic-resistant organisms. Although this feature has not been fully tested for each antibiotic, tetracyclines and sulfa drugs will clearly inhibit bactericidal reactions when present in therapeutic concentrations. Antibiotics do not seem to affect intrinsic neutrophil antibacterial function, but therapeutic concentrations of many of them depress the responsiveness of lymphocytes to phytomitogens in vitro. Despite the adverse effects, there are some positive interactions. When some organisms are first treated with subinhibitory concentrations of some antibiotics, they become more susceptible to the lytic action of complement and to the intracellular killing activity of neutrophils. How these balance out in vivo depends upon many things, including the antibiotic used, immune reserve of the host, and susceptibility of the organism.

There is an important lesson to be learned from the early experience with attempts to use prophylactic antibiotics to prevent wound infections in surgery. When prophylactic antibiotics were first evaluated, the initial dose was customarily given after surgery was completed. Using this schedule, the incidence of wound infection either was not altered or was actually increased. Later, it was learned that the immediate preoperative, intraoperative, and postoperative administration of antibiotics would strikingly reduce infection rates in contaminated wounds. However, when given similarly to patients with clean wounds where the expected incidence of infection was less than 3 per cent, variable results were obtained, sometimes with an increased incidence in patients receiving prophylactic antibiotics in well controlled studies. Experience in the treatment of seriously burned patients with prophylactic antibiotics has also been instructive. Rather than decreasing the incidence of infections, prophylactic antibiotics altered the types of infection to more virulent and antibiotic-resistant ones (Fig. 13–1). A synergistic effect may occur with certain drugs, since the occurrence of "opportunistic" infections is much higher in man and experimental animals receiving both steroids and antibiotics than in either alone. At least a part of this adverse influence of antibiotics can be attributed to interference with the protection afforded by normal flora that may be susceptible to the antimicrobial agent. As an example, *E. coli* produces a substance that suppresses the growth of *C. albicans* in the intestine.

It should be apparent that the decision to use prophylactic systemic antibiotics must be based on a careful evaluation of the potential benefits weighed against potential adverse effects, including influences on the immune system. While each case must be individualized, some general recommendations can be made, as shown in Table 13–2. Prophylactic systemic antibiotics are indicated only when exposure is sufficiently great that an infection is likely to occur and when the exposure does not continue. Since exposure to bacteria continues in immunodepressed patients, the use of prophylactic antibiotics is usually not justified except for the same indications used for nonimmunodepressed patients.

As an alternative to the use of prophylactic antibiotics, topical antimicrobial agents have been proved effective in many instances and have the advantage that they do not produce an adverse effect on the systemic immune system. Several well controlled clinical trials and laboratory studies have demonstrated that wound infection can be significantly reduced by using topical antibiotics in patients with potentially contaminated wounds. It is unproven at the present time whether a combination of topical and systemic prophylactic antibiotics will provide results superior to either alone. Topical therapy also has been shown to be effective in controlling surface infection in patients with thermal burn injury. In this instance, the agents used are ones that cannot be administered systemically. Therefore, emergence of resistant strains does not have an adverse effect on the entire hospital popula-

TABLE 13–2. RECOMMENDATIONS FOR USE OF PROPHYLACTIC SYSTEMIC ANTIBIOTICS

RECOMMENDED	NOT RECOMMENDED	COMMENT
Contaminated wounds; e.g., colon resection, vaginal hysterectomy, traumatic wounds	Clean wounds such as herniorrhaphy, where the incidence of infection should be less than 2 per cent	Wounds contaminated with $<10^5$ bacteria seldom become infected when good surgical technique is used
Brief limited exposure to highly contagious antibiotic-sensitive bacteria; e.g., exposure to gonorrhea	Tracheostomy Open wounds Urinary catheters Indwelling IV lines	Where the opportunity for continued exposure to new pathogens exists, antibiotics produce a selective pressure for infection with resistant strains
For prevention of a single type of infection in susceptible patients; e.g., streptococcus infections in patients with rheumatic heart disease or for tooth extraction in patients with prosthetic valve implants	Generalized or selective immunodeficiency	Some antibiotics further reduce immune function and may actually increase susceptibility, in addition to providing pressure for the emergence of resistant infections

tion and can usually be controlled by the alternative use of several currently available drugs.

INTRACELLULAR PATHOGENS

Some bacteria cause infections characterized by intracellular survival of the organism after phagocytosis. Listeria, brucella, and mycobacteria are typical examples of intracellular pathogens. In general, after challenge with these bacteria, the initial processes of resistance, including development of an acute inflammatory response, opsonization, and phagocytosis by neutrophils, occur in an orderly manner, but instead of being killed, these bacteria resist intracellular digestion and many outlive the neutrophils—only to be ingested later by scavenger macrophages. These bacteria are all eventually ingested by macrophages, in which they may reside for long periods of time. Because of this, infections caused by intracellular bacterial pathogens are usually chronic, and recovery from infection is dependent on mechanisms different from those involved in recovery from extracellular bacterial pathogens, namely, cell-mediated immune responses involving macrophage activation by T lymphocytes (Chapters 3 and 4). Because of this, such infections characteristically occur in patients with T cell defects, including inherited deficiencies of T cell function; virus-infected patients; malnourished patients; and patients receiving steroids, ALG, and cytotoxic drugs.

Correction of defects in T cell function will increase resistance to intracellular bacteria. Nutrition is one of the most important aids to immune resistance to infection, and this will be described in more detail in Chapter 20. Since T cell immunity is usually long-lived, vaccination procedures appear to be worthwhile. Immunization with BCG, for instance, will provide long-lasting immunity against tuberculosis. Perhaps of even more practical importance, stimulation of a T lymphycyte–dependent immune response by antigens of one organism will generate the production of lymphokines, which will cause a generalized nonspecific stimulation and activation of macrophages (Fig. 13–7). Such macrophages provide an increased resistance to infection by intracellular pathogens other than the one responsible for the initial response. BCG has been used extensively for this purpose, but more as a nonspecific immunoadjuvant for cancer therapy than for the treatment of infections. The process obviously works best when T cells are capable of being stimulated, but for some reason have not been stimulated by the existing infection. In this regard, the drug levamisole offers promise since, at least in certain instances, it can restore impaired T cell responsiveness. Unfortunately, the immunopotentiators have not been evaluated sufficiently in human infections. The mechanism responsible for increased resistance for most of the immunopotentiators lies in the stimulation of the synthesis of intracellular lysosomal enzymes by activated macrophages. In athymic (nude) mice, there seems to be a powerful compensatory mechanism for activating macrophages not involving T cells since these mice actually have an increased early resistance to infection by *Listeria monocytogenes*. However,

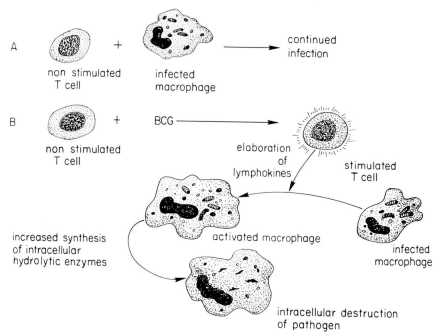

Figure 13–7. One mechanism for increasing resistance to intracellular infection by immunopotentiators. Macrophages may also be activated directly.

such mice cannot effectively terminate chronic infections unless they are given T cells.

While antibiotics do not appear to penetrate neutrophils in sufficient amounts to affect intracellular survival of bacteria, they do enter macrophages, albeit slowly, by the process of pinocytosis. Survival of the intracellular pathogens may therefore be affected by certain antibiotics, but it is well to remember that intracellular antibiotic concentrations never reach extracellular concentrations and that most antibiotics either become degraded or have reduced activity within the acidic milieu of the intracellular lysosome.

Leprosy. Infections with *Mycobacterium leprae* are of great importance immunologically. It is a classical disease, well known even in biblical times, which still produces disease and suffering in 12 to 20 million people around the world. In spite of antibacterial drugs and antibiotics which can affect the organism, control of this disease in many areas has been most difficult. Two polar forms of leprosy occur, and between the two are many intermediate forms. At one pole are the patients with the tuberculoid form of leprosy, who respond well with T cell immunity to the organisms. Such patients are able to keep the organisms within narrow confines, and the disease, although troublesome by producing nerve injury and localized inflammatory lesions, usually is not a threat to life. At the other pole of the clinical spectrum are patients with the lepromatous form of leprosy. These patient initially lack reactivity of T cell immune functions to antigens of *M. leprae.* As the disease progresses, there is progressive anergy to unrelated antigens and finally a decrease in the numbers of T lymphocytes and their response to antigens other than those of *M. leprae*. Increased immunoglobulins, autoantibodies, and rheumatoid factors appear in the serum as the infection extends, apparently unchecked by phagocytic functions. The tuberculoid form of leprosy is featured microscopically by granulomatous infiltrates showing abundant lymphocytes and many epithelioid and giant cells. Organisms of *M. leprae* have been difficult to find in such lesions. In contrast, the inflammation in the lepromatous form of the disease is confined largely to foamy macrophages, which become filled with organisms that the macrophages appear unable to destroy.

Recently, evidence has been presented to indicate that the capacity to exhibit cell-mediated immunity to the leprae bacillus and its products can be restored by the administration of transfer factor and that inflammatory tissue reactions develop in such patients. The threat of serious reversal reactions and failure to significantly reduce the bacterial load have thus far limited the clinical usefulness of this approach. Another group of patients suffering from lepromatous leprosy has been infused at weekly intervals with viable leukocytes from donors mismatched with each other and with the patient at the major histocompatibility determinants. The results were dramatic. T cell-mediated specific and nonspecific immune reactions were progressively corrected and the burden of organisms in the tissues progressively decreased. Chemotherapy and antibiotic therapy previously not tolerated could be given and dramatic clinical improvement ensued. Similar results were then obtained in previously untreated patients as in the treatment failures, using leukocyte infusion therapy followed by antibacterial treatment. These rather astonishing clinical and bacterial observations have subsequently been confirmed in studies in both India and South America.

A recent set of experiments from Norway has provided models of lepromatous and tuberculoid leprosy in inbred mice with polar forms of disturbed immunologic function, tissue involvement, and clinical course. That differences between strains of mice may reflect differences of intrinsic resistance that are controlled at the major histocompatibility locus has been suggested, but thus far has not been proved. This model should provide the basis for investigations to establish or reject the exciting possibility of controlling the intracellular parasitism of the leprobacillus through immunotherapy. Very much needed at the present time is effective immunization with either an attenuated or killed vaccine to permit reduction of the ravages of leprosy. Such an advance awaits development of the ability to culture *M. leprae* in vitro, a process that should be possible using modern tissue culture techniques.

Variant Forms of Bacteria

Variant forms of bacteria were first described in 1935 and, since then, protoplasts, spheroplasts, and L-forms have been demonstrated for almost every species of bacteria. Their importance in clinical infections has only recently begun to be appreciated.

Protoplasts differ from L-forms in that they can increase in mass but cannot divide as such, although they may revert to L-forms. Both characteristically lack a rigid cell wall and are soft, fragile, and pleomorphic. Osmotically fragile, spherical bodies are sometimes obtained from gram-negative organisms that retain some of the cell wall structure, and these are often called spheroplasts. The appearance of these atypical forms of bacteria can often be induced in cultures or tissues by lysozyme or by an inhibitor of cell wall synthesis such as penicillin or one of the cephalosporins. The infectious units of L-forms may be quite small (0.3 μ or less), and elementary bodies may be even smaller (0.05 μ).

Morphologically, L-forms may present an amazing variety of shapes and sizes, ranging in the light microscope from tiny dots to large structures that resemble degenerated leukocytes or erythrocytes. Other forms, even from the same culture, may be filamentous, club-shaped, oval, or irregular. The morphology of L-forms may vary considerably with the media and conditions of culture and is never characteristic for the parent strain. Their resemblance to PPLO (pleuropneumonia-like organisms) or mycoplasma is striking. The actual relationship between PPLO and bacterial L-forms is unknown, but the ability to induce permanent, nonreverting cultures of L-forms from bacteria which closely resemble PPLO suggests that many and perhaps all PPLO may have arisen as stable L-forms from a variety of bacterial species.

L-forms may form spontaneously from the parent bacteria in vivo and may retain exotoxin- and endotoxin-producing properties, thus displaying most if not all of the pathogenic properties of the original form. The persistence of L-forms in vivo may contribute significantly to the establishment of subclinical or chronic infections in the host at sites where ordinary bacterial forms would be destroyed. Reversion of bacteria to L-forms is classically promoted in vivo with antibiotic therapy, particularly the penicillins.

Clinical infections with L-forms have only recently been recognized because of the difficulties of culturing these variants, which will not grow using standard techniques for bacterial culture. L-forms have now been demonstrated to be associated with a range of bacterial infections, including septicemia, meningitis, thrombophlebitis, endocarditis, breast abscess, and pyelonephritis. In some cases, the L-forms seem to have been important in the development of chronic, indolent infections, but at other times the infections have been fulminant, especially in patients with abnormalities of host defense. However, precise mechanisms for resistance against variant forms are not clear.

Several cases of brain abscess and soft tissue infections have been shown to be caused by an L-form of one of the *Bacteroides* species in which ordinary cultures have been sterile. Of particular interest is the demonstration that L-forms of *Sphaerophorus* or *Bacteroides* species can often be cultured from blood or clots of patients who have recurrent or massive thrombophlebitis, particularly when a relative resistance to heparin has developed. In such cases, antibiotic therapy, usually a tetracycline and sulfadiazine, must often be administered for several months before a cure is effected.

VIRAL INFECTIONS

Viruses differ fundamentally from the pathogenic bacteria in several respects. Most importantly, they cannot replicate unless they infect living cells. No living type of organism fails to experience disease caused by viruses, and the virus infections are usually specific for that type of organism or a related species. Viruses differ considerably in their composition, varying from the extremes of naked molecules of nucleic acid to complex structures that also contain lipids, carbohydrates, proteins, and enzymes which are sometimes of host cellular origin. The nucleic acid of viruses may contain either DNA or RNA and be single stranded or double stranded, linear or cyclic. Some may cause generalized infection in the host, while others may affect only certain tissues or organs. Some viral infections are brief and self-limited; others may cause life-long infection and may even be transmitted vertically from parent to child. Some viral infections cause no evidence of disease whereas some cause disease in some infected individuals, but not others. Some are usually latent, some cause intermittent or recurrent disease owing to persistent infection, and some almost always cause overt disease. From this, it becomes apparent that there will be exceptions to any generalizations that may be made concerning viral infections. In spite of this difficulty, an attempt will be made to make our discussion as general as possible, to emphasize mechanisms of viral infections and their relationship to host immunity.

MECHANISMS OF INFECTION

The viruses that infect mammalian cells do so in a manner similar to that by which bacteriophages infect bacteria. The virus first attaches to the cell wall (membrane) and extrudes infectious nucleic acid into the cytoplasm of the host cell. It also seems possible that the infectious nucleic acid can enter the cytoplasm through the membrane of a phagolysosome following phagocytosis of a viral particle. Once inside the cytoplasm, infectious viral nucleic acid either commandeers the use of ribosomal structures for the synthesis of new viral particles or enters into a more permanent and intimate relationship with the nucleic acid of the host cell (lysogeny or insertion). It is in this latter instance that the host cell is often changed to become a more autonomous clone, sometimes with the characteristics of a neoplasm. In many virus-induced malignancies, transformed cells retain antigenic properties characteristic for all tumors produced by that virus, but other traces of viral residence or influence may be lost.

RNA viruses differ from DNA viruses in that they may translate information directly from viral genomes to polypeptides, or synthesize polypeptides via the RNA transcribed from the genome with the aid of virion-induced transcriptase. Alternatively, they may transcribe DNA homologous to the RNA base sequence of the virus RNA that can enter the cell nucleus and function like the DNA of DNA viruses. The DNA viruses enter the nucleus of the cell where they transcribe, replicate, and assemble virus and its components in the nucleus.

Polypeptides synthesized under control of the virus genome are usually virus specific, but polypeptides coded by host cell DNA can also sometimes be induced by virus infection. The virus specific polypeptides may be expressed as antigens primarily on the cell surface, but also may be found in the cytoplasm. Even when virus infection is not productive of virus, either RNA or DNA genome can function to contribute constituents of cell or cell surfaces. Because of this, neoplasms caused by the same type of virus, but originating in different tissues or different animals, often share a common antigenic specificity.

In productive and lytic viral infections, assembly of viral genome and structural proteins occurs shortly before rupture of the cell releases newly formed virions. In some viral infections, the infectious particles are passed from cell to cell by cytoplasmic bridges (horizontal transmission). Whenever the viral genome is incorporated into the host nucleic acid without concurrent cell damage, the infection may be transmitted vertically, i.e., to the progeny of cells during mitotic division. When such virus infection involves the germ line, transmission may occur from parent to offspring and true vertical transmission is the consequence.

ANTIGENS INDUCED BY VIRAL INFECTION

Proteins induced by viral infection may remain unchanged or they may be altered by the host through glycosylation or attachment to membrane lipids. The location and specificity of these new proteins determine whether they become important as viral antigens. They can generally be classified as being virion or nonvirion. Both may appear on the surfaces of viruses or in or on infected cells and play an important role in the immune response to viral infections.

Viral Surface Antigens. Not all virus proteins are important antigens since they may be buried within the interior of the virion and not accessible to immunologic attack. Even when they are on the cell or virus surface, they may not aid the host much if there is little or no immune response to them, such as with the neuraminidase protein on the surface or influenza virus particles. Other distinct virion surface molecules, however, interact with antibody to permit virus neutralization.

One thing that has made immunization against certain viruses (e.g., influenza) difficult is that the important external antigens may undergo extensive antigenic changes (shifts) as a result of recombination and selective immunologic pressures. Thus, immunization of a population against the strain causing an outbreak one year may not protect against next year's mutant.

Theories concerning the basis of frequent mutation of certain viruses are numerous. One of the most attractive for the influenza virus is that more than one form of this complex virus frequently infects both man and animals. When two such viruses involve the same cell, they may experience fusion of nucleic acids, and by a process akin to sexual hybridization, may develop a new strain with new antigenic potentialities to which the population has not been immunized.

Cell Surface Antigens Induced by Virus Infection.   Most but not all virus infections result in the appearance of new antigens on the membranes of the infected cell, often with amazing rapidity, sometimes within one hour. Most of the new antigens are virus specific and require the synthesis of new proteins generated by nucleic acids of the virus. Nucleic acid synthesis may not be required. Some of the new antigens induced by virus infection result from unmasking of existing antigens on the membrane surface, and others result from "depression" of host genes to synthesize host antigens no longer being produced (e.g., embryonic antigens). Since protein synthesis may be altered by the infection, sometimes by gene repression, normal membrane antigens may disappear or be diminished (antigenic deletion).

THE IMMUNE RESPONSE TO VIRUSES

Both humoral and cell-mediated immune responses are important in resistance to viral infections (Table 13–3), but the precise contribution of T cell immunity is not as clear as the role for antibody. T cell function is very likely required, however, for a truly effective humoral response to many of the viruses, including herpes and mumps. In other virus infections studied in nude mice, T cell function seems to be necessary for switching from IgM to IgG production. Thus, one major role of T cell immunity to viral infections appears to be a helper function in antibody production and in differentiation of antibody-producing cells. Another obvious but less well studied role of T cells in providing resistance to viruses probably involves activation of macrophages. Direct killing of virions by T cells by the mechanism of cell-mediated cytotoxicity is not felt to be an important form of antiviral defense. Nonetheless, the cell-mediated inflammatory reactions may play important roles in bringing inflammatory cells and viricidal agents and processes to destroy the infectious virus.

TABLE 13–3.   PARTIAL LIST OF VIRUS INFECTIONS OF MAN AND THEIR RELATIONSHIP TO PREDOMINANT TYPE OF IMMUNE RESISTANCE

T CELL IMMUNITY IMPORTANT	ANTIBODY IMPORTANT
Smallpox	Hepatitis B
Vaccinia	Polio
CMV	Influenza
Varicella-Zoster	Measles
Herpes	Yellow fever
Mumps	Rabies
Measles	

In most instances, both humoral and cellular immunity are important in bodily defense against viruses.

Systemic introduction of virus particles (or antigens) results in a classical humoral immune response with an initial rise in IgM antibody, later giving way to IgG and IgA antibodies. Long-lasting immunity is related to IgG and probably to persistence of virus. Systemic immunization gives rise to both systemic and local immunity.

In contrast, introduction of a viral challenge on a mucosal surface may result in a localized immunity limited to the area coming in contact with the virus, particularly when the virus is nonreplicating. Other mucosal surfaces may remain susceptible. Even the distal half of the colon may develop immunity whereas the proximal half may not, if an appropriate challenge is introduced into the fecal stream at midcolon. The localized immunity is very much a result of the synthesis of IgA antibody secreted onto the surfaces of the bowel. Secretory IgA appears to control virus infections primarily by limiting colonization. Interestingly, patients with selective IgA deficiency, although often susceptible to respiratory and bowel infections, may not have an increased susceptibility to viral infections. In these instances, the function usually assumed by secretory IgA seems to be filled by mucosal IgG and IgM.

Local immunity may also involve sensitization of T lymphocytes that may be produced after antigenic stimulation via the Peyer's patches and yield an enteroenteric local cellular immunity system involving T cells that is a parallel to the local enteroenteric humoral immunity system that operates through the IgA immunity functions. Similarly, antigenic stimulation via the pulmonic route can yield a T cell immunity confined largely to the lungs. How much these local immunity systems are involved in defense against or recovery from virus infections is not clear and needs much further study. When replicating viruses are used for mucosal immunization, viruses may reach internal lymphoid structures, and, depending upon the amount of antigen, a variable degree of systemic immunization may occur.

VIRUS NEUTRALIZATION

The ability of antibody to initiate events leading to loss of infectivity of a virus is called neutralization. Aggregation of virus particles does not fully explain neutralization, since certain viruses can be neutralized with Fab fragments or after absorption to the cell. The process, therefore, may involved one or many "critical sites" on the virion surface and it may interfere with the processes of attachment, penetration, or uncoating of the virus, all of which are necessary for infection. The distribution of "critical sites" on the virion particles and the affinity of the antibody both seem to play a role in the effectiveness of neutralization by antibody. Even in the presence of large amounts of antibody, however, there is usually a persistent fraction of a virus inoculum that remains ineffective. This may result from inability of available antibody to coat all of the critical sites. Here, steric factors may be important.

While many viruses can be neutralized by coating with antibody alone, the presence of complement components markedly enhances neutralization of many others. For example, *Herpes simplex* virus (HSV) is not neutralized by IgM antibody, and when C1 is added, neutralization does not occur. However, addition of C4 to the HSV-IgM-C1 mixture causes partial neutralization, which is potentiated by C2 and even more when C3 is subsequently added. Neutralization of HSV occurs perfectly well in C5- and C6-deficient sera, but neutralization of other virus particles may be potentiated by the late-acting complement components, and these components may be required to neutralize others. In vivo, viral lysis may be an important factor in acquired resistance. Nonspecific inhibitors in serum have been described, and some of these undoubtedly relate to the alternative pathway of complement. However, the relative role of the alternative pathway as opposed to the classical pathway in virus neutralization is still uncertain.

Since neutralization may prevent infection of cells by virions, the process may be of importance both for the prevention of virus infections via immunization or for natural infection and recovery from them.

INTERFERON

Interferon is a term used to designate a group of inducible proteins capable of increasing resistance of mammalian cells to many viruses. Interferons are a heterogeneous group of proteins with molecular weights varying roughly from 22,000 to greater than 100,000, but usually around 30,000. They are induced by viral infections and certain other substances, including endotoxin, pyran, PHA, and double-stranded polyribonucleotides. The inducing agent may influence the properties of the interferon to some extent. An even greater factor in determining the physical characteristics of interferons, however, is the tissue by which they are produced. Most of the interferons have tissue and species specificity, especially the latter, although species specificity in not absolute. Lymphocytes are an important site of interferon production in vivo. As proteins, the interferons are sensitive to proteolytic enzymes, but are relatively stable to low pH and heat. Mammalian interferons have a lower thermostability than avian interferons. Perhaps the most important property of the interferons is a lack of virus specificity, i.e., interferon induced by one virus may provide protection against infection by an unrelated virus.

Interferons inhibit both RNA and DNA viruses by interfering with intracellular replication. Synthesis of a new antiviral protein is induced that may interfere with transcription or translation of viral messenger RNA, or both.

Viral infection causes a rapid synthesis and release of interferon — within hours both in vitro and in vivo. The released interferon appears to aid in protecting both adjacent and distant cells from infection. In vivo, peak interferon levels are achieved about three days after challenge with influenza virus, just before the onset of recovery from the infection. However, the precise role of the interferons is still not well delineated for most viral infections nor is its relative importance to specific antibody and other nonspecific variables. Very recently, an important role for human interferon in treatment of chronic active hepatitis and a possible role for human leukocyte interferon in treatment of patients with cytomegalovirus infection have been reported.

DESTRUCTION OF VIRUS-INFECTED CELLS BY THE HOST

As mentioned earlier, viral infection can and usually does elicit the early formation of new antigens on the surface of infected cells, often long before mature virions are released. These new antigens can be recognized by the host as foreign, and they may elicit a substantial immune response of both humoral and cell-mediated types. Thus, immunologic destruction of virus-infected cells is common and may occur by antibody–complement-mediated cytolysis, antibody-macrophage cell destruction, antibody dependent–K cell-mediated cytolysis, and T cell-mediated cytolysis. The degree to which virus-induced antigen is expressed on the surface of infected cells and their antigenic "strength" and specificity obviously play important roles in the degree and type of host response to infected cells.

IMMUNOLOGIC DAMAGE IN VIRUS INFECTIONS

The host immune response to virus-induced cell surface antigens appears to be both beneficial and harmful. Destruction of the affected cell may prevent the release of mature virions if this occurs early in the replicative cycle, before the stage of assembly, and thereby limits spread of the infection. It may be even more important in limiting virus infections that do not cause cell death. On the other hand, cell lysis, activation of the complement system, and activation of macrophages and T cells can cause intense inflammatory responses which may, in fact, be responsible for the major pathologic changes associated with infection. Infection with the virus of lymphocytic choriomeningitis (LCM) provides a classic example in which infection by the virus causes minimal disease, but the cell-mediated immune response to virus-infected cells may cause intense inflammation with death. In contrast, infection of mice early in life with the LCM virus produces a chronic, persistent viral infection in a host virtually lacking in cell-mediated immunity to the virus. Antibody production is accomplished, and the continued production of antibody in the face of persisting antigen yields an ideal circumstance for antigen-antibody complex injury. Such animals infected with this virus early in development experience little overt evidence of virus infection, but ultimately die with lymphoproliferative diseases and antigen-antibody–induced vascular and renal damage. There are thus major differences in the type of response and degree and type of immunopathology induced by this virus in different inbred strains of mice. It must be be emphasized that the consequences of this persisting infection with LCM virus that destroys the host by one immunopathologic reaction, i.e., antigen-antibody complex injury or cancer, is very different from acute lymphocytic choriomeningitis in which the acute immunologic reaction to the virus may be destructive to the host by another immunopathologic mechanism, namely, acute inflammation of the brain and meninges.

Other examples in which the immune response plays a vigorous role in pathogenesis of the virus-induced disease include Aleutian mink disease, hepatitis, measles, mumps, and herpes. In Aleutian mink disease, formation of antigen-antibody complexes in the circulation leads to deposition in the liver, systemic blood vessels, and vessels of the kidneys resulting in forms of chronic persistent hepatitis, vasculitis, and glomerulonephritis. In hepatitis B infection, a disease of great importance to man, the virus itself appears to have limited cytopathologic potential, and most of the clinical disease appears to result from the host's immune response to the infection. Immune complexes associated with vasculitis and renal disease may occur. Even more important in hepatitis B is the liver lesion, which appears to result from inflammation caused both by T cell-mediated mechanisms and antigen-antibody complex injury. The former may be of even greater significance than the latter. In most acute viral infections of man, the onset of myalgia, joint pain, rash, lethargy, and behavioral disturbances correlates well with the appearance of viral-antibody immune complexes in the circulation and development of a hypersensitive state.

PERSISTENT VIRAL INFECTIONS

A number of viruses may persist for extended periods in the infected host, and even for a lifetime in some. In man, infections caused by cytomegalovirus, rubella, herpesvirus and hepatitis B virus are classic examples. Persistent oncogenic virus infection, thus far documented only in experimental animals, is another striking example. Some persistent virus infections may cause severe and fatal disease, while others cause subclinical infections with minimal injury and no apparent disease. Some of the persistent viruses, such as that responsible for kuru, have an extremely long latent period before the onset of clinical infections. These have been called slow viruses. Some viruses may infect almost every member of a species. As an example, virtually all mice carry the genetic information for oncornaviruses in their genomes, and the vast majority of humans carry *Herpes simplex* or cytomegalovirus by the time of adulthood. *Herpes simplex* appears to persist in the neurons of the sensory ganglia. The immune response can modulate this ganglionic infection and reactivation can occur by either neuronal insult or immunosuppression. IgG antibodies can terminate productive infection by the ganglion cell in vitro.

Persistent viral infections are only partly understood. It is obvious that certain viruses may enter the host cell genome in a more or less stable relationship. If virus-induced surface antigens do not result in immune destruction of the cell, infected cells will persist. It is less obvious why some viruses cause persistent viremia in the presence of neutralizing antibody and apparent intact immune defenses. In some instances, genetic factors specifically permissive to certain viruses appear to predispose individuals to persistent infection. However, a wide variety of other mechanisms may be involved in persistent infections, including abnormal immune responses.

Of special interest is the relationship of measles virus to subacute sclerosing panencephalitis (SSPE), a progressive neurological deterioration associated with extremely high levels of antibody to measles virus in the cerebrospinal fluid. The victims of SSPE have viral inclusion bodies in brain cells, and measles virus can sometimes be cultured using special techniques. Patients usually develop this disease during childhood or adolescence. Over one half of the affected children have a past history of measles before the age of two, and some investigators feel that immunologic immaturity may play an important role in establishment of the persistent infection. Variant forms of virus may also play a role, and this has been of particular interest since measles vaccine is produced from a temperature sensitive (ts) mutant. However, there is no evidence that the use of measles vaccine causes SSPE. Indeed, it may well protect against this disease.

The degree to which the ts mutant of measles virus persists in vaccinated individuals is unknown and therefore of some concern. The same is true for most live vaccines and following infection with many wild viruses. Long-lasting immunity suggests persistence of virus, which in turn causes continued stimulation of the immune response. That persistence of virus may not always be bad is exemplified by recent experiences with Marek's disease of chickens. Marek's disease is produced by infection with a cell-associated herpes virus, which causes a high incidence of lymphomas that appear at an early age. Immunization of newly hatched chicks with a related attenuated virus derived from turkeys prevents the lymphomas and has caused a 97 per cent reduction in mortality from this economically important disease. However, the immunized chicks become chronically infected with both the Marek's disease virus and the turkey virus, but no disease that has been recognized thus far results in this dual infection.

EFFECT OF VIRAL INFECTIONS ON THE IMMUNE SYSTEM

The interaction between viruses and the immune system is complex, to say the least. Many viruses nonspecifically alter the immune response, usually by depressing it. Cell-mediated immune responses are more often involved than humoral ones, and such disturbances are, in fact, common. Delayed hypersensitivity responses are inhibited by rubella, rubeola, mumps, influenza, herpesvirus, cytomegalovirus, and others. The oncogenic viruses as a group characteristically depress delayed hypersensitivity. A striking effect has been shown in mice neonatally infected with the Gross leukemia virus. Such animals become unable to reject allografts differing at non-H2 loci long before leukemia develops. The mechanisms involved are not well understood but could involve suppression of lymphocyte antigen-binding or blastogenesis, destruction of lymphocytes, stimulation of suppressor cells, or alteration of traffic patterns of T cell. In this regard, interferon may have an inhibitory effect on lymphocyte proliferation.

In a few instances, the immune response appears to be enhanced by virus infection.

VIRAL INFECTIONS AND AUTOIMMUNITY

The host's response to self-antigens is commonplace in viral infections. While the mechanisms responsible for such autoimmune phenomena are sometimes not clear, study of animal model systems has provided considerable insight into the problem. Both the afferent and efferent limbs of the immune response may be involved, and several mechanisms may be operative in a single individual.

Perhaps the most obvious of the mechanisms involving the afferent arcs is cross-reactivity between viral and host antigens. Since viral replication often involves incorporation of host antigens into the coat during assembly, such antigens may act as carrier molecules for antigenic specificities of the virus, or vice versa. In some instances, direct similarity may exist between antigens of the host and those which are strictly virus-derived. Also obvious and perhaps even more important are virus-induced antigenic changes in the host cell membrane. Derepression of genes coding for developmental (embryonic) antigens and enzymatic exposure of hidden surface antigens are both important mechanisms. The former, for example, by induction of an embryonic antigen, is responsible for cold autoimmune hemolytic anemia associated with infection with Epstein-Barr virus or cytomegalovirus. Lastly, cellular disruption as a result of infection may release usually sequestered antigens. This accounts for the development of antinuclear antibodies and immune complex glomerulonephritis in virus-infected NZB mice; indirect evidence suggests an important role for this in human systemic lupus erythematosus (SLE) since clinical exacerbations are frequently preceded by viral infections and appearance of free nucleic acids in the blood.

The efferent arc of the response to virus infections may cause autoimmune response by termination of tolerance, inhibition of suppressor T cells, or stimulation of effector cell mechanisms. It seems a likely possibility that immunologically based tissue damage resulting from chronic virus infection occurs in all manner of human diseases. The latter ranges from autoimmune diseases, like thyroiditis, to cancer and probably include a wide variety of vasculitides, lupus erythematosus, autoimmune hemolytic anemias, pancytopenia, amyloidosis, arthritis, multiple sclerosis, and several forms of progressive glomerulonephritis. One corollary to the concept is that immunologic injuries and autoimmunity are often caused by responses to forbidden antigens introduced by persisting virus infections and not to forbidden clones. A second corollary is that improved methods for defining these putative persisting virus infections and methods for their treatment and/or prevention will yield great dividends in management of many human diseases.

IMMUNOPROPHYLAXIS AND IMMUNOTHERAPY

It is obvious that no one approach to immunotherapy of viral infections will be successful in all cases, but little doubt remains that the most successful of all vaccines have been those used against viral pathogens. Live attenuated vaccines are presently available for smallpox, yellow fever, measles, polio, mumps, rubella, and rubeola, but even with considerable evidence of their great effectiveness, there remains a lingering concern about possible long-term adverse effects since there may be viral persistence, as suggested by long-lasting immunity. Only three killed viral vaccines — against rabies, polio, and influenza — are licensed in the United States.

Passive administration of pooled normal gammaglobulin or immune gammaglobulin can prevent measles, mumps, polio, varicella-zoster, and viral hepatitis to some extent. The potential of such specific human globulin preparations for therapy is promising, but has not been fully investigated. Recently, however, when a form of thrombocytopenic purpura was shown to be attributable to persistent infection with hepatitis B virus, passive administration of gammaglobulin containing antibody to the virus dramatically corrected the thrombocytopenia purpura.

Immunopotentiation in virus infection has also been inadequately studied, even though such therapy holds great promise. For example, repeated immunization with smallpox vaccine will sometimes aid in controlling *Herpes simplex* infection. The consequences of greatly increased antibody response to virus that might be induced with powerful chemically defined adjuvants or to specific virus components that have been appropriately selected are exciting to consider. Furthermore, the therapeutic consequences to be anticipated from the use of large to massive amounts of human leukocyte interferon in persisting virus infection are of great interest. Recent observations showing that both active and passive immunity can be used to perturb the virus-host relationships that lead to leukemia to MuLV-infected AKR mice, thus preventing the leukemia, can be used as an illustration of the potential for future developments in this field.

FUNGAL INFECTIONS

The participation of humoral and cellular defense mechanisms against fungal diseases appears to be even more complex than that for bacteria or viruses, although these mechanisms have not yet been studied as well.

Infections caused by *Candida* are the most common among the fungi, and such infections affect many individuals. These include people with inborn immunodeficiencies, patients with chronic mucocutaneous candidiasis or diabetes, and those receiving hyperalimentation therapy, broad spectrum antibiotic therapy, and various forms of immunosuppression and cancer chemotherapy. Epithelial and mucosal barriers obviously play a major role in early defense against these fungi, and factors elaborated by the normal epithelial and mucosal flora are inhibitory to candidal growth. Thus, when the normal ecology is altered by antibiotic therapy, overgrowth by *Candida* may occur, with invasion of the mucosa. Even in normal persons, ingestion of large amounts of *Candida* may result in a transient candidemia.

These organisms are rapidly removed by the RES, especially in the liver and lungs, although some may be removed by the kidney and excreted in the urine. In vitro, *Candida* are ingested and killed by normal neutrophils, but neutrophils from patients with chronic granulomatous disease of childhood and those with myeloperoxidase deficiency have diminished ability to kill *Candida*. Both antibody and other serum factors promote phagocytosis of *Candida*, but candidal infections do not seem to be associated with hypogammaglobulinemia and the antibody deficiency syndrome per se. On the other hand, patients with C5 deficiency or abnormality have an increased susceptibility to candidal infection, and C5 is required for efficient opsonization of *Candida* in some in vitro systems. The precise role of thymus-dependent immunity is equally confusing. Patients with abnormalities of T cell immunity often develop candidal infections, and patients with chronic mucocutaneous candidiasis often have depressed delayed hypersensitivity responses. These may be generalized or limited to deficient responses to candidal antigen. Also, treatment of patients with chronic mucocutaneous candidiasis with lymphocyte transfusions or transfer factor has resulted in remarkable resolution of the disease in approximately 50 per cent of the patients. Neonatal thymectomized mice are rendered extremely susceptible to fatal visceral infection with *Candida*. In contrast, in one experiment, nude mice who had no T cell function seemed to resist candidal infection better than conventional mice when challenged with *Candida*. Patients with candidal infection often have perfectly normal T cell responses. These rather conflicting findings, when taken together, suggest that the macrophage plays the dominant role in resistance to candidal infections, with neutrophils, T cells, and B cells participating in a lesser but often meaningful way.

It is probable that macrophage function plays the major role in other fungal diseases as well. Steroids, which significantly interfere with macrophage function, will increase susceptibility to most, if not all, fungal pathogens. Most patients with fungal infections have defective T cell function, which could in turn directly affect macrophage activation. Therapy with transfer factor has been reported to be of benefit in patients with disseminated coccidioidomycosis, who are often T cell-immunodeficient. It will be of great importance to evaluate the roles of immunopotentiators and cellular and macromolecular engineering that manipulate the immune response in control of these diseases.

PARASITIC INFECTIONS

Humoral mechanisms seem to play a relatively minor role in protection of a host against this broad group of pathogens. In fact, the formation of antibody may be deleterious, and frank IgE-mediated allergic responses are responsible for much of the symptomatology in many parasitic infections. Recent studies indicate, however, that T cell functions and locally based immunity involving the IgA and IgE local systems may be important in resistance to some parasitic diseases. Also, maximal resistance to certain parasites requires both antibody and cell-mediated functions.

Malaria is still of grave importance worldwide. Both humoral and phagocytic responses seem to be associated with initial resistance to malarial infection. Antibody to a plasmodium may coat free parasites (sporozoites) in the blood and result in their removal and rapid destruction by phagocytic cells, and passive antibody has been clearly effective in preventing experimental infections. However, immune serum has no effect on the growth of intracellular parasites, and cell-mediated immune responses seem to be more closely associated with resolution of chronic infection. Macrophages are clearly important in this disease, both from the standpoint of resistance and because of suppression of their activity by persisting malarial activity. Animals with depressed RES activity have an increased susceptibility to malarial infection. Soluble antigens have been demonstrated in patients with high degrees of malarial parasitemia, and some of the progressive nephropathies associated with malarial infection appear to result from antigen-antibody immune complex deposition in the glomeruli. In this regard, increased levels of complement components are found early after malarial infection, but complement levels are diminished late in infection.

Resistance against trypanosomes, leishmania, and other protozoa appears to be similar, but macrophages probably play a more direct role in recovery. Recent experiments show that *Trypanosoma cruzi* are killed much more effectively by activated macrophages than by normal macrophages, suggesting that the immunopotentiating drugs may play an important role in control of this disease. Also, transfer factor has some effectiveness experimentally against coccidiosis in rats. *Pneumocystis carinii* is an important pathogen in immunodepressed patients. Cell-mediated deficiencies appear to be of great importance in resistance to this organism, as revealed by lack of T cell responsiveness of some patients who develop these infections and the great susceptibility to this infection in patients who lack T cell or T cell functions. However, humoral immune mechanisms may also play a vital role in the bodily defenses against *Pneumocystis carinii* infection, which is indicated by the fact that patients with Bruton's X-linked infantile agammaglobulinemia, who have well developed T cell immunologic defenses, have often succumbed to infection with this ubiquitous agent. Clinical toxoplasmosis also appears to be associated with deficiencies of cell-mediated immunity. It is of interest that infections by one protozoal organism often result in generalized resistance to other intracellular pathogens. The mechanisms underlying such resistance have not yet been fully elucidated but presumably involve release of lymphokines from activated T cells.

Cell-mediated immunity has also been shown to play a role in resistance to infections caused by nematodes (round worms), cestodes (tapeworms), and trematodes (flukes). Cell transfer experiments provide clear evidence that antibody response to nematodes may alter the organism and the host-parasite interaction somewhat, but is not a major factor in elimination of these organisms from the host. Likewise, thymus dependent immunity to tapeworms or flukes prevents the disease, and ALG or steroids can worsen such infestations. It is probable that the drug levamisole, which strikingly influences such parasitism has a primary effect in control of worms by its nonspecific potentiation of delayed hypersensitivity mechanisms, although its direct antiparasitic action to inhibit metabolism of the parasites is also well established.

14

Cancer

Cancer is the second leading cause of death in the United States, directly responsible for 16 per cent of all deaths. Approximately one third of the general population over the age of 60 will develop a malignant neoplasm (excluding those of the skin), and at least one half of those who get cancer will die from their disease. In those who survive after successful treatment, increasing numbers of multiple primary malignancies of the same or different type are being discovered. Early detection and appropriate therapy are important to successful management in this group of diseases, but of even greater importance to recovery of an individual patient are the biological characteristics of his neoplasm and his immunologic response as a tumor-bearing host.

Surgery and irradiation are normally effective when the cancer is still localized, but when cancer cells have extended beyond the initial site of origin, treatment methods are required that can destroy cancer cells throughout the body. Because of this, chemotherapy is being used with increasing frequency and effectiveness. However, the fact that all chemotherapeutic agents used in the treatment of cancer are toxic to many normal cells limits their usefulness, and treatment methods that are less toxic and more specific for disseminated cancers are needed. Methods are also badly needed that can prevent the initial appearance of neoplasms, the development of secondary primary cancers of the same or different type, and the spread of metastases.

For these reasons, it is not surprising that intense interest and hope centers on the ultimate possibility of harnessing the powerful immunologic processes to fight cancer in humans. The historical success of using immunization as a basis for prevention and treatment of many infectious diseases has further encouraged physicians and scientists to seek means of applying immunologic approaches to cancer. Perhaps because of high hopes generated by the prospects of such application, great waves of enthusiasm and contrapuntal pessimism have featured efforts to develop this potentiality, but substantial progress has nevertheless been made. For scientific analysis, no area is more popular today than cancer immunology. The crucial issue is whether or not cancer cells have antigens at their surface that can be recognized as being foreign to the host. If this is indeed the case, it will be possible to develop effective methods to provoke specific assault on neoplastic cells. By contrast, if most human cancers lack antigens foreign to the host, the immunologic approach to cancer will remain nonspecific, and therapeutic use will necessarily be indirect and lack specificity.

Malignancies may result from a variety of etiologic influences, all of which involve alteration of the genetic code or its expression. These changes are manifested by proliferative advantage, independence of controlling influences, ability to invade, and ability to metastasize. Numerous cell components could be immunogenic under proper conditions, but it is especially the cell surface components that seem most important as antigens. These could be involved as the crucial characteristics of cancer cells and also subject to manipulations that might have an influence on the outcome of cancer. Thus, the enigma of cancer and truly effective means of cancer control may ultimately be understood in terms of changes at the cell surface that underlie disordered local growth, invasiveness, and metastases. Since regulatory signals that control proliferation of normal cells are known to reside at the cell surface, one can readily appreciate that cell surface changes profoundly influence where cells go and how they respond to their environment (e.g., to hormones or to other influences affecting differentiation and development).

In this chapter we will consider the relationship of cancer to immunity and attempt to visualize the directions this field is taking that hold promise for ultimate practical application to diagnosis, therapy, and prophylaxis.

IS THERE IMMUNE RESISTANCE TO CANCER?

THE EVIDENCE IN MAN

In man, strong evidence for immune resistance to cancer has been both sparse and circumstantial.

Particularly noteworthy in this body of evidence are exceptions to the rule that well-established malignancies characteristically grow progressively to cause death in untreated patients. Every clinician has observed malignancies that have remained dormant for long periods, only later to grow and spread rapidly. In numerous patients, metastases have appeared as long as 10 to 20 years after removal of a primary neoplasm. The reasons for prolonged dormancy of malignant tumors in these patients often remain unclear, but it may sometimes result from immunologic resistance.

Complete spontaneous regression of established malignancies in humans is even less common, but numerous cases are well documented. Four types of tumor—adenocarcinoma of the kidney, neuroblastoma, malignant melanoma, and choriocarcinoma—comprise more than 50 per cent of the collected cases. In some of these cases, an immune mechanism appears related to the regression. "Spontaneous" regression of malignant melanoma has occurred following injections of rabies vaccine, the administration of radioiodinated antibodies, blood transfusion from a patient who previously had spontaneous regression of a malignant melanoma, blood transfusion from a patient who had survived the removal of a malignant melanoma, and even blood transfusion from a normal patient. In several cases of choriocarcinoma, metastases have regressed after removal of the primary tumor. Regression of neuroblastoma has followed inadequate surgical removal or incisional biopsy of the neoplasm, and regression of pulmonary metastases has been observed several times in patients with adenocarcinoma of the kidney.

A number of experiments in man using autotransplantation of tumors have shown that patients are often quite resistant to subcutaneous transplantation of their own tumor cells. The degree of resistance may sometimes be enhanced further by preincubation of the isolated tumor cells with autologous leukocytes before they are injected. Human tumors which have been injected into normal, nonrelated volunteers invariably have been rejected, but in patients having abnormalities of their immune response, growth of tumors and even metastases from the subcutaneous inoculations have been observed.

Histologic study of many human tumors reveals evidence of ongoing immunologic events in the vicinity of tumors or in the regional lymph nodes. For example, combinations of lymphocytes, histiocytes, and plasma cells (those cellular indicators of an immunologic reaction) are frequently present in and around many human tumors, and controlled double blind retrospective analyses have shown that the outcome of uterine cancer, breast cancer, colon cancer, epithelial tumors of the head and neck region, and bladder cancer are closely linked to the degree of histologic evidence for immunologic stimulation in both the regional lymph nodes and primary tumor.

Another indication that immunologic reactions are often occurring in patients with cancer has come from frequent demonstration of antigen-antibody complexes in their plasma and with evidence that the complement system has been activated. In one study of approximately 7000 cancer patients, more than 60 per cent showed evidence of antigen-antibody complexes in the circulating blood. The presence of such immune complexes has been demonstrated by a number of different tests, including C1q deviation tests and competition with aggregated gamma globulin for receptors on cells of the Raji lymphoblastoid cell line. In another study that used a somewhat more sensitive technique for detection of such complexes, 85 per cent of cancer patients were shown to be experiencing these indications of an ongoing immunologic reaction. Thus, indirect evidence of several types suggests that immunologic processes accompany many malignancies.

THE EVIDENCE IN EXPERIMENTAL ANIMALS

Shortly after the turn of the century, it was found that animals injected with an experimental tumor often exhibited a remarkable degree of resistance to that tumor and, if they resisted a first tumor challenge, were particularly resistant to subsequent challenges. In some instances, the sera from animals that had spontaneously rejected tumors were found to prevent or retard the growth of transplanted tumors in other animals. As interest grew, a variety of immunizing procedures was used with great success in experimental tumors, and this encouraged application of immunologic manipulation for the treatment of cancer in man. Therapeutic efforts in man, however, led to disheartening failure. When genetically pure strains of animals became available for study, experiments on tumor immunity with the techniques employed in the earlier studies showed that previous success was related primarily to the presence of genetically incompatible histocompatibility antigens in the tumor of the original host, and tumor regression, when it occurred, was a result of allograft injection rather than immunity to tumor-specific antigens.

Interest in tumor immunity waned until it was discovered that cancers can be antigenic whether they are induced by viruses or by chemical carcinogens when transplanted, even within members of highly inbred strains of mice. The basic experiments were to transplant tumors in syngeneic animals and then remove the transplanted tumor entirely after a period of growth. Subsequent challenge with tumor cells showed that the host could eliminate the transplanted cancer cells and prevent their growth. Irradiated tumor cells or tumor cells treated with chemicals which prevent their replication could be used as a vaccine to raise immunity against the tumor. It was then shown that immunity to a tumor could be developed in the host of origin—autochthonous immunity. Since these pioneering discoveries, tumor immunity has been studied in many different systems, and tumor immunology has developed as a specialty.

Although there are a number of exceptions, chemical carcinogens tend to induce tumors with antigenicity characteristic for the particular malignant deviation. Even different tumors in the same animal may have antigens that are distinct from each other and from host antigens. The nature of these antigens has not been precisely defined, nor has the basis for the specific antigenicity of chemical carcinogen–induced tumors. Reexpression during adult life of genes normally expressed only in fetal life, or gene mutation as a consequence of the carcinogenic influence or as a consequence of the cell transformation are among the best possibilities.

Even physical agents like ultraviolet light or x-irradiation, which can induce transplantable cancers, induce tumors with individual antigens of this type. Many DNA and RNA viruses are now known to cause experimental cancers, including leukemias, lymphomas, sarcomas, and mammary cancer. Experimental cancers induced by viruses generally possess surface antigens which characterize the influence of the individual virus inducing the cancer. In certain instances, as with the polyoma DNA virus, infection with the virus in neonatal mice will produce tumors of many different organs and tissues. Ordinarily this virus will not infect or produce cancer when injected in adult animals. If the animal is immunodeficient, however, virus infection produces multiple cancers, involving many different organs and tissues. When live virus is introduced into immunocompetent adult animals, cancer does not occur and the host develops immunity to polyoma-induced, transplantable cancer cells, which would ordinarily produce widely disseminated lethal cancer if the animals have not been exposed to virus antigen. Thus, immunization against virus can yield immunity to tumor cells.

Other DNA and RNA tumor viruses induce malignancies of different organs and tissues with common antigenicity. The antigenicity of cancers induced by different chemical, physical, and virus agents in mice may range from very weak to very strong. Tumors occurring as apparently spontaneous tumors in aged mice have been studied and are said to lack antigenicity. However, it is clear that some spontaneous animal cancers are highly immunogenic.

SEROLOGY OF CANCER

ANIMAL CANCERS

In addition to tumor immunology that involves cell-mediated immunity, tumor immunogenicity can be evaluated using the same serologic methods that permitted definitions of infectious agents, analysis of the surface antigens of red blood cells, and characterization of the histocompatibility antigens. This methodology permits a most discriminative dissection of the specificity of antigens and the nature of immune reactions to them. Classical methods include cytotoxic tests, agglutinin reactions, complement fixation, hemadsorption, and precipitin and immunoprecipitation analyses. There are sensitive newer tools like mixed hemadsorption, radioimmunoassay, and precipitin diffusion. All these methods have been used to dissect the serology of cancer-causing viruses and virus components, virus-induced cell surface antigens, virus-coded cancer-specific antigens, chemical carcinogen-induced antigens, differentiation alloantigens, and oncoembryonic antigens, each of which is now known to be represented among cancer-associated antigens in experimental malignancy.

In addition, these methods can be and have been used to analyze the expression of components in host and virus genome and to dissect the role of viruses and expression of cancer-associated antigens with the malignant or premalignant state of the cell in experimental tumor systems. An extraordinary body of knowledge has already been developed which has yielded important information about the nature of many different experimental cancers and cancer viruses, and the role of chemical and physical agents in experimental oncogenesis. Carcinoembryonic antigens like the alpha fetoprotein have been discovered, and their value in making a diagnosis of cancer, establishing prognosis, and detecting persistent tumor has been demonstrated.

From these experimental beginnings, it is clear that the same precision must be applied to human tumor immunology in order to understand the malignant process, detect human tumors immunologically, and develop immunologic methods to treat or prevent cancer.

HUMAN CANCERS

It is encouraging that chemically induced cancers, cancers caused by viruses, and at least some spontaneous cancers in animals possess antigens at their cell surfaces that are readily identifiable. These antigens behave as though they were foreign to the host and can be recognized as such by the immunologic system if it is properly stimulated. It is further encouraging that studies of human tumors are likewise beginning to reveal antigens foreign to the host, which are characteristic of the tumor or of subclasses of one kind of tumor that can be examined by critical serologic analysis.

However, few of the putative tumor antigens described for human tumors to date have been defined in sufficiently precise and clear serologic terms. In Burkitt's lymphoma and in nasopharyngeal carcinoma, tumor-specific antigens induced by the EB virus are present in and on cancer cells. Also, recent studies have shown that tumor-specific antigens are present on human malignant melanomas. One class of antigens is specific for the individual melanoma and can be recognized by autoantibody. These antibodies reflect the immune response of the patient against his own tumor. Another class of autoantibody identifies surface antigens on some but not all melanomas. Similarly, tumor-specific surface antigens seem to exist on tumor cells in acute myeloid leukemia, hypernephroma, and some forms of bladder cancers. Less well-defined antigens associated with lung cancer are being studied.

Improvements in methods to permit culturing human cancer cells in vitro have been most useful in establishing the existence of these antigens and in uncovering the evidence of immunity to these spontaneous autochthonous human tumors. The use of autochthonous serum as a reagent to demonstrate the tumor-associated antigens avoids complexities that attend analyses of such antigens when heteroantisera or alloantisera must be used. Further, culturing the tumor cells away from the influence of a putative anticancer immune response helps to eliminate confusion which may derive from certain escape mechanisms, such as antigenic modulations, that tumor cells use to circumvent the immunologic response of the host.

In man as in experimental animals, alpha fetoprotein, an oncoembryonic antigen, is regularly produced by human liver tumors. This fact has already been found useful as the basis of an immunologic screening method to detect hepatic cancers early enough in their development to permit surgical cure. Important new information also indicates that illegitimate blood group antigens may act as tumor-associated antigens capable of being recognized as foreign by the tumor-bearing host. For example, antigens related to A blood groups are associated with stomach cancer, Thompson-Friedenreich antigens of the MN blood group sequence are found on breast cancer, and illegitimate antigens of the P system on stomach cancer. These serologic findings seem certain to represent an opening wedge that could lead to progressive immunologic approaches to earlier diagnosis, effective immunotherapy, immunologically directed chemotherapy, and more incisive cancer immunobiology for man.

ESCAPE MECHANISMS IN TUMOR IMMUNOLOGY

Listed in Table 14–1 are escape mechanisms by which tumor cells might be able to grow progressively even in the face of effective host immune response directed against tumor antigens.

The first and most deceptive of these has been called sneaking through.

**TABLE 14-1.   ESCAPE MECHANISMS FOR TUMORS
AGAINST TUMOR IMMUNITY**

Sneaking through
Immune modulation
Capping of cell surface antigens
Tolerance or unresponsiveness to tumor antigen or virus antigen
Immunologic blindfolding or smoke screen effect
    (Ag, Ag-Ab or blocking Ab)
Immunoselection for low antigenicity or lack of antigenicity
Host immunodeficiency
    genetic
    infection
    suppression
    induction of suppressor cells
    aging
Limitation of amplification or effector processes of host

With the establishment of a neoplasm featured by relatively weak antigenicity, the tumor may grow to considerable size before it is able to initiate an immune response by the host. By that time, its size alone may render it aloof to immune elimination. Recent observations that some tumors are actually stimulated to grow and metastasize by weak immunologic reactions might be looked upon as a tumor adaptation to facilitate sneaking through.

Immune modulation and surface capping of tumor cells are related but distinct means by which tumor cells can protect themselves from immunologic destruction. When grown in the presence of cytotoxic antibodies in vivo or in vitro, certain tumor cells modulate or lose their tumor-specific surface antigens by a now much studied process that involves movement of the antigens in the fluid surface membrane. These antigens may be internalized and then the cell ceases to produce them. When, however, the tumor cells grow in the absence of immune assault, the characteristic tumor antigens reappear. Capping has been extensively studied as a characteristic of normal lymphocytes and lymphoblasts and, like modulation, could be a mechanism used by tumor cells to accomplish defense against cytotoxic immunity.

Viral-coded viral protein and tumor-specific antigens may be presented to the host in a manner that induces unresponsiveness rather than an effective immune response against the malignancy. Conditions favoring development of a tolerant or unresponsive state may relate to the nature and strength of antigen, the method of presentation of antigen to the host's immune system, the dose of antigen delivered, and concomitant suppression of the host immune response. Simply acting as a consumer, coupled with suppression of production of substances essential to the amplification of immunity or effector responses, tumor cells can escape from effectiveness of an immune response. In AKR complement-deficient mice, as well as in cats and dogs, treatment with nonimmune serum or complement components has frequently led to dramatic destruction of cancer cells. These studies have revealed that factors engaged secondarily in the immune response may critically limit effective immunity against certain tumors. Recently, means of suppressing the immune response that involve specific and nonspecific immunosuppressive lymphocytes or adherent mononuclear cells have been defined. These have been found to be important in lack of effective immune responses to certain tumors. In addition, there is evidence that certain antigen-antibody complexes, sometimes acting through a suppressor cell mechanism, can interfere with or suppress killer T cell activities directed toward tumors.

Blindfolding or smoke screen effects refers to the shedding of antigen by the tumor or to the presence of antigen-antibody complexes that combine with free antibody directed against the tumor cell surface or that combine with combining sites on killer T cells to interfere with these immunologic effector mechanisms. Blocking or enhancing antibody, e.g., of a class which does not fix complement, can also protect tumor cells from effective immunity. Such blocking or enhancing antibodies may be able to stimulate tumor cells to proliferate and can, by combining with tumor cell surface antigen, compete with cytotoxic antibody, with the third population lymphocytes (K cells), or with monocytes armed with antibody. Noncomplement-fixing IgG or IgA antibodies can act in this way.

The ultimate in escape mechanisms may operate by immunoselection of a tumor cell population to one of minimal antigenicity. The ultimate extension of this escape mechanism would be to select a population of tumor cells completely lacking in surface antigens. However, the potential great importance of other escape mechanisms in tumor immunology is reflected in the fact that there are no examples to date of well-studied tumor systems in the inbred mouse in which total lack of tumor-specific antigen has been established. Furthermore, presence of these escape mechanisms permits the conclusion that progressive tumor growth does not indicate absence of tumor-specific antigens or immune reaction against cancerous tumors.

The concept of immunosurveillance was first clearly stated by Ehrlich and has been repeatedly reiterated in the modern era. This postulates that tumors arise frequently but that in most instances, immunologic responses of the host eliminate the malignant clone. The tenets of the immunosurveillance concept are listed in Table 14–2. Although much circumstantial evidence seems to be consonant with this view, some major challenges put forth are listed in Table 14–3. However, none of these arguments is absolutely definitive, and the immunosurveillance hypothesis remains a possibility, although perhaps less attractive today than it was a few years ago.

Much has been made of the fact that nu/nu mutant mice, characterized by thymic dysplasia and failure to develop T lymphocytes and T cell immunity, are most susceptible to viral oncogens but do not experience spontaneous cancer in great frequency, and do not appear inordinately susceptible to

TABLE 14–2. TENETS OF THE IMMUNOSURVEILLANCE
CONCEPT IN CANCER

Neoplastic cells have unique antigens.
These antigens provoke immune response.
This immune response is destructive of tumor cells.
Tumors arise when immunocompetence is depressed.

TABLE 14–3. CHALLENGES OF THE IMMUNOSURVEILLANCE
CONCEPT IN CANCER

Nude mice and B mice have few tumors without causative infection — may resist chemical carcinogen.
Some tumors prevented by T cell deficiency.
Immunosuppression without infection does not necessarily lead to increased cancer.
In situ cancer can become large without initiating immune reaction.
Spontaneous and carcinogen-induced cancers may have no demonstrable immunogens.
Immunity may be required for development and metastases of some cancers.
Genetic immunodeficiencies — narrow range of cancers.
Chemical immunosuppression — narrow range of cancers.

induction of cancer with many chemical carcinogens. Nude mice, however, do not lack immunity, and powerful immunologic mechanisms for resisting cancer have been demonstrated in such mice. Likewise, the finding that only certain cancers occur with inordinate frequency in patients who suffer from primary immunodeficiency syndromes and in patients experiencing secondary immunosuppression, as in transplantation, is of interest, but, like most of the arguments against immunosurveillance, is by no means conclusive.

What these findings do suggest is that immunosurveillance against cancer is a function of macrophages or other cells associated with primary recognition rather than T cells. That spontaneous tumors quite regularly seem to have weak antigens could be taken as an argument in favor of rather than as an argument against the concept of immunosurveillance. It would seem that additional, more critical analyses are necessary before this hypothesis, which has already generated much new information about cancer, is discarded.

Intensive suppression of the immune response, particularly for renal transplantation, has only recently been used in humans. Malignancies transferred as a metastasis in the kidney from the donor have sometimes grown progressively in the recipient, in contrast to normal persons in whom allogeneic grafting of tumor tissue is uniformly unsuccessful. In addition, patients who have been on immunosuppressive regimens for renal transplantation have developed spontaneous malignancies with an incidence 2 to 400 times as great as an age-related population, depending upon the type of tumor.

The possible effect of chemotherapy or radiation therapy upon immunologic resistance to cancer is an important consideration which must be remembered by all who treat patients with malignancies. In most instances, these methods of treatment have a more deleterious effect on the tumor than on the host, but it is the relative resistance of the two to the therapy that is of importance.

DEVELOPMENTAL LINK BETWEEN THE LYMPHOID SYSTEM AND CANCER

Recent phylogenetic studies suggest that an important developmental relationship underlies the intimate association between the development of malignancy and failure of normal function of the lymphoid apparatus. The lymphoid system, as we recognize it in mammals, developed in ancestors of the primitive fishes. All animals phylogenetically distal to the forms in which this development occurred have a lymphoid system, signaling its survival advantage. All animals possessing a lymphoid system also show a high degree of susceptibility to total body irradiation, alkylating agents, and carcinogens. By contrast, the invertebrates lack an organized lymphoid system and are extraordinarily resistant to x-irradiation, chemical carcinogens, and alkylating agents. Furthermore, it appears that they rarely develop malignancies. It seems likely that the lymphoid cells developed from cells capable of somatic mutation, susceptible to irradiation, and vulnerable to carcinogens. The intimate link between failure of lymphoid function and malignancy, which has been demonstrated in so many ways, may reflect the fact that the evolution of a lymphoid system made it possible for higher forms to take advantage of a characteristic of nuclear metabolism which would have been a major disadvantage to a host lacking the ability to express adaptive immunity.

CANCER IN PATIENTS WITH PRIMARY IMMUNODEFICIENCY

Patients with primary immunodeficiency, e.g., common variable immunodeficiency, ataxia telangiectasia, Wiskott-Aldrich syndrome, and Chediak-Higashi syndrome, experience cancer between 100 and 1000 times more frequently than members of the general population of comparable age. This relationship was predicted by Thomas in his modern expression of the concept of immunosurveillance in 1958. It has turned out, however, that not all cancers occur with such great frequency in immunodeficient patients. Wilms' tumor, neuroblastoma, bone tumors, and embryomas, relatively common among cancers occurring in children in the general population, do not occur in the same high proportion among the immunodeficient patients. Instead, cancers of the lymphoid tissues—lymphomas, reticulum cell sarcomas—tumors of the stomach, head and neck epitheliomas, and bowel carcinomas are encountered with excess frequency in patients with primary immunodeficiency diseases. This finding can be taken as an argument against the general concept of immunosurveillance and has also been taken as an argument in support of a possible virus etiology of these types of malignancy. These and consonant observations in experimental animals have provoked others to postulate that the immunologic system in patients with primary immunodeficiency disease may be developing malignancy because it has been stimulated to proliferate by excessive antigenic stimulation.

None of these findings explain the high frequency of pernicious anemia, achlorhydria, gastric malfunction, and gastric and colonic cancer that seem to occur in some populations in immunodeficient patients. A possible basis in chromosomal instability and nucleic acid dysmetabolism underlying the cancers of the rapidly dividing cell systems of the gastrointestinal tract and the immunologic lymphoid system has recently been postulated which could be unifying.

Neonatal animals are inordinately susceptible to viral oncogenesis, as they are to transplantation of many tumors. Neonatal thymectomy predisposes to viral oncogenesis but much less to chemical carcinogen–induced malignancy. Neonatal thymectomy, however, protects against many leukemias and lymphomas that develop in the thymus and also against MT virus–induced mammary adenocarcinoma. Restoration of immunologic capacity with thymus transplants restores capacity to develop both virus-induced cancers. Reconstruction of immunocompetence by injection of differentiated lymphoid cells restores capacity to develop mammary adenocarcinoma but not capacity to develop leukemias in athymic animals. These findings indicate that virus-induced mammary adenocarcinoma in some ways involves normal immunologic function for its development.

Most if not all carcinogens are both oncogenic and immunosuppressive, and many are anticancer drugs. However, the immunosuppressive doses and carcinogenic doses of these agents are not concordant. Carcinogenesis may be produced by doses of these agents that are ten times less than the dose required to produce measurable immunosuppression.

In aged animals, there is a marked decline in immune functions, which is attributable to a sharply declining thymic function and involution of the T cell system. Decline of B cell functions occurs later. In aging animals, an increased incidence of both spontaneous and induced malignancies is also seen, which is temporally correlated with susceptibility to tumor transplantation, decreasing activity of the lymphoreticular system, and diminished immunologic responses in general.

IMMUNOLOGIC DEFICIENCIES IN CANCER PATIENTS

Malignancies involving the lymphoid organs characteristically produce immunologic deficiencies which are related to the extent and type of involvement. In patients with Hodgkin's disease, the thymic dependent system of lymphocytes characteristically functions less well than in normal persons. Early in the course of the disease, prolongation of allogeneic graft survival and a marked suppression of delayed hypersensitivity reactions may be present, but gamma globulin levels and antibody synthesis are normal. Not surprisingly, patients with Hodgkin's disease have a high incidence of tuberculosis and fungus infection. In contrast to Hodgkin's disease, multiple myeloma involves primarily the system of lymphocytes associated with the production of circulating antibodies (the B cells), and early in its course, chronic lymphocytic leukemia appears to involve deficiencies of both the T cell and B cell lymphoid systems. Decreased levels of the normal immunoglobulins are frequently found in the myeloma patients, but delayed hypersensitivity reactions are characteristically normal until the disease has reached an advanced stage.

Patients with other forms of cancer may also show immunologic abnormalities. In some cancers, like epitheliomas of the head and neck region, T cell immunities are deficient early in the course. The freedom from recurrences of cancer after surgery correlates with the extent of T cell immunodeficiency, as revealed by capacity to develop and express delayed allergic reactions. The deficiency of T cell dependent immunities also correlates with the extent of malignancies and presence or absence of metastases in many cancers. In a few cancers, like lung cancer, immunodeficiency secondary to the malignant process is very much delayed and not seen until the most advanced stages. However, a number of significant immunologic deficiencies may be noted which can be positively correlated with the extent of the malignancy. The reasons for the appearance of these deficiencies are unclear at the present time, but the tumor itself or the agent inducing the malignant transformation may be responsible. Similar abnormalities have not been demonstrable in patients with similar degrees of debility from many nonmalignant causes.

The ability to produce circulating antibody is usually preserved, even in far-advanced cases of malignancy, but the same patients often have prolonged survival of allogeneic skin grafts, a decrease in the quantity of macrophages that can be recruited to sites of inflammation, a loss of their ability to develop delayed hypersensitivity reactions, a decreased ability to reject transplants of their own or allogeneic tumors, and an abnormality in the response to lymphocytes that have been injected intradermally.

In experimental tumor systems, it has been shown that secondary neoplasms will develop when tumor implants have been made at the time of removal of a primary tumor. Similar animals reject tumor grafts when challenged at a later time (for example, one month after resection of the primary tumor), suggesting that the ability to express cellular immunity has been depressed by the presence of the tumor.

It has now been found, in a variety of malignancies in several different species of experimental animals, that the host may have serious deficits of his immunologic mechanism during the period of incubation in the development of virus-induced malignancies. These deficiencies, which are particularly of the cell-mediated type, may be a consequence of either direct or indirect influence by the virus on the lymphoid cells of the host. Whatever their nature, they may contribute to the establishment of the malignant process by decreasing the capacity of the host to exercise a normally vigorous immunologic resistance. Viruses which are not directly involved in the process of malignant adaptation may also have an indirect influence on oncogenesis by causing abnormalities of immunologic function.

The question of whether specific immunologic tolerance develops to human tumors remains unanswered. When a tumor-inducing virus is introduced during the neonatal period in animals, specific tolerance to the virus can develop, and the virus can remain in the host to exert its oncogenic effect later in life, usually during adulthood. Tolerance is more difficult to establish in adult animals, but it may be established if the antigen is weak, if there is a suppression of the immunologic response of the host, or if large doses of antigen are administered. Since all three of these conditions are often met by self-replicating neoplasms, they might be expected to produce a state of tolerance in adult animals. Tolerance seems to play an important role in the continued development and growth of some malignancies but not in others.

IMMUNOPOTENTIATION

The discovery that treatment of experimental animals with BCG would increase resistance to certain tumors raised the possibility that enhancement of immune responses might be used to prevent or treat human cancer. Much has been learned since that time, and these immunopotentiators are discussed at length in Chapter 10. Both immunopotentiators and some immunomodulators act primarily on macrophages, which become more active in phagocytosis and may be stimulated to divide and develop abundant digestive enzymes in their cytoplasm.

In experimental studies in animals, such activated macrophages have been shown to kill cancer cells in tissue culture while not damaging normal noncancerous cells. The experiments with immunopotentiators and the considerations discussed in the section on immunosurveillance now make it relatively clear that immune surveillance against cancer is primarily a function of macrophages rather than lymphocytes, and that the role of lymphocytes in this disease is primarily to expand macrophage activity.

TUMOR NECROSIS FACTOR

In pursuit of the action of two immunopotentiators, BCG and bacterial endotoxin, a substance called tumor necrosis factor was discovered, which seems to be capable of destroying certain cancer cells in culture while not damaging normal cells. Lipopolysaccharide endotoxins from gram-negative bacteria produce hemorrhagic necrosis in certain tumors, an effect originally attributed to damage to blood vessels of tumors. However, it was recently discovered that plasma 24 to 48 hours following endotoxin treatment is capable of killing cancer cells directly in vitro. This effect of serum is very much greater if the animals have been treated with BCG prior to being given endotoxin. A glycoprotein of 150,000 MW seems to contain the active principle.

IMMUNOTHERAPY OF CANCER

In experimental animals, immunotherapy based on stimulation of the immune system with immunopotentiators alone, or using immunopotentiation plus cancer cells or antigens, can prevent cancer, prevent metastasis, or treat cancer, causing regression of both primary cancer and metastases. Expectations for this approach to cancer therapy are high, even though the scientific development at present must be considered to be in its earliest phase. Preliminary results already indicate that immunotherapy of cancer can work. One impressive achievement has been the capacity to use contact allergic reactions induced in the vicinity of skin cancer to treat and even prevent it from occurring in susceptible persons.

Local injections of BCG vaccine have induced regression of most melanomas treated and have proved effective enough to become a clinically useful tool. Even more encouraging is the fact that, following such local treatment, an apparent immune reaction often leads to regression of distant skin metastases of the malignant melanoma. Treatment using BCG injection of skin and systemic BCG as an adjunct to surgical operation and chemotherapy has also apparently improved the outcome of melanoma in some series. Intrapleural injections with BCG appear to prolong the disease-free interval in relatively early lung cancer, from one well-controlled clinical trial. Prolongation of life and improvement in remissions of lung, breast, colon, and other cancers in advanced stages by treatment with BCG, *Corynebacterium parvum*, or levamisole have been observed. Immunotherapy has also been coupled with chemotherapy or irradiation therapy to apparent advantage for patients with cancer, especially leukemia, and active immunization with neuraminidase-treated allogeneic leukemic cells has appeared to improve the outlook of acute myeloid leukemia in some studies. Similarly, *Pseudomonas* vaccine, with or after chemotherapy, has yielded long-term survival in acute leukemia where chemotherapy alone has usually failed.

It is encouraging that these crude immunotherapeutic measures that have been used up to now work at all. The future holds promise of increasingly precise chemical management using immunostimulation, immunopotentiation and immunomodulation, and a real understanding and improved control of immunoeffector mechanisms. In addition, specific immunotherapy and immunodirected chemotherapy may be anticipated for at least some cancers in the future.

15

Transplantation

The successful alleviation of disease by transplantation of organs or tissues is one of the most exciting advances in the history of medicine. Replacement of diseased parts was first considered in Greek mythology but, in the light of present knowledge, such procedures were neither technically nor biologically possible for many centuries, and it is certain that the early stories of successful transplants were not true. For example, Saints Cosmas and Damian reportedly transplanted the leg of a deceased Ethiopian to a white patient in the third century A.D., as popularized by many paintings of the Renaissance.

Although many of the early surgeons most certainly thought about the transplantation of human tissues, even primitive scientific efforts did not begin until the nineteenth century, and no real progress was made until the earliest part of the twentieth century when Carrell and his colleague, Guthrie, developed the sound techniques still used for vascular anastomosis. Most of the technical problems of organ grafting were soon solved, but it became painfully obvious that failure was an inevitable consequence of organs grafted to unrelated individuals. Many of the early workers of the twentieth century perceived that some sort of mechanism of nonself recognition was responsible for this failure, but it remained for Medawar and his colleagues in the 1940's to provide unequivocal evidence that the rejection of grafted tissues resulted from an immunologic reaction. From this improved understanding of the biological nature of graft rejection grew a renewed interest in the possibility of transplanting human organs.

The first long-term success following transplantation of a human kidney was in 1954, when the organ was donated by a genetically identical sibling. However, attempts to transplant kidneys from relatives other than nonidentical twins, or from cadavers, met with uniform failure until the development of immunosuppressive drugs and their application to prevent rejection of allografts (a graft between members of the same species). Results began to improve, and many patients who received both living donor and cadaveric renal allografts in the early 1960s are still alive with functioning grafts.

The greatest experience in clinical transplantation has been with kidney allografts for the treatment of chronic renal failure. In 1963, such cases from all over the world began to be reported to the Human Renal Transplant Registry, and by 1976, over 25,000 kidney transplants had been reported from 301 institutions, 165 of them in the United States of America. The accumulated results in terms of graft and patient survival are shown in Fig. 15–1. It is noteworthy that during the past five years, functional survival of transplanted kidneys has actually decreased slightly while patient survival has had a steady increase. This trend reflects several factors which include improved supportive services; an older patient population; transplantation of more patients with a higher risk, such as those with diabetes or who are highly sensitized; and of most importance, a willingness to remove poorly functioning kidneys and return patients to dialysis. The survival of patients receiving cadaveric kidneys and of those who remain on chronic hemodialysis is not significantly different at the present time for patients under the age of 50, unless there are specific associated conditions that increase the risk for one or the other type of treatment. Over the age of 55, most patients have better survival when treated by chronic hemodialysis. Therefore, considering economic factors, quality of life, patient comfort, and survival, almost all patients under the age of 45 should be treated primarily by transplantation and those over 55 by dialysis. Patients of intermediate age or with complicating diseases must be individualized.

Clinical transplantation has also been extended to the heart, lung, liver, pancreas, endocrine organs, cancellous bone, bone marrow, cornea, heart valves, blood vessels, skin, and fibrous tissues. The reported results for some of these are summarized in Table 15–1. Corneal transplants are routinely performed and have been highly successful because they are less vulnerable to immune recognition. Skin transplants are also used routinely in the care of burn patients, but no serious attempts have been made to obtain permanent survival.

From the results achieved thus far, it is clear that much progress has been made, but it is equally clear that we are far from a complete understanding of the processes involving recognition, cellular interaction, and dif-

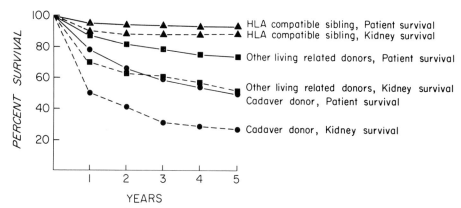

Figure 15–1. Patient and kidney survival following human renal transplantation. Data based on world experience as reported by the Human Renal Transplant Registry.

TABLE 15-1. TRANSPLANTATION OF ORGANS OTHER THAN THE
KIDNEY AS REPORTED BY TRANSPLANT REGISTRY (JANUARY, 1977)

UPDATE ON ORGAN TRANSPLANTATION IN THE WORLD	HEART	LIVER	LUNG	PANCREAS
Transplant teams	64	41	22	15
Transplants	328	288	37	52
Recipients	320	273	37	50
Alive with functioning grafts	70	36	0	0
Longest survival with functioning graft	8.2 yr	6.9 yr	10 mo	4.2 yr

ferentiation. Already, transplantations' interface with other fields has led to a
better understanding of autoimmunity, infection, renal disease, genetics,
cancer, and aging. Solving the remaining problems of transplantation will
have an additional profound impact not only upon these fields but also on all
of clinical medicine since it will expose and unravel the most elementary biological processes of life and lead to their control. This is a not so distant
goal, and we anticipate that by the end of this century, it will be possible to
successfully transplant most organs with regularity.

TYPES OF GRAFTS

It is well to review the terminology used to designate the genetic relationship between the graft (donor) and recipient.

Isografts (isogeneic grafts) are those free grafts which are transferred
from one individual to another who is genetically identical. Grafts between
identical twins and grafts between members of the same inbred strain of
animals account for this group. Immunologic rejection does not occur, with
the possible exception of those grafts from males to females, since minor histocompatibility antigens may be expressed as a result of their being carried
by the Y chromosome.

Allografts or allogeneic grafts (once called homografts) are those grafts
which are transferred from one individual to another of different genetic con-
stitution within the same species, for example, grafts from man to man or dog
to dog, excluding identical twins. The vast majority of human organ transplants are allogeneic grafts. Within this classification one may encounter a
wide range of genetic disparity, varying from those with almost identical inheritance of histocompatibility antigens to those with extreme differences. It
is with this type of graft that testing for histocompatibility differences
becomes of critical importance, since success or failure depends largely
upon these differences.

Xenografts or xenogeneic grafts (once called heterografts) are those
grafts which are transferred from a member of one species to an individual of
another species. Examples are the transplantation of a chimpanzee's kidney

to man or the transplantation of a dog's heart to a pig. These types of grafts may be expected to fail quickly because of extreme differences in histocompatibility. Antibodies reacting with the tissue antigens of disparate species often are already present in the host, and their presence results in immediate rejection.

REJECTION

Failure of function of a vascularized allograft or xenograft occurs primarily as the result of one or more immunologic processes leading to permanent damage or death of the transplant. Virtually all of the mechanisms discussed in Chapter 8 may be involved at one time or another, but only three types of rejection are recognized clinically, based both on the time of appearance and the lesion produced.

HYPERACUTE REJECTION

Hyperacute or immediate rejection occurs within minutes to hours after revascularization of a transplanted organ. Its development is associated with the presence of preexisting (preformed) antibodies in the blood of the recipient, which react with antigens present in the donor tissues, especially HLA antigens and endothelial cell specific antigens of the intima of blood vessels. This antigen-antibody reaction activates the complement system, which causes endothelial cell disruption, exposure of the basement membranes, adherence of neutrophils and platelets, and activation of the clotting mechanism. When examined microscopically, the lesions are primarily vascular, and the classical features are platelet aggregation (Fig. 15–2); fibrin deposition and plugs, which are especially prominent in the glomeruli; and a marked increase in neutrophils adhering to the walls of small and medium-sized vessels. By immunofluorescence, IgG, complement, and sometimes IgM are found in heavy concentrations in the vessels and glomeruli. The gross appearance of the kidney may be altered significantly, depending upon the concentration of the antibody in the recipient and its ability to activate complement.

In the most severe instances, the kidney becomes swollen and blue within minutes of establishment of the circulation because of obvious engorgement with blood. However, the renal vein is usually collapsed or at least not tense. Upon compression of the vein, there is either no or a markedly delayed increase in tenseness of the kidney, indicating an intrarenal venous blockade. The extrarenal arterial pulsations are vigorous, but the kidney does not pulsate. The gross changes of hyperacute rejection are not always so striking, and some affected kidneys may become flaccid or at first appear normal. Eventually, however, all acquire a bluish discoloration and fill poorly upon compression of the renal vein. Occasionally, venous spasm or hypovolemia without hypotension may produce a similar ap-

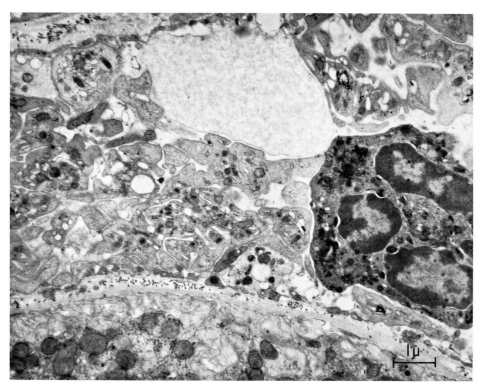

Figure 15–2.   Electron micrograph of a biopsy specimen removed from a dog kidney 5 hours after allogeneic transplantation, showing features of the immediate type of rejection. The host had been presensitized by two sets of skin grafts and a kidney graft from the specific donor. The vessel in the figure is completely obstructed by a platelet thrombus. Degranulation of the platelets and extensive fusion are evident, A neutrophil is seen at the edge of the figure. (From Lowenhaupt, R., and Nathan, P., Nature, 220:822, 1968.)

perance, and a gross diagnosis of hyperacute rejection should always be supported by a frozen section before removal of a kidney.

   With present methods of prescreening for preformed antibodies, typical hyperacute rejection is not commonly seen. However, a milder form of the same basic process frequently occurs, which is characterized by initial normal appearance of the kidney, initial good urine output (often over one liter the first day) decreasing progressively to significant oliguria by days three or four, and falling platelet counts. Biopsy of the kidney will reveal collections of neutrophils, platelets, and fibrin in glomeruli and vessels, similar to but less severe than the lesions of hyperacute rejection. This variant, called accelerated rejection, is mediated by circulating antibodies which either activate complement less well or are in sufficiently low concentration that they are not detected by lymphocytotoxicity. In contrast to the clear futility of treating hyperacute rejection, the lesion caused by accelerated rejection may reverse with time on immunosuppressive therapy.

   Acute immunologic injury can also occur when a kidney is transplanted to a patient with circulating antibodies against glomerular basement membranes, but the lesions produced are clearly different from those caused by antibody-mediated rejection.

ACUTE REJECTION

Acute rejection is the term applied to a primary rejection occurring in a nonsensitized recipient. In the unmodified recipient, initial good function of a transplanted organ is followed by a gradual decline of function, accelerating within hours to an abrupt cessation by the sixth to tenth posttransplant day. In individuals receiving immunosuppressive therapy, acute rejection can occur at any time, even years after the transplant.

The early pathologic lesion of acute rejection is characterized by infiltration of the affected tissue by both neutrophils and mononuclear cells. Later, mononuclear cells clearly predominate (Fig. 15–3). Most of the infiltrating mononuclear cells are immature lymphocytes, but plasma cells and macrophages also abound. Lymphocytic infiltration is especially prominent about the small and medium-sized blood vessels, sometimes accompanied by disruption of the media and intima of arterioles and complete destruction of

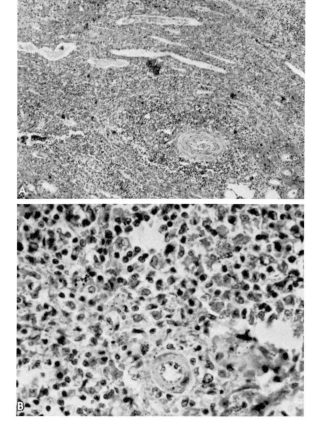

Figure 15–3. Microscopic appearance of a dog kidney late in acute rejection. There is extensive infiltration of the interstitial tissues with mononuclear cells and extensive hemorrhage. A, × 25, B, × 160.

venular walls. Platelet thrombi and small vessel thrombi form progressively to curtail blood flow, sometimes leading to extensive hemorrhage within the parenchyma or to sequential infarctions. Diagnosis of acute rejection by microscopic examination alone is not always an easy task, however, because a variable degree of lymphocytic infiltration can be found in most allografts, and the intensity of the cellular infiltrate often does not correlate with functional changes.

While both humoral and cellular components play an obvious role in acute rejection episodes, cellular processes probably predominate. Direct killing by T lymphocytes and activation of macrophages by lymphokines to act as aggressor cells appear to be primary mechanisms, but the formation of cytotoxic antibody and antibody which participates in antibody-dependent cell-mediated cytotoxicity have also been found to play important roles.

The clinical manifestations of acute rejection might be predicted by the pathologic findings. The immunologic damage causes abnormalities of function, and the most reliable indicator of acute rejection following renal transplantation is a decrease in function unexplained by other findings. Infiltration of the kidney by cells and the associated edema may cause gross enlargement of the organ, associated with tenseness. Sometimes the swelling becomes so great that flow is curtailed by enclosure within a tight capsule sufficient to cause acute renal failure, which may persist for several days after resolution of the rejection episode. The diminution of blood flow may be detected by radioisotopic scans or even angiograms. Also, hypertension may occur because of the elaboration of renin. Inflammation of the kidney may involve the surrounding tissue to cause pain, especially upon palpation, and the patient may become febrile, occasionally with temperatures as high as 104°F, making the decision to treat with intensified immunosuppression even more difficult. Blood changes may include elevated LDH, lymphocytosis and elevated ESR, all nonspecific findings. Decreased urinary sodium, elevated urinary lysozyme (and other enzymes) and lymphocyte rosetting about tubular epithelial cells in the urine are more suggestive, but still not diagnostic of acute rejection. At the present time, no one test or finding is diagnostic of rejection and the clinician must carefully weigh the evidence for or against rejection, with decreased renal function assuming major importance.

The manifestations of acute rejection of other organs or tissues are similar to those found with the kidney, with a diminution of function being the most reliable, although a late, finding.

Chronic Rejection

In this type of rejection, loss of function is more gradual, sometimes occurring over months to years with renal allografts, and it is of relatively late onset.

The pathologic lesion of chronic rejection is primarily one of progressive vascular occlusion. The arterioles are involved to the greatest degree, developing a markedly contracted lumen associated with subintimal thickening, en-

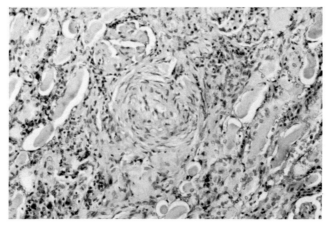

Figure 15–4. Microscopic appearance of a dog kidney showing vascular lesions often found in chronic rejection. The artery in the center is almost completely obliterated. ×63.

dothelial cell proliferation, disruption of the internal elastic lamina, and defects of the media (Fig. 15–4). Since these vessels are largely terminal without collateral circulation, focal ischemic areas develop, which progress to fibrosis.

Most authorities feel that chronic rejection is mediated by humoral processes, but there is little direct evidence to support this view. At least in some cases, the lesions of chronic rejection may simply represent healing lesions of acute rejection. The cellular infiltrate is usually not impressive in the chronic lesions, but they also do not always show the presence of immunoglobulins. Both sensitized T cells and antibody with specificity directed against donor cells may be found in the blood of the recipient. Recently, there has been a good correlation reported between the presence of lymphocyte dependent antibody and chronic rejection in patients. The development of chronic vascular lesions in allogeneic transplants given to athymic, T cell-depleted animals provides perhaps the best evidence that chronic rejection is antibody-mediated.

The clinical manifestations of chronic rejection of the kidney include hypertension, proteinuria, and a slow but progressive decrease in function.

HISTOCOMPATIBILITY TESTING

It has long been obvious from both early human kidney transplants and animal experiments that grafts between closely related individuals survive considerably longer than grafts from unrelated individuals. Further refinement of these observations led to extensive investigations of the relationship between genetic factors and graft survival. Both the questions asked and the answers obtained have been extraordinarily complex, and many relationships between genetics and transplantation are still far from clear. In fact, the picture is only now beginning to emerge in sufficient detail that orderly analyses can begin to be made.

Histocompatibility is a term used to designate antigenic individuality within members of a species. It is determined by the presence of histocompatibility antigens (also called transplantation antigens) expressed primarily on the surface of nucleated cells. The presence of these antigens is determined by genes at several loci, but the ones of major importance are clustered together on a single chromosome. This region is called the major histocompatibility complex (MHC). The MHC in man is located on chromosome 6 and has been designated the HLA region (for human leukocyte antigen). In mice, this region is referred to as the H2 region; in chickens, as the B region; and in rats, it is the AgB region. The H2 region of mice and the HLA region of man, which are the best studied, have a remarkable similarity.

THE HLA REGION

The HLA region has been partially mapped, and at least four genetic loci hve been established, which bear a major relationship to histocompatibility (Fig. 15–5). In addition, other loci have important relationships to other aspects of the immune processes, in particular, the presence of loci for coding for certain complement components and for determining the ability of an individual to respond to certain antigens (the Ir loci). It is indeed amazing that nearly all of the genes in the complex appear to be involved as a functional unit in the immune response in one way or another.

The four major HLA loci each have several known antigenic specificities (alleles), as indicated in Table 15–2, as well as many more probable antigens yet to be defined. The HLA-A, HLA-B and HLA-C loci all code for antigens which are usually defined by serologic methods, and because of this, they are sometimes called serologically defined (SD) antigens. These antigens have several specificities, much like blood group antigens, which may be "public" (i.e., shared) or "private" (i.e., specific). In addition, serologic testing shows considerable cross-reactivity between specific antigens (e.g., between A29, AW30, AW31, AW32, and AW33; A9, AW23, and AW24; and B7, BW22, and B27). The HLA-D region codes for antigens that are located on

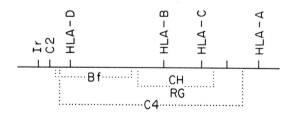

Figure 15–5. Conceptual diagram of the HLA region.

Bf Factor B
CH Chido Blood group
RG Rogers Blood group
Ir Immunoregulatory region

TABLE 15–2. ANTIGENIC SPECIFICITIES OF HLA*

HLA-A	HLA-B	HLA-C	HLA-D
A1	B5	CW1	DW1
A2	B7	CW2	DW2
A3	B8	CW3	DW3
A9	B12	CW4	DW4
A10	B13	CW5	DW5
A11	B14		DW6
A28	B18		
A29	B27		
AW23	BW15		
AW24	BW16		
AW25	BW17		
AW26	BW21		
AW30	BW22		
AW31	BW35		
AW32	BW37		
AW33	BW38		
AW34	BW39		
AW36	BW40		
AW43	BW41		
	BW42		

*Presence of a W means the specificities are still tentative.

lymphocytes, and their presence can be determined by mixed lymphocyte culture. Therefore, they are sometimes called lymphocyte-defined (LD) antigens. Recent evidence indicates that the LD antigens may be expressed on B lymphocytes, but not very well on T lymphocytes. Because of this, sera have been developed which have B cell specificity, and it appears that at least some of these may be able to define LD specificities (i.e., HLA-D antigens). If so, rapid typing of cadaveric donors will be possible to allow better matching at this locus. HLA-D antigens have also been demonstrated on sperm, macrophages, skin cells, and perhaps others.

RELATIONSHIP OF HISTOCOMPATIBILITY TESTING IN GRAFT SURVIVAL

Extensive experience has shown that for living related donors, renal allograft survival is closely linked to histocompatibility. Siblings who share identical HLA-A and HLA-B antigens and who do not stimulate in mixed lymphocyte cultures (MLC negative) have excellent long-term results with almost no loss from rejection (Fig. 15–1). On the other hand, HLA-A and HLA-B identical, MLC nonstimulating, living related, sibling donor grafts have been reported (rarely) that have vigorously rejected, indicating that the HLA determinants are not the only important variables of histocompatibility. Grafts from many thousands of cadaveric donors have now been analyzed statistically for the relationship of SD antigens and long-term organ survival. These analyses provide clear indication that a well matched graft has a better chance for ultimate acceptance than a poorly matched one, about 10 to 15 per cent better for four antigen matches (no mismatches at HLA-A and HLA-

B loci) compared to complete (four antigen) mismatches, with intermediate degrees of success varying with the number of shared antigens.

In retrospective studies, compatibility of HLA-D locus, as evidenced by MLC reactivity, has been associated with considerably better results than incompatibility for both living donor and cadaveric grafts. This type of test is not suitable for selection of cadaveric donors at the present time, but if B cell typing can be developed which correlates well with MLC to measure HLA-D specificity, a great advance will have been made for improved selection of cadveric donor–recipient combinations. Another technique to detect HLA-D specificities has recently been introduced that utilizes "primed" lymphocytes or PHA-induced blasts from the prospective recipient. Further refinement of such tests may allow HLA-D typing within 36 to 48 hours to permit prospective selection of cadaveric donor–receipient combinations. At the present time, the MLC test appears to be the most discriminating index of compatibility for selecting the best among several potential living related donors who are incompatible for HLA, HLA-B or HLA-C. Since HLA-D is closer to the HLA-B locus than the HLA-A locus in the major histocompatibility complex, it might be expected that compatibility for antigens in the HLA-B locus would be more important than compatibility at the HLA-A locus, and this seems to be borne out by clinical experience. Thus, it is better to share haplotype specificity for the B locus than the A locus for both living related and cadaveric donors.

There have been many attempts to determine whether or not some of the SD specificities are antigenically stronger than others, with somewhat varying results. Only the common antigen HLA-A2 has emerged as one which may be significantly more important than the others when there is incompatibility between donor and recipient.

It is also important to recognize the relationship between the histocompatibility antigens and erythrocyte antigens of man. The ABO antigens are widely distributed throughout the body and appear to be on the surface of most if not all types of cells. Since isohemagglutinins for the ABO antigens are almost invariably present in the serum of normal individuals, ABO incompatibilities of prospective donors must be excluded before histocompatibility testing is undertaken, since they will not be suitable donors. The Rh, MNS, and Lewis antigens are not present in significant quantities on the surface of leukocytes, platelets, and other cells, but the Kell, Duffy, and P antigens do appear to be present. Conversely, the histocompatibility antigens are not present in significant concentration on the surface of human erythrocytes. The histocompatibility antigens are well represented on the surface of leukocytes and platelets which can be obtained easily for examination. For this reason examination of leukocytes and platelets for the presence of histocompatibility antigens has formed the backbone for histcompatibility analysis.

Leukocyte Typing. A variety of serologic techniques for the detection of antigen-antibody reactions between appropriate antisera and leukocytes or platelets has been devised. These include complement fixation tests, lymphocyte cytotoxicity tests, leukoagglutination tests, immunofluorescence tests, mixed hemagglutination tests, antiglobulin consumption tetsts, and immune adherence tests.

Using the same sets of sera and cells, occasional and sometimes striking discrepancies occur between the results from lymphoagglutination tests and lymphocyte cytotoxicity tests. Negative agglutination tests when there is a positive cytotoxicity test could best be explained by location of the antigen deep within folds of the surface membrane, and negative cytotoxicity tests in the presence of a positive agglutination test might be explained by either a low antigenic density on the membrane or by the presence of antibodies which do not fix complement. Lymphocyte cytotoxicity tests are most used at the present time.

Antisera for the detection of leukocyte antibodies are most frequently obtained from patients who have received multiple transfusions or from multiparous women. Approximately one third of these women, after the fourth or fifth pregnancy, develop detectable serum antibody against histocompatibility antigens of the fetus, which have been inherited from the father. Of these antisera, only a few have been found to be monospecific. Useful antisera for typing can sometimes be obtained from persons who have rejected grafts. The results of the lymphocyte cytotoxicity tests are analyzed, after the lymphocyte antigens have been identified, by reacting the cells with groups of antisera (Fig. 15–6).

Mixed Lymphocyte Culture. When antigens are added to cultures of lymphocytes, they may stimulate cellular division and transformation of the lymphocytes into more primitive or blast-like forms. The degree of reactivity of the lymphocytes in these tests can be estimated by visual counting of the percentage of lymphocytes that have undergone transformation, but a more accurate and less laborious estimate of transformation can be obtained by measurement of the incorporation of a radioisotope-labeled DNA precursor into the cell. DNA synthesis is usually estimated using the incorporation of tritiated thymidine as an indicator, and similar measures of transformation can be made by studying RNA and protein synthesis with appropriate isotopes.

Since stronger antigens elicit a greater in vitro immune response than do weaker ones, early workers reasoned that the lymphocyte stimulation tests would be a practical way to measure directly the degree of histocompatibility differences between lymphoid cells. Tests were soon devised in which the lymphocytes of a prospective recipient were mixed in cultures with the lymphocytes of each of several prospective donors. At the end of the period of incubation (usually four to seven days) tritiated thymidine was added, and counts were made for the incorporation of the radioisotope by lymphocytes. Those tests with low counts indicated that minor antigenic differences existed between the two individuals. These tests, however, proved to be imperfect because the lymphocytes of both recipient and donor stimulated each other, and falsely high counts were often obtained. This problem has been circumvented by treating the cells of the donor in such a way that they become unable to divide and incorporate thymidine, but they continue to live and retain antigenicity. Two methods have been used to

Lymphocyte Antigens

D or R	Name	RBC	Relation	A				AW		A	AW		A			AW —19—							B								BW												CW					XM	Grade
				1	2	3	9	23	24	10	25	26	11	28	29	30	31	32	33	34	36	43	5	7	8	12	13	14	18	27	15	16	17	21	22	35	37	38	39	40	41	42	1	2	3	4	5		
	Recipient	0			+														+											+										+				+					
	Donor 1	0	M		+														+							⊕				+													⊕					Neg	C
	Donor 2	0	F							⊕									+																					+				+				Neg	C
	Donor 3	0	Bro		+														+											+										+				+				Neg	A
	Donor 4	0	Sis							⊕									+							⊕																						Neg	D

A = 1st Locus B = 2nd Locus C = 3rd Locus W = Tentative Designation

Figure 15–6. Representative example of a tissue typing report used for selection of a living related donor from the recipient's immediate family. Occasionally, mother and father have a common antigen or either may have inherited the same antigen from their mother and father, as appears to be the case in this example. Donor 4 has only three antigens for the HLA-A and HLA-B loci, with a "double dose" of AW33. Donor 3 has inherited identical antigens to the recipient and clearly would be the best among the donors available.

TABLE 15–3.   EXAMPLE OF MLC TEST FOR SELECTION OF
MOST SUITABLE DONOR

Donor or Recipient Name	Relationship	Stimulation Index°
Recipient		
Donor 1	Brother (A match)	1.4
Donor 2	Sister (D match)	2.5
Donor 3	Mother (D match)	9.8
Donor 4	Unrelated	26.1
Donor 5	Unrelated	18.0

$$°\text{The Stimulation Index} = \frac{\text{CPM recipient cells + irradiated donor cells}}{\text{CPM recipient cells + irradiated recipient cells}}.$$

produce this influence: treatment of the cells with mitomycin-C, and irradiation. Both of these modifications of the mixed lymphocyte culture provide a one-way stimulation of the recipient's lymphocytes that seems satisfactory. It is of critical importance to standarize the number of lymphocytes from various donors, and comparisons between prospective donors must be run on the same day to obtain identical conditions. Enough macrophages from the recipient must be included in the cultures to ensure processing of the antigen. Good correlation between length of skin graft survival and ranking by the one-way mixed lymphocyte culture has been obtained. This has been most dramatically demonstrated among related family members. An example of application of an MLC test for selection of suitable donor is given in Table 15–3.

PREOPERATIVE EVALUATION OF IMMUNE RESPONSIVENESS

In addition to histocompatibility differences between donor and recipient, there are other variables of importance in determining graft survival. One of these is the innate ability of the recipient to respond to an immune stimulus. Cell-mediated responses and the ability to synthesize cytotoxic antibody seem to be of importance.

When the ability to become sensitized to DNCB was used as a measure of integrity of delayed hypersensitivity mechanisms, one study showed a graft survival rate three times higher in DNCB negative patients compared to DNCB positive patients (76 versus 23 per cent). Responsiveness to recall antigens showed a less spectacular trend in the same direction. Preoperative responsiveness of recipient lymphocytes to in vitro stimulation with PHA or Con-A has also correlated well with graft survival, high responders having a 44 per cent one-year graft survival versus 83 per cent for low responders.

Patients on hemodialysis often develop in their serum antibodies that are cytotoxic to lymphocytes from random donors. It has been demonstrated by some investigators that the results became progressively worse in patients who had increasing amounts of cytotoxic antibody. However, others have shown that most of such losses are a result of hyperacute or accelerated rejection and that by the use of very sensitive cross-match techniques to test all available sera against cells of potential donors and to exclude positive donors, transplantation can be accomplished with success equal to that obtained in recipients not having cytotoxic antibodies in their sera. Unfortunately, no other measure of B cell function has been correlated with subsequent graft survival.

STANDARD IMMUNOSUPPRESSION

The effect of immunosuppressive drugs on the immune system and other means for achieving negative immunologic adaptation were discussed at length in Chapter 9. Among the numerous immunosuppressive drugs available, only azathioprine and prednisone are used with great regularity. However, there is significant variability from center to center concerning dosage and timing.

In patients with good renal function, it is customary in most centers to give azathioprine once daily in a dose of 2.0 to 2.5 mgm per kg indefinitely, decreasing the dose only for leukopenia or in patients with kidneys from histocompatible donors. Lesser doses result in an increased loss from rejection. There is some evidence that splenectomy in selected patients may allow tolerance of a higher maintenance dose of azathioprine. In the presence of severe renal failure, the daily dose should be decreased to no more than 1.5 mgm per kg per day, to avoid a cumulative affect which may result in severe leukopenia two to three weeks later. The dose of azathioprine is not increased for the treatment of acute rejection episodes. In patients who are intolerant of azathioprine because of an exaggerated effect on the bone marrow or (rarely) a drug-induced nephritis, cyclophosphamide is sometimes substituted with clinical results comparable to those obtained with azathioprine.

Adrenocortical steroids form the backbone of immunosuppressive therapy for most patients. At our center, adult patients of 60 to 80 kg who receive cadaveric renal allografts are initially given prednisone 200 mgm preoperatively, then methylprednisolone, 500 mgm IV during the operation. On the first postoperative day, 400 mgm of methylprednisolone or prednisone is given IV or orally, and on each subsequent day, there is a reduction in daily dosage of 50 mgm per day until a dosage of 200 mgm per day is reached. Then the dosage is reduced 10 mgm per day until a daily dosage of 100 mgm per day is reached, with further reduction of 5 mgm per day until 60 mgm per day is reached. Stepwise reduction is then slowed, to achieve a dose of about 35 mgm per day by 90 days and 15 to 20 mgm per day by the end of a year. Maintenance steroid dosages are reduced more rapidly for living related donors, especially when they are histocompatible. Rejection episodes may require treatment with an increase in the maintenance dosage and the administration of intermittent intravenous "pulses" of methyl prednisolone, 250 to 500 mgm daily for a total dose of no more than 3000 mgm.

Antilymphocyte globulin has been used in many transplant centers, but the beneficial effects of routine use are still somewhat in question because various lots of it have been shown to be clinically inactive. Nevertheless, with at least some lots of ALG, cadaveric allograft survival at one year has been improved by about 20 per cent in well controlled studies.

X-irradiation of the graft to destroy immunocytes has been used frequently as an adjunct for the treatment of acute rejection episodes. Usually, 150 rads are given to the graft daily or every other day for a total of up to four times for a single rejection episode, with no more than 1050 rads total for the kidney.

Since vascular occlusion and platelet deposition are significant events in the rejection process, antiplatelet drugs or anticoagulants or both have been advocated by some investigators to lessen the pathologic consequences of rejection episodes. Reported success of such programs has been variable, but their use has resulted in no detectable benefit in patients treated at our institutions. Certainly, this type of treatment has no significant effect on the basic immune mechanism.

OTHER METHODS FOR MODIFICATION OF HOST RESPONSIVENESS

BLOOD TRANSFUSIONS

During the past few years, there has been increasing evidence that patients who receive multiple blood transfusions while they are on dialysis have better graft survival than those who have received none, despite the fact that many patients given multiple transfusions develop cytotoxic antibodies. One proposed explanation was that the transfusions had divided the patients into two groups: a low responder group without cytotoxic antibodies who were not likely to develop a hyperacute or accelerated rejection, and a high responder group with cytotoxic antibody who were difficult to match with a suitable kidney and had an increased likelihood for an antibody-mediated rejection. Many of the latter group may not have been transplanted thereby removing more immunologically competent individuals from the analysis. No such segregation could take place in nontransfused patients. This explanation did not completely explain the observations, however, and it is now believed that enhancing antibodies or a type of low dose tolerance induced by histocompatibility antigens in blood contributed to the observed improvement in success. Still another explanation, which has not been fully evaluated, is that patients requiring multiple transfusions are sicker, with a greater acquired depression of their cellular immune responses.

ENHANCEMENT

Enhancement is used to describe prolongation of graft survival by the presence of specific antidonor antibody. The immunobiology of this important mechanism is discussed more completely in Chapter 9. It has a very important role in transplantation, and it has been repeatedly demonstrated that the presence of blocking (enhancing) antibody will significantly prolong graft survival. In one group of experiments in rats with major histocompatible differences, the passive administration of blocking antibody as the sole immunosuppressive agent achieved long-lasting graft survival in most animals and permanent survival in some. Low doses of antigen to achieve enhancement have also been quite successful in the laboratory in a variety of experimental animals, but on occasion, sensitization rather than enhancement occurs, and the technique is not yet safe for clinical application. In recent studies, enhancement has been achieved by giving blood-associated antigens and also by antigen-antibody complexes.

There has recently been interest in the use of retroplacental source gamma globulin (RPGG) as a biologically active agent to achieve immunosuppression. RPGG has been found to inhibit MLC responses and responses of T cells to phytomitogens. It also has some lymphocytotoxicity in high concentrations. Early clinical trials suggest improved graft survival after its administration, probably by a mechanism of enhancement.

ANTIRECEPTOR ANTIBODY

One of the most exciting new areas of research in the field of transplantation relates to the immunosuppressive effects of antireceptor antibody. In reality, this is antiidiotypic antibody, as discussed earlier in Chapter 9, and arises as a result of an immune response of an individual against the combining site of an antibody, especially when complexed to antigen in antibody excess. Grafting of kidneys in animals with high levels of actively or passively induced specific antireceptor antibody often results in long-lasting or permanent survival. This may be and probably is the primary mechanism operative in enhancement and may be important in the regulation of many immune responses. In some experiments, even antibody against crude or nonspecific IgG, given passively, has prolonged graft survival. Procedures to enhance the synthesis of antiidiotypic antibody still need refinement before the principles can be applied to clinical transplantation, but there is little doubt that they will someday be of significant value.

STEM CELL TRANSPLANTATION

One of the most exciting areas of current research involves the transplantation of stem cells from fetal liver to replace a destroyed bone marrow. In this technique, lethal doses of total body irradiation or cyclophosphamide are given to an animal, which is then given fetal liver cells from a genetically unrelated, histoincompatible donor to provide a source of stem cells. Such animals do not reject the engrafted cells, nor do they develop graft versus host reactions. Instead, their bone marrow becomes populated with normal functional cells of the donor. Such animals can subsequently be grafted with adult skin from the donor strain without rejection, even when immunosuppression is not given, but skin from donors of other strains is readily rejected. This technique has now been applied with equal success to a few humans, but the supply of appropriate stem cells without postthymic cells is a major limiting factor in its widespread application. Once the techniques for isolation and cultivation of stem cells are worked out, it may be possible to use bone marrow stem cell transplantation as a prelude to transplantation of solid organs from the same donor.

IMMUNOLOGIC ADAPTATION OF LONG-LASTING GRAFTS

Many allogeneic grafts develop a special relationship to the hostile environment of their host, which permits long-term survival, and in some instances, even complete discontinuance of immunosuppressive therapy does not result in rejection. Studies in such patients with long-lasting grafts show that cell-mediated immune responses of the hosts' lymphocytes against donor cells persist indefinitely, but that this reaction is blocked by factors in the recipient's serum. At least some and perhaps all of this blocking activity is composed of IgG antibody, but it has not yet been determined whether the important fraction has antiidiotypic specificity or donor antigenic specificity. In most patients with long-standing grafts, there is also a decreased ability to generate cytotoxic T cells in vitro when stimulated when donor antigen. The role of the suppressor T cell in graft maintenance has not been sufficiently studied, and it would appear at the present time that a form of enhancement is the most important mechanism for long-term graft adaptation. Future studies of suppressor cell influences may yield practical approaches to control graft rejection.

POSTOPERATIVE IMMUNOLOGIC MONITORING

Many investigators now feel that monitoring a patient's immune response following transplantation will aid in detection and management of rejection episodes and diminish the incidence and severity of infection through directed use of immunosuppression. Such goals can now be only partially achieved, but several observations of importance have already been made: (1) The appearance of blocking IgG antibody that will inhibit mixed lymphocyte reactions is consistent with an excellent posttransplant course and few rejections. (2) The appearance of endothelial cell antibody or antibody that participates in antibody dependent cell-mediated cytotoxicity reactions is associated with chronic progressive rejection. (3) The appearance of cytotoxic antibody in the serum is often associated with acute rejection episodes. (4) Lymphocyte responsiveness to donor cells (MLC), circulating levels of T cells, and responsiveness of recipient lymphocyte to PHA have not correlated well with rejection episodes or eventual success. (5) A depression in the generation of cytotoxic effector cells when recipient cells are stimulated in vitro with donor cells has been associated with immunologic adaptation of the graft. (6) Rejection episodes are associated with the appearance of increased numbers of tubular cells in the urine which have lymphocytes rosetted about them. (7) Decreased T cell numbers and function are significantly associated with the appearance of viral, protozoal, and fungal infections. (8) Abnormalities of the antibacterial function of neutrophils or depressed levels of complement lead to an increased susceptibility to bacterial infections.

The tests that will be of greatest practical importance in the day-to-day management of transplant patients remain to be determined.

MODIFICATION OF GRAFT ANTIGENICITY

For several years it has been known that a graft could be modified in such a way that acceptance could be prolonged when it was transplanted to an antigenically incompatible host. Perhaps the first such evidence came from experiments with skin grafts. In vitro treatment of grafts with steroids, antilymphocyte globulin, antidonor antibody, x-irradiation, and even formalin could delay rejection. At first the reason for this delay was thought to be simple modification of antigens expressed on cells of the graft. However, another group of experiments using donor skin from lethally irradiated rats suggested that "passenger leukocytes" present in the graft might be largely responsible for induction of the immune response against transplanted tissues. In these experiments, skin taken soon after the lethal irradiation and transplanted to normal rats rejected at the expected time. However, as the length of time between irradiation and taking of the skin for grafting increased, so did the length of graft survival in an unrelated normal recipient. The effect on graft survival was marked when skin was taken a week or more after irradiation and correlated well with the disappearance of lymphocytes from the blood and tissues.

Perhaps the most compelling evidence of a role for passenger leukocytes comes from a recent experiment in which thyroid allografts modified by long-term tissue culture could be transplanted beneath the renal capsule with prolonged graft survival. However, when fresh donor lymph node cells from the donor strain were injected on the day of transplantation, the effects of organ culture were abolished. Even this experiment does not clearly distinguish between the induction effects of antigens on passenger leukocytes and the induction effects of antigens expressed primarily on vascular and parenchymal cells of the graft, since the effector response remained intact.

Organ culture has been the method of modification of graft antigenicity that has been the most popularized and controversial, largely because of the now infamous misdirected efforts of a single investigator. This young man showed that survival of skin allografts could be significantly prolonged by in vitro culture, but he misinterpreted some of his experiments to reach the conclusion that permanent survival could be achieved with cultured skin transplanted across major histocompatible barriers. In his effort to prove this interpretation correct, experimental data were falsified; exposure of this fact in both the scientific and lay press quickly led to abandonment of experiments on organ culture by the majority of the scientific community interested in the problem. However, it is now clear that long-term culture of some tissues in vitro can regularly result in a degree of modification of graft antigenicity and prolonged, albeit not permanent, take of subsequent grafts to an unrelated incompatible recipient. This finding promises to be of benefit in transplantation of certain endocrine organs, pancreatic islet cells, cornea, thymus, and possibly even bone marrow and skin. Furthermore, subsequent experiments should lead to a better understanding of how "transplantation" antigens are expressed by cells of vascularized grafts.

The compelling interpretation of the above experiments is that short-lived and radiosensitive cells, probably lymphoid in origin, are primarily responsible for the inductive phase of the immune response following transplantation of vascularized grafts. Recently, this "principle" has been put to practice in clinical organ transplantation. At least two centers are treating heart-beating cadaveric donors with lethal doses of cyclophosphamide before harvesting of the kidneys, in an effort to kill "passenger leukocytes." Preliminary results suggest improved long-term survival of the transplanted kidneys. However, these initial studies are not sufficiently controlled to be conclusive. Pharmacologic doses of steroids have also been given to prospective cadaveric donors, but the improved results seem to be related more to protection from ischemic damage of the organ than to modification of graft antigenicity.

The use of RNA and concanavallin A in solutions used to flush kidneys before transplantation has also been reported to prolong graft survival, but the mechanisms involved are not yet clear.

PRESERVATION AND IMMUNOLOGIC INJURY

It has now been conclusively demonstrated that preservation by pulsatile perfusion using cryoprecipitated plasma may result in immunologic damage of the preserved organ if specific antibodies directed against histocompatibility antigens or other antigens expressed on the vascular endothelium are present in the perfusate. Such antibodies can cause damage by absorption to the graft during perfusion and activation of complement upon revascularization in the host. The type of damage that may occur, therefore, closely resembles hyperacute or accelerated rejection. This complication can be reduced markedly by using only AB positive or type specific plasma from male donors not previously transfused, who are prescreened for the absence of antibodies against HLA and erythrocyte antigens, and who have low titers of cold hemagglutinins. By additionally using plasma from only a single donor and routinely performing a cross-match between the perfusate plasma and donor lymphocytes, the incidence of immunologic damage from perfusion can be virtually eliminated.

MATERNAL-FETAL RELATIONSHIPS

The developing fetus represents the most successful of all transplants. Yet, the fetus possesses antigens of paternal origin that are fully capable of stimulating a vigorous response in the mother. In fact, there is good evidence that sensitivity to fetal antigens develops regularly during pregnancy. Cell-mediated immune reactivity against paternal antigens following pregnancy has been demonstrated regularly in nearly all patients studied, and cytotoxic antibody can often be demonstrated as well.

Blocking factors may play an important role in the maternal acceptance of a fetus. One of these blocking factors, human chorionic gonadotropin (HCG), is a potent inhibitor of mixed lymphocyte reactions in vitro. Alpha fetoprotein, another glycoprotein, has been implicated as an inhibitor of the immune response during pregnancy. It is produced by the fetus, largely in the liver but perhaps also by the placenta. Levels in the maternal circulation are probably not high enough to produce a suppressive effect, but placental levels and fetal levels are high. In addition, eluates from placentas have blocking factors that appear to be IgG in nature, but the specificity is not against HLA antigens. Maternal serum also contains a blocking IgG antibody that can be removed by absorption with paternal lymphocytes, but not random platelets, which would remove HLA-A, HLA-B and HLA-C specificities. Patients with chronic abortion have been found to lack this blocking factor in their serum. Also, female animals hypersensitized by repeated skin grafts from paternal strains have a high incidence of stillbirths and neonatal deaths, and the placentas of such offspring show marked inflammatory changes. There is some evidence that nonspecific suppressor lymphocytes are capable of inhibiting expression of cell-mediated immunity of the maternal cells toward fetal antigens.

All in all, the important relationships between immunologic responses of the mother to her offspring are still not clearly defined, but progress in this area promises to aid the search for methods to establish successful long-term maintenance of other incompatible grafts.

16

Autoimmune Diseases

Autoimmune phenomena designate those immune responses of an individual to antigens normally present in the self. Autoimmune disease refers to the pathologic and physiologic alterations caused by autoimmune phenomena. Not surprisingly, autoimmune phenomena, although they must usually be considered to be abnormal, often do not produce disease and frequently occur in otherwise healthy individuals. Several examples exist where autoantibodies are found almost ubiquitously and include the presence of T agglutinin and anti-I cold autoantibody. About 12 per cent of normal persons have antibodies to smooth muscle, and this may increase to 80 per cent following viral infection. In addition, they are found in very frequent association with autoimmune diseases to specificities not associated with the disease. Further autoimmune phenomena often occur with infections or following tissue injury. Indeed, many authorities feel that autoimmune phenomena are part of the normal immunoregulatory process and that autoimmune disease results primarily from disorders of immunoregulation.

The autoimmune process can be initiated in a number of ways (Table 16–1). Viral infection and malignant transformation may result in the induction of new antigens, which may be released from the cell or expressed on the cell surface. Cellular injury or infection can produce enzymatic changes that can alter existing antigens to expose new antigenic sites or alter cell membranes to expose previously hidden antigens. Aging can also be associated with the appearance of new antigens or expression of previously hidden ones. Very often, small molecular haptens introduced into the body by a variety of means may become attached to normal tissue proteins which then act as carrier proteins, and an immune response is developed against both the hapten and its conjugated carrier protein. Antigens of bacterial viruses or foods entering the body may cross-react with antigens of the host and induce immune responses reactive with host antigenic constituents. Hereditary changes or genetic alterations may result in the expression of new antigens. Finally, the immune apparatus itself may become altered so that

234

**TABLE 16–1. POSSIBLE MECHANISMS IN INITIATION OF
AUTOIMMUNE PROCESS**

Expression of new antigens
    Virus infections, occasionally other forms of infection
    Malignant transformation
    Hereditary
    Genetic alteration (somatic mutation)

Exposure (unmasking) of hidden antigens
    Injury
    Infection

Alteration of normal antigens by haptens
    Drugs
    Environmental substances
    Infection, especially by viruses

Loss of tolerance of self-antigens

an abnormal response is elicited to antigens normally expressed on cells or tissues that in the healthy person do not initiate an immune response. Some investigators have felt that such types of autoimmunity may result from a failure of T cells to regulate lymphocyte function, either via a loss of suppressor T cell function or loss of tolerance of helper T cells to autoantigens. Both primary and secondary immunodeficiency states are associated with a higher incidence of autoimmune disease than might be expected. This observation also implicates aberrations of normal immune mechanisms in the pathogenesis. There is clearly a higher incidence of autoimmune disease in women and in family members of persons who have autoimmune diseases.

Regardless of the initial mechanism by which an autoantigen becomes an immunogenic substance, the subsequent immune response is similar to any other. Both cell-mediated and humoral immunity may be stimulated, often with one proportionally more vigorous than the other. All of the mechanisms of immunologic injury discussed in Chapter 8, with the possible exception of anaphylactic reactions and IgE-mediated responses, may occur as a result of this autoimmune process. Depending upon the antigen, its distribution, and the type of immunity which has been stimulated, all portions of the body and all major organ tissues and cellular systems may be affected. In some instances, the disease process is highly localized while in others, systemic disease results. To better illustrate the immunopathology and clinical relationships, only selected diseases of autoimmunity will be discussed. However, a listing of others is provided.

AUTOIMMUNE DISEASES OF A SYSTEMIC NATURE

Systemic manifestations may occur with many autoimmune diseases, but they are particularly prevalent in the so-called collagen diseases, many of which have autoimmune processes as a significant component of their pathogenesis (Table 16–2).

TABLE 16–2. AUTOIMMUNE DISEASES PRIMARILY OF A SYSTEMIC NATURE

Disease[*]	Probable Antigens	Experimental Model	Clinical Lesions	Comments on Immunopathology
Rheumatoid arthritis	IgG	Porcine arthritis by *Erysipelothrix insidiosa* infection Adjuvant arthritis	Arthritis Synovitis Vasculitis Amyloidosis Rheumatoid nodules	Rheumatoid factor is an IgM antibody reactive against native IgG. Some have Gm specificity. High synthesis in synovial tissues. Reaction with complement in joints causes accumulation of neutrophils, which cause joint damage by discharge of lysosomal enzymes.
Dermatomyositis (polymyositis)	Myosin?	Experimental allergic myositis	Muscle weakness, pain. Inflammation of muscle and sometimes skin	Elevated gamma globulin, rheumatoid factor, and ANA. May follow viral illness. May have vasculitis. Muscle infiltrated with lymphocytes. Major part of disease may be cell-mediated.
Sjögren's syndrome	Antigens of salivary glandular tissue?	?	Lymphoid infiltration of salivary and lacrimal gland. Sometimes involves lungs, kidneys. Decreased glandular secretions (sicca)	Association with rheumatoid disease. Rheumatoid factor often present, as are antinuclear antibodies.

Scleroderma	?	Sclerosis of dermis, esophagus, GI tract, kidney inflammation. Many with vasculitis	?	Hypergammaglobulinemia. Often ANA (40–70%). Occasionally associated hemolytic anemia and/or antimitochondrial antibody.
Polyarteritis nodosa	?	Fever, generalized pain, weakness, vascular insufficiency, hypertension, kidney failure	?	ANA or rheumatoid factor sometimes present.
Rheumatic fever	Sarcolemma and sarcoplasm in cardiac myofibrils and skeletal muscles, smooth muscle of vessel walls, and endocardium	Primarily vasculitis, carditis, serositis. Late cardiac valvular lesions	None suitable	M protein of group A *Streptococcus pyogenes* is the inciting antigen but secondary antigens may be involved. Some streptococcal antigens cross-react with histocompatibility antigens.

*SLE is discussed in the text.

Systemic Lupus Erythematosus (SLE)

SLE is a disease characterized by multisystemic involvement by a variety of autoimmune processes. There is an increased prevalence of other connective tissue diseases and asymptomatic autoimmune phenomena in families of affected patients. SLE affects females six to nine times more frequently than males and occurs primarily in young adults (10 to 35 yrs). Its relationship to virus disease is disputed, but many lupus patients have demonstrable C type viral particles in their cells on electron microscopy, and the disease both follows and is exacerbated by acute viral infections. However, bacterial infections, emotional stress, and ultraviolet irradiation can also trigger the acute onset of SLE. Several drugs, including hydralazine, hydantoins and procainamide, can cause a syndrome which has striking similarities to SLE of idiopathic nature. However, drug-induced lupus in contradistinction to idiopathic lupus, usually regresses upon withdrawal of the drug.

Clinically, SLE is associated with arthritis and arthralgia (95 per cent), cutaneous manifestations (81 per cent) which include a butterfly rash, maculopapular lesions, urticaria, alopecia, and photosensitivity, fever (77 per cent), neurologic and neuropsychiatric disorders (59 per cent), renal disease (53 per cent), cardiac manifestations (38 per cent), pulmonary disease (48 per cent), hemolytic anemia (5 per cent), leukopenia, thrombocytopenia, bleeding, susceptibility to infection, weight loss, hypertension, gastrointestinal complaints, hepatomegaly, splenomegaly, and ocular problems. Much of the clinical disease is attributable to deposition of complexes of antigen-antibody and complement in the tissues and blood vessels. These immune complexes are frequently deposited in the endothelium of small vessels. Irregular masses of antigen-antibody complexes can be demonstrated on the basement membrane of the kidney. These consist of antigen, antibody, complement, and fibrinogen. However, immune complex vasculitis in this disease can involve any organ or tissue, and this widely distributed process accounts for many of the protean manifestations. Pathologically, LE (hematoxylin) bodies, composed of collections of nuclei or nuclear components, form in tissues, especially in lymph nodes and peripherally in areas where necrosis has occurred. These LE bodies are the residue of phagocytized nuclei and cells. Complement is consumed in the process, inciting an inflammatory process by the release of mediators. Fibrinoid deposition is another important pathologic feature, the end result of an immunologic reaction against damaged cells. Fibrinoid can result in collagen formation and fibrosis.

Basic to the underlying immunologic mechanism of the disease is the formation of autoantibody to double-stranded DNA, single-stranded DNA, RNA, histone, and other nuclear components. These are responsible for the major symptom complexes (Fig. 16–1). However, autoantibodies may also occur against erythrocytes, platelets, lymphocytes, neutrophils, thyroglobulin, muscle, and clotting factors. Anti-IgG antibodies (rheumatoid factors) are found in about one third of patients with SLE, and they may play a role in the disease process. Thus, the disease is caused largely by antigen-antibody interactions which activate complement and cause inflammation, but autoim-

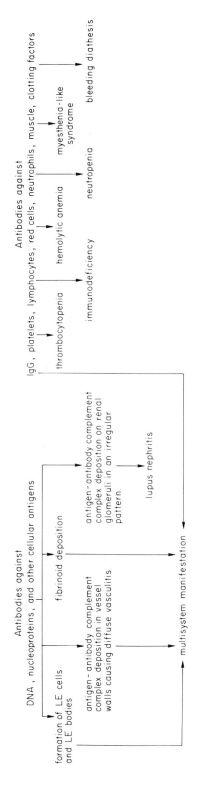

Figure 16–1. Mechanisms of immunopathology in SLE.

mune antibodies against specific nonnuclear antigens may result in additional clinical manifestations.

The laboratory diagnosis of SLE depends largely upon the demonstration of antibodies against nuclear components. While antibodies to both single-stranded and double-stranded DNA have been demonstrated, only those to the latter have diagnostic value. These can be demonstrated by a variety of tests. High titers of anti-DNA are highly associated with SLE, but low titers of anti-DNA are found in a variety of other diseases. The test for LE cells is performed on peripheral blood. IgG antibody to DNA-nucleoprotein enters dead cells and they are opsonized in the presence of complement. These are then phagocytized by normal cells, usually neutrophils, giving rise to the LE inclusion. On occasion, rosette formation occurs around an opsonized dead cell. Strong reactions (5 to 10 per cent of cells involved) indicate a high probability of SLE, but, like the presence of anti-DNA antibodies, the LE cell phenomenon may occur in association with other diseases.

Fortunately, an excellent animal model for human SLE exists in the New Zealand mouse, especially NZB/NZW hybrids. Antinuclear antibodies appear at about three months of age and subsequently appear in large amounts in virtually all animals. Renal disease follows in one to two months, and most of the animals die from renal disease before reaching one year of age. The occurrence of SLE in a colony of dogs has also been described.

Treatment of SLE depends primarily upon suppression of inflammatory reactions and the immune response. For this, corticosteroids have been the most useful drug. Many patients exhibit exacerbations and recurrences after remission of varying lengths of time and require treatment again. Both azathioprine and cyclophosphamide have been used, alone and in combination with corticosteroids, with varied results. From the standpoint of antibody suppression, cyclophosphamide should be superior to azathioprine, but this theoretical advantage has not been demonstrated clinically in controlled studies. The immunopotentiator levamisole has apparently caused remission in some patients. This finding might be interpreted to implicate an abnormal depression of T cell function in the pathogenesis of some cases of SLE.

AUTOIMMUNE DISEASES OF THE BLOOD

All of the formed elements of the blood may be involved in autoimmune reactions. These diseases are summarized in Table 16–3. Only the warm type of autoimmune hemolytic anemia will be discussed in detail.

Acquired hemolytic anemias were the first of the autoimmune diseases to be recognized and are the best studied. About 70 per cent of the time, these processes are associated with another disease of autoimmunity. Autoimmune hemolytic anemias have been separated into those caused by antibodies reacting best at warm temperatures (warm type) and those which react best at cold temperatures (cold type). The warm type is the most frequent.

TABLE 16–3. AUTOIMMUNE DISEASES OF THE FORMED ELEMENTS OF THE BLOOD

DISEASE[*]	PROBABLE ANTIGENS	CLINICAL LESIONS	EXPERIMENTAL MODEL	COMMENTS ON IMMUNOPATHOLOGY
Cold hemagglutinin disease	I or i, rarely Sp$_1$	Anemia, severity depends on thermal activity of the antibody. Renal failure from hemolysis rare. Disease associated with cirrhosis, malignancies, infectious mononucleosis, mycoplasma infections, sarcoidosis. Some patients later develop overt lymphoma	Immunization of rabbits with *Listeria monocytogenes*	Caused by IgM antibodies reacting best at 0–4° C with lesser avidities at higher temps. Usually dissociated at 37° C. Complement is fixed to red cell.
Paroxysmal cold hemoglobinuria	P	Hemolysis occurs when a body part is cooled below critical temp. (15–20° C). Hemolysis may occur with hemoglobinuria, fever, chills, hypotension, and abdominal and back pain. Associated with congenital syphilis and viral infections	?	Caused by cold antibodies of the IgG class, which strongly fix complement.
Idiopathic thrombocytopenic purpura	Surface antigens of platelet	Usually preceded by viral illness. Thrombocytopenia may respond to steroids, splenectomy, or cytotoxic drugs	Experimental thrombocytopenia	Serological tests not very good for detection of antibody. IgG antibody involved.
Neutropenia	Surface antigens of neutrophil	Susceptibility to infection	Experimental neutropenia	Antibody detected by anti-globulin consumption test.
Lymphopenia	Lymphocyte specific surface antigens	Secondary immunodeficiency	ALG administration in animals	Antibody much like heterologous antilymphocyte globulin.
Autoimmune aplastic anemia	Probably stem cell cell specific antigens	Hypoplasia of bone marrow	?	Seems to be T cell-mediated immunity. Occurs in about $\frac{1}{3}$ of all patients with aplastic anemia.

[*]Warm-type AIHA is discussed in the text.

WARM-TYPE AUTOIMMUNE HEMOLYTIC ANEMIA (AIHA)

Warm-type AIHA affects all ages and both sexes. This anemia nearly always involves antibodies of the IgG type although sometimes IgA or IgM occurs; the vast majority of these antibodies react with Rh or En antigens. Some fix complement, but many do not. Intravascular hemolysis occurs rarely. The patients' cells become coated only with IgG in 30 to 40 per cent, with IgG and complement in 50 per cent, and apparently only with complement in 10 to 20 per cent. In each case, IgG and/or complement may be readily detected by the direct antiglobulin (Coombs') test.

Erythrocytes coated with IgG are preferentially removed by the spleen, and splenectomy may be of benefit early in the disease. Because broader specificity often develops later in the disease with more fixation of complement, splenectomy becomes of less benefit. Transfusion tends to aggravate the disease and should be avoided whenever possible to prevent additional stimulation of the immune system by red cell antigens and to prevent further formation of autoantibody. Steroids may be of benefit, especially when given for a long time to suppress antibody formation. Cyclophosphamide or azathioprine should be considered in those patients refractory to treatment with adrenal steroids. Not infrequently, spontaneous regression occurs after weeks to years. In important recent studies, it has been shown that the autoantibodies in AIHA can be differentiated from those in lupus or malignant disease by an analysis that uses polybrene to eliminate electrostatic forces that keep the cells apart. When the divalent antibodies have attached, the polybrene is removed and heat applied, and a measurement of avidity of antibody is made. Greater energy of combination of the antibody to red cells is regularly observed with AIHA than with lupus or malignancy. This analysis has been completely automated and is often most helpful in differential diagnosis of hemolytic anemias associated with autoantibodies. The method increases the sensitivity of conventional analysis of autoantibodies to red blood cells as much as 1000-fold.

AUTOIMMUNE DISEASES OF THE KIDNEY

The kidney is frequently involved in autoimmune disease, both as the primary organ of attack and as an innocent bystander.

AUTOIMMUNITY AGAINST GLOMERULAR BASEMENT MEMBRANES

Goodpasture's syndrome is an uncommon disease of man that illustrates a directed immunologic assault. It regularly begins with respiratory infection, variable pulmonary infiltrations, and occasional hemoptysis, followed by a rapidly progressive renal disease in which hematuria, proteinuria, hypertension, and progressive azotemia are features. The untreated disease is characterized by a rapidly fatal course. In one collection of early cases, 50

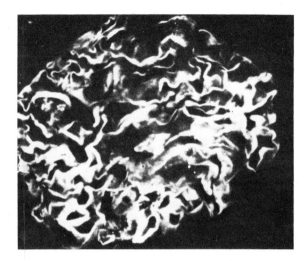

Figure 16–2. Linear deposits of IgG antibody and complement on the glomerular basement membrane in Goodpasture's syndrome,

of 52 patients died within a year of onset of the renal lesions. In contrast to lupus, the immunologic assault on the kidneys appears to be directed toward the basement membranes, similar to the immunologic assault in Masugi nephritis and in the Steblay model. Immunofluorescent examination of the kidneys and lungs in these patients shows that IgG and complement are deposited in a fine linear distribution along the basement membranes (Fig. 16–2). Just as in the Steblay model, nephrotoxic antibody can be eluted from the glomerular membranes of kidneys from patients with Goodpasture's syndrome. This nephrotoxic antibody has been shown to be capable of producing lethal glomerulonephritis upon intravenous injection into a monkey. Extraction of the gamma globulin from the kidney or lung of patients with Goodpasture's syndrome yields an antibody which is specific for the basement membranes of these two organs and which does not react with basement membranes in other parts of the body. Thus, certain of the pulmonary components and the entire renal disease in Goodpasture's syndrome can be attributed to an autoimmune assault in which immunologic injury is directed toward antigenic components in the basement membranes. Although the treatment of Goodpasture's syndrome is not entirely satisfactory at the present time, therapy with immunosuppressive regimens has led to cessation of progression in several instances and disappearance of the gamma globulin from the glomeruli. Transplantation is often an effective form of therapy when chronic renal failure develops, and bilateral nephrectomy is often effective in arresting the pulmonary hemorrhage.

IMMUNE COMPLEX NEPHRITIS

Deposition of immune complexes formed in the blood in the glomeruli of kidneys is the basis for the vast majority of autoimmune damage to the kidney even though the immunologic specificity is not directed toward antigens of the kidney.

A classic example of immune complex disease of the kidney is provided by SLE. Complexes of antigen-antibody–complement form in the blood and become deposited in the glomeruli, appearing in a granular distribution both by electron and fluorescent microscopy (Fig. 16–3). Complement is activated in the process, inducing inflammation and activating the clotting system. The lesions may regress with immunosuppressive treatment.

Acute poststreptococcal glomerulonephritis deserves consideration as an example of another form of immune complex disease. Infections with certain group A beta hemolytic streptococci, particularly types 12 and 49, are frequently followed by the onset of acute glomerulonephritis after an incubation period of 10 to 18 days. This disease is characterized by acute inflammation in the glomeruli, proliferation of endothelial cells, hypertension, and transient renal failure in many instances. Immunologic analysis of this renal disease reveals that gamma globulin and complement are deposited on the glomerular membranes, usually in a granular distribution, but occasionally in an interrupted linear distribution. Serum complement levels are low, and intravenously injected isotope-labeled C3 disappears rapidly from the blood, reflecting an excessive utilization of this complement component in the active phase of acute nephritis. Figure 16–4 shows the characteristic distribution of gamma globulin and complement on the glomeruli in this disease, and Figure 16–5 shows the typical large granular deposits on the epithelial side of the basement membrane, which are demonstrable by electron microscopy.

The complement profile in acute nephritis is quite different from that

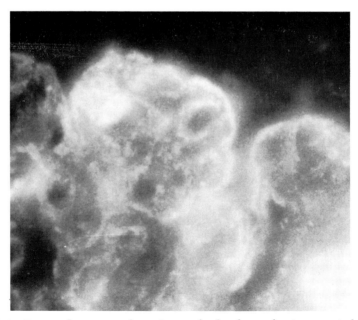

Figure 16–3. Immunofluorescent photomicrograph of a glomerulus in systemic lupus erythematosus (SLE) showing granular deposition of human IgG. (From Michael, A. F., et al., N. Engl. J. Med., 276:817–828, 1967.)

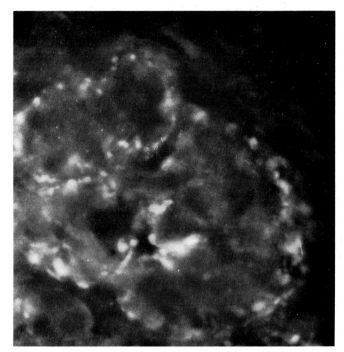

Figure 16–4. Immunofluorescent photomicrograph of a portion of a glomerulus in a patient with acute poststreptococcal glomerulonephritis, showing nodular deposits of β_{IC} globulin. (Courtesy of Dr. A. J. Fish.)

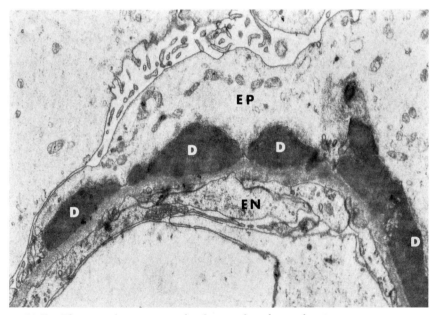

Figure 16–5. Electron photomicrograph of part of a glomerulus in acute poststreptococcal glomerulonephritis showing endothelial cell (EN) swelling and many electron-dense deposits (D) projecting from the epithelial (EP) side of the glomerular basement membrane. (From Fish, A. J., et al., Am. J. Pathol., 49:997–1022, 1966.)

observed in lupus, in which all complement components are depressed. Total complement levels are low with depression of C3 and the more terminal complement components, but there is a distinct sparing of C1 and C4. During acute glomerulonephritis, a heat labile factor can be demonstrated in the serum, which has the capacity to preferentially activate the system at the C3 step via the alternative pathway, much as occurs with endotoxin. Most patients with acute glomerulonephritis recover spontaneously, and recovery is preceded by return of serum complement and complement components to normal levels. With recovery, there is gradual disappearance of the deposits of gamma globulin and complement from the glomerular membranes.

In those few patients who do not recover from acute glomerulonephritis and proceed to develop chronic glomerulonephritis, the nature of the immunologic assault seems to change, and immunologic injury attributable to antibody directed toward the glomerular basement membrane has been demonstrated. Recently, investigators have observed that streptococcal antigen or an antigen that is cross-reactive with streptococci can regularly be demonstrated at the sites of gamma globulin and complement deposition in the kidney. This antigen can be demonstrated by antibodies present in the serum of normal persons and patients with glomerulonephritis, suggesting that the original antigen-antibody complex in the kidney was formed and deposited in antigen excess, as in serum sickness. The findings are compatible with the view that membrane damage and cellular proliferation in acute glomerulonephritis could be consequent to combination of circulating antibody with streptococcal antigen even following deposition of the antigen on the renal membranes.

In hypocomplementemic chronic progressive glomerulonephritis of childhood, progressive glomerulonephritis, hematuria, proteinuria, and a mild to moderate nephrotic syndrome are associated with the persistent presence of elevated levels of a heat labile activator of the complement system (NeF), which is similar to that found during acute glomerulonephritis. However, no evidence of prior infection with a nephritogenic strain of group A streptococcus exists, and instead of a short-lived period of indirect immunologic assault on the kidneys, which is characteristic of acute glomerulonephritis, one observes persistent and progressive renal disease over several years. The rate of progression is variable, and in a few patients the process seems to have arrested spontaneously. As in acute glomerulonephritis, this form of renal disease is associated with a decrease in total serum complement levels. The serum complement component profile reveals sparing of C1, C4, and to some extent, C2, with great depression of C3 and the terminal components. Irregular granular and lumpy deposits of gamma globulin and complement components in the kidney reflect the immunologic nature of the assault. The antigenic determinants of C3 that are deposited in the kidney are largely the A and D components, which reflects an immunologic activation of C3. The presence of properdin indicates activation of the alternative pathway. The immunohistochemical evidence of deposition of these complement components is regularly much more striking than is deposition of IgG or IgM. The half-life of β_{1c} (C3) in the serum is significantly shorter than normal in these patients.

It would seem that hypocomplementemic nephritis is a chronic progressive nephritis of older children resulting from an indirect assault on the kidneys by an antigen-antibody complex of unusual nature. The latter seems capable of preferential activation of the complement system at the C3 step. This immunologic amplification produces a unique complement profile, reflected in preferential accumulation of C3 components on the renal membranes. Progression of the disease is associated with persistence of the macromolecular complement inhibitor (or activator) in the blood. Deposition of fibrinogen in the kidneys has often been a feature of disease in these patients. Treatment has been unsatisfactory, but some patients have responded at least temporarily to cytotoxic and immunosuppressive regimens, and heparin has frequently produced return of complement levels toward normal, with improvement of renal function.

AUTOIMMUNE DISEASES OF ENDOCRINE ORGANS

All of the endocrine organs have been associated with autoimmune disease of one type or another. In fact, our knowledge about many endocrine diseases has been revolutionized during the past few years by the demonstration of these autoimmune phenomena.

THYROID DISEASE

Lymphocytic Thyroiditis. This disease, typified by Hashimoto's goiter, is characterized by diffuse infiltration of lymphocytes in the thyroid, which occasionally form germinal centers and replace normal structures. Common multifocal thyroiditis, severe atrophic thyroiditis, adult primary myxedema, and fibrosing thyroiditis are all considered variants of lymphocytic thyroiditis. This disease occurs much more frequently in women than men and is commonly associated with other autoimmune diseases.

Antibodies to at least four antigens are involved in the immune process: microsomal antigens, thyroid cell surface antigen, thyroglobulin, and a second colloid antigen. Antibodies to thyroglobulin increase with age and can be found in some 20 per cent of both sexes over the age of 70, about the same incidence as focal thyroiditis at autopsy. Cell-mediated immunity also occurs in Hashimoto's disease, and antibody dependent cell-mediated reactions have been demonstrated.

Treatment of the disease is relatively simple since replacement with thyroid hormone is quite effective for correction of hypothyroidism, and symptomatic goiters may be removed surgically.

Thyrotoxicosis. Graves' disease is another autoimmune disorder of the thyroid and occurs in the same families as patients with Hashimoto's goiter and myxedema. Studies of twins show a 60 per cent concordance rate of Graves' disease in monozygotic pairs, compared to 9 per cent in dizygotic twins. Focal thyroiditis is found in nearly all thyrotoxic glands. Its association with other autoimmune disorders is also well known.

At least three types of autoantibody occur in association with thyrotoxicosis. The first of these, long-acting thyroid stimulator (LATS), is a monoclonal IgG detectable by a mouse assay in 20 to 40 per cent of patients. The placental transfer of LATS during pregnancy can result in neonatal thyrotoxicosis, which subsides within weeks after birth. LATS apparently acts by binding at or near the TSH sensitive site where it activates the adenyl-cyclase-cyclic AMP system. Another IgG autoantibody, LATS protector, has been found in thyrotoxic sera. It blocks the absorption of LATS onto thyroid microsomes in vitro. Its role in the disease is unknown, but it may be responsible for negative bioassays for LATS. The third autoantibody in Graves' disease is called human specific thyroid stimulator (HTS). HTS will stimulate endocytosis and droplet formation. In addition to these, there may be a fourth autoantibody, which has the capacity to increase binding of TSH to retroorbital tissues to cause exophthalmos, thus completing the clinical picture with a nonthyroid complication that may be most difficult to manage.

AUTOIMMUNE DISEASES OF OTHER ENDOCRINE SYSTEMS

An abbreviated summary of these conditions is given in Table 16–4. Only those conditions are presented for which reasonably clear evidence of autoimmune mechanisms in the pathogenesis has been presented.

AUTOIMMUNE DISEASES OF THE NERVOUS SYSTEM

This group comprises a spectrum of diseases, not all of which have proven autoimmune etiology, although autoimmune phenomena seem to play a role in each. The best-studied of these diseases, from both a clinical and an experimental standpoint, is acute disseminated encephalomyelitis. Other autoimmune conditions of the nervous system are shown in Table 16–5.

ACUTE DISSEMINATED ENCEPHALOMYELITIS

This condition may develop following infection by either bacterial or viral agents. However, viral infections are a much more common predisposing cause, and these may include measles, mumps, rubella, influenza, vaccinia, smallpox, herpes, and infectious mononucleosis. There is usually a latent period of 5 to 30 days following the infection. Various immunizations may also precipitate acute disseminated encephalomyelitis. This complication most often occurs after vaccination for smallpox or, especially, rabies. The clinical manifestations include fever, photophobia, blindness, muscle

TABLE 16-4. AUTOIMMUNE DISEASES OF ENDOCRINE ORGANS (EXCLUSIVE OF THE THYROID)

DISEASE	PROBABLE ANTIGENS	CLINICAL LESIONS	EXPERIMENTAL MODEL	COMMENTS ON IMMUNOPATHOLOGY
Autoimmune adrenalitis (idiopathic Addison's disease)	Zona fasciculata microsomes and mitochondria	Female/male ratio 2.5:1. High ACTH, acute or chronic adrenal insufficiency	Experimental adrenalitis after injection of adrenal tissue with Freund's adjuvant. Can be passively transferred with lymphoid cells	Antiadrenal antibodies demonstrated by complement fixation + immunofluoresence in 65%. Association with primary ovarian failure, diabetes, hypoparathyroidism, thyroid diseases, and pernicious anemia.
Premature gonadal failure	Theca interna and corpus luteum of ovaries. Interstitial cells of testes (steroid-producing cells)	Gonadal failure	Immunization with gonadal tissues	Frequent association with idiopathic Addison's disease and idiopathic hypoparathyroidism. Frequent lymphocytic infiltration of organ.
Autoimmune diabetes mellitus	May be three types: insulin, insulin receptor, or islet cells	Primarily of juvenile onset. Usually insulin dependent and often insulin resistant	Experimental insulinitis	Early may have lymphocytic infiltration in pancreas. Onset may follow viral infection.
Idiopathic hypoparathyroidism	Parathyroid cells	Primarily in young people	Experimental immune hypoparathyroidism	Atrophy and lymphocytic infiltration.

TABLE 16–5. AUTOIMMUNE DISEASES OF THE NERVOUS SYSTEM

DISEASE*	PROBABLE ANTIGENS	CLINICAL LESIONS	EXPERIMENTAL MODEL	COMMENTS ON IMMUNOPATHOLOGY
Acute idiopathic polyneuritis (Guillain-Barré syndrome, Landry's paralysis)	Peripheral nerve myelin	Paresthesia and weakness. Ascending motor paralysis. Progressive for 1–2 weeks, then slow recovery when not fatal. Cranial nerve involvement	Allergic neuritis	60% have history of viral infection. Increased CSF protein without cells. May develop nephrotic syndrome or acute glomerulonephritis. Histological features and precipitating causes same as acute disseminated encephalomyelitis.
Multiple sclerosis	?	Paralysis	None	Not proved to be autoimmune in nature.

*Acute disseminated encephalomyelitis is discussed in the text.

weakness, decreased consciousness, seizures, paresis, paralysis, loss of appetite, and sphincter disturbance. Examination of the CSF shows increased protein and lymphocytosis.

Much of our understanding of this disease has come from the animal model called experimental allergic encephalomyelitis (EAE). Injection of brain tissue alone or, more recently, use of a purified peptide with complete Freund's adjuvant results in the development of an allergic disease of the brain after a latent period of about two weeks, with pathologic and clinical counterparts very similar to that seen in the human disease. Recent investigations concerning the specific antigen involved have resulted in the preparation of encephalitogenic factors (EF), the majority of which are highly basic and related to histones. Even the amino acid sequence for the antigenic specificity of EF has been determined. Gross examination of the brains of affected animals usually shows only hyperemia, but microscopic examination shows focal collections of T lymphocytes and disseminated perivascular lymphocytic infiltration. The first changes are in the axis cylinders, with demyelination occurring as a secondary feature.

While circulating antibody to EF has been demonstrated by a number of techniques, there is now rather clear evidence that at least the major pathology in EAE is mediated by sensitized lymphocytes, since the disease can be transferred by lymphocyte preparations but not by serum. In keeping with these findings, x-irradiation, neonatal thymectomy, immunosuppressive drugs, and postconvalescent (EAE) serum will prevent or favorably influence the disease. Steroid treatment has probably benefited "rabies immunization encephalomyelitis" when given during or following immunization for rabies using vaccines that employ central nervous tissue. This disease in man appears to be the exact counterpart of the experimental encephalomyelitis of experimental animals.

AUTOIMMUNE DISEASES OF THE STOMACH, INTESTINE, AND LIVER

GASTRIC ATROPHY AND PERNICIOUS ANEMIA

Atrophic gastritis, as evidenced by biopsy, affects about 20 to 30 per cent of an adult population, but occurs with increasing frequency with age, apparently progressing from a lesion of superficial gastritis. Gastric autoantibodies also increase with the age of a population (from 2 to 16 per cent), but are less common than the atrophic changes in the stomach. Pernicious anemia occurring as a clinical disease, of course, is much less common. Thus, parietal cell antibodies and intrinsic factor antibody can occur without causing pernicious anemia. Their presence is particularly associated with other diseases of autoimmunity, such as Graves' disease, myxedema, insulin dependent diabetes, and Addison's disease, and they occur with increased frequency in the families of patients with pernicious anemia, thyroid diseases, and other autoimmune disorders.

Pernicious anemia, however, is characteristically associated with the presence of parietal cell antibody, intrinsic factor antibody, or both, in patients with atrophic gastritis. Thus, it appears that the functional lesion depends upon lack of production of intrinsic factor or sufficient binding by antibody to prevent B_{12} absorption. In addition to the clear link between the presence of these antibodies and the clinical disease, the fact that pernicious anemia may respond to steroid therapy and will recur when steroids are withdrawn lends further support to the autoimmune nature of the disease. Also, infants born of mothers with intrinsic factor antibody may have suppression of intrinsic factor production for one to two months after birth, concurrent with disappearance of the placentally transferred antibody from the infant's circulation.

Autoimmune diseases of the intestine and liver are summarized in Table 16–6.

AUTOIMMUNE DISEASES OF MUSCLE

Polymyositis (dermatomyositis) has already been considered with the systemic autoimmune conditions. The other muscular disorder considered to be autoimmune in nature is myasthenia gravis. This disease is of particular interest because of its association with thymic abnormalities.

Myasthenia is characterized by muscle weakness and easy fatigability. Interestingly, it most commonly affects young females, with a peak incidence in the second decade, while the peak incidence in males is in the sixth decade. About 10 per cent of patients with myasthenia gravis have a thymoma. Another 80 per cent have thymic dysplasia or "thymitis," characterized by a normal-sized thymus with numerous germinal centers in the medulla, increased numbers of mast cells, plasma cells, and macrophages. With fluorescent-tagged antibody for an indicator, IgG can be demonstrated on myoid cells. In the remaining 10 per cent of patients, the thymus appears to be normal. About 80 per cent of patients improve following thymectomy. Muscle lesions are also an important feature of the disease, and they range from simple atrophy of the fibers to acute necrosis.

The precise role of antibody in the pathogenesis of the disease remains unsettled. However, antibodies are certainly present in these patients and react strongly with the striations of skeletal muscle, with heart muscle, and with the myoid cells in the thymus. During acute exacerbations, complement titers may become reduced, and serum from such patients may have a cytolytic effect on frog muscle in vitro. Neuromuscular transmission can also be inhibited by serum or by factors passing transplacentally to the newborn infant. It has recently been shown that some patients have an IgG antibody that reacts with the acetylcholine receptor in the myoneural junction. On the other hand, cell-mediated immunity to striated muscle is felt to be responsible for some of the damage, and the effect of soluble factors of the delayed hypersensitivity response on neuromuscular transmission has been suggested as a potential mechanism in the disease. Also, there is some evi-

TABLE 16–6. AUTOIMMUNE DISEASES OF THE INTESTINE AND LIVER

Disease	Probable Antigens	Clinical Lesions	Experimental Model	Comments on Immunopathology
Ulcerative colitis	Colonic mucosal cell	Diarrhea, mucosal ulceration. Responds to steroids and other immunosuppressive therapy	Animal models minimized with colon mucosa or intestinal bacteria	Possible cross-reactions with antigens of colon cells and *E. coli* may be etiologically important. Lesion heavily infiltrated with lymphocytes. Both autoimmune lymphocytotoxicity and autoimmune antibodies to colon have been demonstrated.
Chronic active hepatitis	Hepatocytes	Female/male ratio 3–4:1. Features of hepatitis. Disease often progressive but may respond to steroids. One form associated with hepatitis B infection, another associated with prior infection with hepatitis A	None satisfactory	Associated with arthritis, vasculitis, ulcerative colitis, hemolytic anemia, Sjögren's syndrome, diabetes, and thyroid disease. Hepatocellular necrosis associated with infiltration of lymphocytes and plasma cells. LE cells and antibody to nuclei, smooth muscle, ductal cells, hepatocytes, and mitochondria often present. Hypergammaglobulinemia.
Primary biliary cirrhosis	Bile ductal cells. Mitochondria	Intrahepatic cholestasis, obstructive jaundice, hepatosplenomegaly. More common in females. Steroids not effective	Rat model	Early inflammatory periportal infiltrate with lymphocytes, plasma cells, and eosinophils. Granulomatous reaction in some. Mitochondrial antibody present in 90%.

dence that the thymus itself elaborates a polypeptide that depresses neuro-muscular transmission, and this is supported clinically by the benefit of thymectomy.

In addition to thymectomy, myasthenia has been treated successfully with immunosuppressive drugs, including steroids, azathioprine, cyclophosphamide and others. That myasthenia gravis is a disease of autoimmunity is further evidenced by the ability to induce the disease in experimental animals. Repeated injections of either thymus or skeletal muscle extracts into guinea pigs or rats with FCA results in the development of a thymitis, defective neuromuscular transmission, and the appearance of antibodies against striated muscle, heart muscle, and thymic myoid cells. In addition, the South African rodent mastomys has a high incidence of thymomas associated with myositis, muscle atrophy, and myocarditis.

AUTOIMMUNE DISEASES OF THE EYE

Sympathetic ophthalmia typically follows penetrating injuries of the globe. Several days to weeks later, the injured eye may develop an endophthalmitis characterized by diffuse lymphocytic infiltration of the uvea. Weeks to years later, the other eye may spontaneously develop a similar lesion. Antiuveal antibody has been demonstrated in some patients. The disease can be induced experimentally by the injection of homologous uveal tissue with adjuvant.

Phacogenic uveitis (also called endophthalmitis phacoanaphylactica) may occur as a consequence of autosensitization to lens antigens as a result of injury, often caused by lens extraction. Reexposure to lens material may result in the development of a uveitis. The disease is easily produced in animals, and one interesting aspect is that the lens antigens appear to be similar or identical among many species.

Both of these diseases respond to steroid therapy.

OTHER DISEASES OF AUTOIMMUNITY

In addition to the above diseases, several others have autoimmune mechanisms as their basis. Included among these are allergic orchitis, which may occur because of autosensitization to spermatozoa. This has particular interest since it may follow operations for vasectomy or vas repair as well as traumatic injury to the testicle. Infertility can occur in this condition because of hypospermia or aspermia and also because of the presence of sperm-immobilizing antibodies excreted into the seminal fluid.

Injury to the myocardium appears to result in subsequent autoimmune disease of the heart in some patients. This condition is often referred to as the postcardiotomy syndrome when it follows surgery or postmyocardial infarction (Dressler's) syndrome when it follows coronary occlusion. In both of these conditions there is an association with autoantibodies against heart muscle. A similar disease can be produced in animals by appropriate immunization against heart tissue antigens.

Pemphigus is another disease that has many of the hallmarks of an autoimmune disease. Here, the loss of intercellular bridges in the epidermis is associated with the presence of autoantibodies directed against antigens located in the intercellular zones between adjacent epidermal cells. The serum titer of these antibodies correlates with activity of the disease and may have some prognostic value. Evidence of activation of the complement system in the blister fluid has been found. Steroids are of value, especially when used with other immunosuppressive drugs. Bullous pemphigoid is another skin disease in which the blisters arise subepidermally and the autoantibodies react with constituents in the zona pellucida of the basement membrane in the epidermis rather than the intercellular cement. Activation of the complement system in the bullous fluid has also been demonstrated.

As mentioned at the outset, many other diseases, especially viral diseases and others associated with tissue destruction, exhibit autoimmune phenomena that may be related to manifestations of illness. Only further study will lead to a full understanding of these complex interrelationships.

17

Transfusion

The development of modern medicine and surgery could not have been possible without the discovery of the major blood group antigens by Landsteiner in 1900. Correctly matched transfusions were used soon thereafter, but modern blood banking did not become a safe and practical reality until the period between World War I and World War II. The first blood bank was not established until 1937, at Cook County Hospital in Chicago. Serologic techniques for the detection of erythrocyte antigens are now used not only for the preparation of safe blood for transfusion, but also in the diagnosis of hemolytic disorders, in forensic medicine, and in genetic analysis. The possible immunologic reactions that can occur with human erythrocytes are unbelievably complex, but only those of general interest will be discussed.

ERYTHROCYTE ANTIGENS

Since the cells of the thymic dependent lymphoid system provide such an extraordinarily effective surveillance against the introduction of allogeneic cells, it is remarkable that blood can be transfused at all. Indeed, success with transfusions is mostly dependent upon the fact that histocompatibility antigens are not expressed on the erythrocyte membrane. However, the antigenic structure of the erythrocyte membrane is complicated enough and almost 400 different red cell antigens have been recognized.

THE MAJOR BLOOD GROUPS

Four major blood group phenotypes exist in man: A, B, O, and AB. They are of overwhelming importance in the safe transfusion of blood. These phenotypic symbols designate the presence or absence of the A and B antigens. Persons with type O blood have an antigen designated by the symbol H. Very rarely, an H-negative person is found and this is called "Bombay" blood type. Since H is a precursor of A and B antigens, persons with Bombay blood also lack A and B antigens even though they may have genes coding for A and B.

256

The A, B, and H groups of antigens are a part of the structure of the surface membranes of virtually all human cells. From the present evidence, it would appear that A and B antigens have arisen as a genetically controlled biochemical modification of the H antigen, which exists unchanged in patients with type O blood.

Two important subgroups of the A antigen exist (A_1 and A_2), as well as other less common variants. Approximately 80 per cent of individuals secrete a water-soluble form of A, B, or H antigen in their saliva and other excretory fluids. Almost all persons who have type A, B, or O blood have demonstrable antibodies (isohemagglutinins) in their serum against A or B antigens if they are not a part of their own cells. Because of variability of natural immunization from antigens with A and B specificity, found ubiquitously in nature, titers of the isohemagglutinins for A and B substances vary widely in different individuals. It is the presence of these naturally occurring antibodies that makes the random transfusion of blood so hazardous. If transfusions were given randomly within the Caucasian population, approximately 25 per cent would develop acute hemolytic transfusion reactions because of anti-A, and 10 per cent would develop transfusion reactions because of anti-B.

A schema for the relatively safe administration of typed but unmatched blood is shown in Figure 17–1. In persons who have not been pregnant and who have not received previous transfusions, the urgent transfusion of blood by such a protocol is surprisingly safe since approximately 1 per cent of such persons have antibodies in their serum to blood group antigens other than those in the ABO system. These are predominantly antibodies against the antigens Le^a, Le^b, P1, M, and N. The incidence of antierythrocyte antibodies rises to approximately 4 per cent in patients who have been pregnant or who have received prior transfusions. In Viet Nam, type O blood was regularly used for urgent transfusions to recipients of any type, and difficulty was encountered only rarely. The use of type-specific blood, however, is preferable in most circumstances to avoid minor transfusion incompatibilities when blood must be administered before complete compatibility testing is performed.

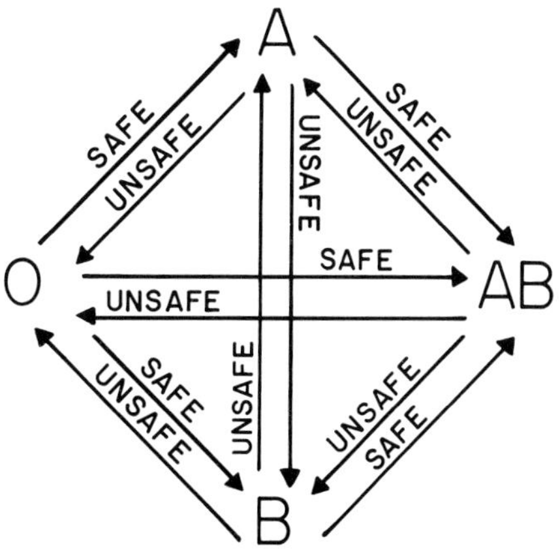

Figure 17–1. Schema for the relatively safe administration of typed but unmatched blood.

TABLE 17–1. APPROXIMATE RISK OF HEMOLYTIC TRANSFUSION REACTIONS FOR DIFFERENT COMPATIBILITY TESTS

TYPE OF TEST	MINIMUM TIME FOR TESTING	RISK OF HEMOLYTIC TRANSFUSION REACTION (%)	
		"Low Risk" Patients*	"High Risk" Patients*
Type specific blood and immediate spin test	15 min.	<1	<4
Emergency compatibility test	50 min.	<0.5	<0.5
Routine compatibility test	80 min.	<0.01	<0.01

*High risk patients are those who have been pregnant or who have had prior transfusions. Low risk patients are those not exposed to such hazards.

Because of the possibility of prior sensitization, a cross-matching procedure should be done prior to the administration of blood, except in the most pressing emergency. In this simple procedure, donor serum is mixed with recipient cells in one test, and the donor cells are mixed with recipient serum in a second test. If agglutination is found in the major cross-match (the test with recipient serum and donor cells), the blood should not be administered. The minor cross-match has relatively less importance, but such blood nevertheless should be given only in urgent situations. Performance of a direct cross-match will eliminate the vast majority of hemolytic transfusion reactions. The approximate risk of hemolytic transfusion reactions for different degrees of compatibility testing is shown in Table 17–1.

THE RH SYSTEM

Unlike the ABO antigens, Rh antigens occur primarily, if not exclusively, on erythrocytes. Antisera are commonly used in testing for five of the Rh antigens (C, D, E, c, and e) but when the terms Rh-positive and Rh-negative are used, the presence or absence of D is implied, since the D antigen is more immunogenic than any of the other Rh antigens. For this reason Rh(D)-negative patients should be transfused with Rh(D)-negative blood except in extreme emergencies. In Rh-negative patients who have already formed anti-D, only Rh-negative blood can be transfused. Within a large group of patients whose sera were examined for unexpected (irregular) antibodies, using the same methods as in major cross-match tests, Rh antibodies were the ones most commonly present. Among these, antibodies to D, made by Rh-negative persons, accounted for approximately 95 per cent of the positive reactions. Antibodies to C were found in less than 20 per cent of the cases and then usually with anti-D in Rh-negatives. Other anti-Rh antibodies (anti-c, -E, -e, and so on) can be made, but their incidence is much lower than the incidence of anti-D made by Rh-negatives. Although Rh-negative blood is usually in short supply and the occasion does not often occur, there are no indications against the transfusion of Rh-positive patients with Rh-negative blood. This is because the two major antigens present in Rh-negative blood (c and e) are also present in the majority of Rh-positive patients. Approximately 85 per cent of the population are Rh(D)-positive. Many genetic variations of the alleles coding for the Rh factors have now been decribed which are of relatively little importance to the clinician except where sensitization has occurred as a result of multiple transfusions or pregnancy.

Rh antibody was once thought to be univalent because it does not cause a typical agglutination reaction in saline. This assumption has since been proved to be false. The Rh antigens of erythrocytes suspended in saline are apparently located spatially on the cell surface in a way that physically prevents cross-linkages between erythrocytes by divalent antibody. Also, a relatively small number of specific sites and the negative charge of the cell surface may not permit effective cross-linking. The presence of Rh antibody bound to its corresponding antigen on the surface of erythrocytes can be detected by reacting it with antibody that is specific for human gamma globulin, causing typical agglutination reactions to occur (Coombs' test). Detection of Rh antibody with enzyme-treated cells or in the presence of 30 per cent bovine serum albumin or positively charged macromolecules are alternative methods of practical importance. In the latter instances, the erythrocyte membranes are sufficiently altered to permit the development of cross-linkages.

The transfusion of blood that is incompatible with an anti-Rh antibody in the recipient's serum (whether it be Rh-positive blood given to a patient with anti-D or Rh-positive blood given to an Rh-positive patient with an antibody such as anti-c or anti-E) does not usually result in immediate hemolysis, since Rh antibodies do not usually fix complement. Instead, the incompatible erythrocytes are removed by macrophage sequestration, predominately in the spleen. This rapid removal of erythrocytes from the circulation by cells of the reticuloendothelial system results in jaundice because of the conversion of hemoglobin to bilirubin during the process of erythrocyte destruction. Although complement-induced hemolysis is uncommon in in vitro tests when either IgM or IgG anti-Rh antibodies are involved, there are sometimes clinical signs of intravascular cell destruction in patients who receive Rh-incompatible blood. It is possible that Rh antibodies behave differently in vivo and in vitro. Alternatively, there is some evidence that the intravascular lysis may be K cell dependent.

OTHER BLOOD GROUPS

Hemolytic transfusion reactions have been reported in patients who have been sensitized to other erythrocyte antigens, notably those in the MN, Kell, Lewis, Duffy, Kidd, P, and Lutheran systems. Fortunately, sensitization to these antigens can be detected by the major cross-match reaction, is uncommon, and is of more concern to those responsible for blood banking procedures than for those administering the blood. Numerous texts are available for those wishing to extend their knowledge of these groups.

TESTING FOR COMPATIBILITY AND BLOOD GROUP SPECIFICITIES

Routine Tests. Donor red cells are routinely tested for the presence of A, B, D, and D^u antigens, and the serum is tested for the presence of antibody against A_1, A_2 and B antigens. It is further screened for the presence of unexpected (irregular) antibodies using O red cells carrying most of the well-known antigens (usually a pool of cells). An indirect Coombs' test is preferred as part of the antibody screen. In donors with group O blood, a check is made for the presence of hemolysins against A and B red cells. O blood without hemolysins is a "universal" donor and may be used in the rare extreme emergencies before type-specific blood is available. Donor blood is also routinely screened for the presence of hepatitis B antigen (HB_SAg), and a serologic test for syphilis is performed.

Recipients are typed for the presence of A, B, and D antigens on the red cells and anti-A, anti-A_1, and anti-B in the serum. A test is made for the presence of irregular antibodies, using individual cells of known specificity. An indirect Coombs' test is done to detect the presence of nonagglutinating antibodies in the serum, and the patient's red cells are tested by a direct Coombs' test to detect autoantibodies.

Finally, routine compatibility tests are performed between patient serum and donor cells at room temperature and at 37° C. Sequentially, the reactivity is tested after incubation with saline, after the addition of albumin, and after the addition of Coombs' reagent. Further incubation is performed after each additive. In many blood banks, the minor cross-match is performed (patient cells and donor serum) as an additional check against ABO incompatibility. Also, the past records of the recipient are routinely checked and comparisons made with past pretransfusion tests before issuance of the blood. Often, mistakes in labelling (by the person drawing the bloods) are discovered by this process and transfusion of incompatible blood thereby avoided.

Blood found to be compatible and held for a recipient longer than 48 hours must be retested for compatibility if the patient has received a transfusion within the preceding 48 hours, because of the possibility that a new antibody response has been stimulated.

Coombs' Test. The direct Coombs' test is often used to detect the presence of surfacebound IgG antibody or complement components (usually C4 or C3). In this test antibody against human IgG or complement (Coombs' reagent) is added to a red cell suspension and the tests observed. Agglutination will occur if the red cells have been coated with antibody and/or complement (Fig. 17–2). The indirect Coombs' test utilizes selected red cells which are first incubated with the serum to be tested and then with Coombs' reagent. If the serum has nonagglutinating antibodies that react with the selected red cell antigens, they will bind, and agglutination will occur with the addition of the antiglobulin reagent. The inclusion of antibodies against complement is important because low affinity antibody may not be present on some cells after the activation of complement has occurred.

Elution of Antibodies. Specificity of antibodies on red cells can often

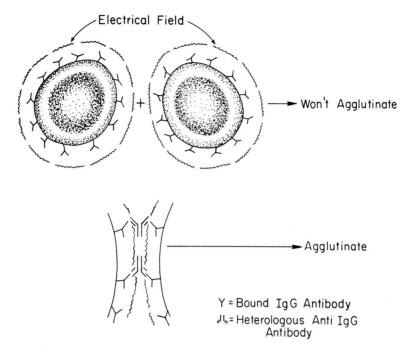

Figure 17-2. Diagrammatic representation of the direct Coombs' test.

be determined by elution, followed by reaction of indicator cells of known specificity.

COMPLICATIONS OF TRANSFUSION WITH BLOOD OR BLOOD PRODUCTS

Many types of adverse reactions may occur following the administration of blood or its components. Most, but not all, have an immune response as their basis.

INTRAVASCULAR HEMOLYTIC TRANSFUSION REACTIONS

Intravascular hemolytic transfusion reactions occur infrequently in modern practice, and when they do, it is usually because of clerical error. Their development may be disastrous, and early recognition of the problem is essential for adequate treatment. When mismatched blood is administered to a patient with incompatible antibodies, an immediate and life-threatening reaction may occur. Only a few ml of incompatible blood may be enough to cause a severe hemolytic reaction. This reaction is characterized by erythrocyte agglutination, capillary plugging, hemolysis, activation of the complement system, and the development of disseminated intravascular coagulation.

The clinical features of an intravascular hemolytic reaction include fever, chills, headache, pain predominately in the lower back, head, and chest, vomiting, diarrhea, cyanosis, shock, loss of consciousness, hemoglobinemia, hemoglobinuria, and oliguria that often progresses to complete renal failure. A bleeding tendency develops in approximately 25 per cent of those with this type of reaction, depending somewhat on its severity. It is a particularly important sign during surgery, since it may be the only clinically obvious manifestation of a transfusion reaction of an anesthetized patient. Suspicion of a transfusion reaction should be aroused whenever any symptoms develop in a patient who has been recently transfused. A blood sample should be taken immediately and checked for the presence of hemolysis, and a urine sample should be checked for the presence of hemoglobin. With the intravascular coagulation are associated decreases in fibrinogen, prothrombin, and platelets; an increase in the bleeding time; and the development of fibrinolysis.

Treatment of a suspected transfusion reaction includes the immediate discontinuance of the transfusion. When a diagnosis is firmly established, adrenocortical steroids may be helpful in controlling the deleterious effects of complement activation, including shock. This is one of the few situations where the administration of a large dose of steroids (30 mg per kg methylprednisolone) is clearly beneficial. Usually, a single dose will suffice. Low molecular weight dextran may help to increase small vessel flow and may also have a beneficial effect as an osmotic diuretic. Administration of mannitol or a diuretic such as furosemide early in the course may be helpful to prevent acute renal failure. When active bleeding is associated with a coagulation defect, administration of fresh plasma or correctly matched whole blood may be life-saving. Specific replacement of fibrinogen may also be helpful, but should probably be given as cryoprecipitate to avoid an undue risk of hepatitis. The abnormally increased fibrinolysis may be controlled with epsilon-aminocaproic acid, but this treatment can result in unchecked disseminated intravascular coagulation. It is therefore recommended that heparin be administered in a dose of approximately 100 units per kg of body weight at the same time that epsilon-aminocaproic acid is given. Many authorities prefer to treat the DIC with heparin alone.

Extravascular Hemolysis

Sometimes, preformed circulating antibody will not cause hemolysis of erythrocytes in vivo; certain Rh incompatibilities are examples. However, the fixed antibody will serve as an opsonin for the RES and the transfused cells may be removed rapidly from the circulation. Massive intracellular destruction of erythrocytes causes jaundice within a few days of the transfusion, and spherocytes are found in the blood smear. The direct Coombs' test becomes positive, though sometimes with a mixed-field pattern (transfused cells coated with antibody, patient's own cells not coated) that may be difficult to interpret. This condition is self-limited and usually does not require treatment.

ALLERGIC REACTIONS

Allergic reactions characterized by urticaria, bronchospasm, and generalized itching are common complications of blood transfusions, but rarely are they severe. The transfer of an antigen or a reaginic antibody into the recipient is the usual cause of these reactions, which occur predominately in persons with a history of atopic allergies. The reactions usually respond well to treatment with antihistaminic drugs, and the blood may continue to be given if the reaction is minimized and there is clearly no evidence of a hemolytic reaction.

FEBRILE REACTIONS

Fever may be associated with major hemolytic transfusion reaction, bacterial contamination, the presence of pyrogens in the preservative, or the presence of leukocyte or platelet antibody. Among these, the presence of antibodies reacting within human leukocyte and platelet antigens in patients who have received multiple transfusions or who have been pregnant is the most common cause, accounting for approximately 75 per cent of all transfusion reactions. The febrile reaction can be prevented by transfusion with washed erythrocytes or deglycerolized frozen blood. Since the symptoms may be very similar to an early intravascular hemolytic reaction, it is mandatory to discontinue the transfusion and perform a work-up for possible incompatibilities.

ACUTE BACTERIAL INFECTIONS

The transfusion of blood or plasma which has been contaminated by bacterial growth is a rare but disastrous complication. It should be suspected when fever and shaking chills develop soon after a transfusion has begun. This iatrogenic disease is often accompanied by the classic picture of septic shock, including vascular collapse and a bleeding tendency. Activation of complement accounts for many of the adverse reactions. The diagnosis cannot always be made by examination of a Gram stain of the transfused blood, but this test may be helpful since greater than 10^5 organisms per ml may be detected in a direct smear, and greater than 10^6 organisms per ml in the contaminated blood are usually necessary to cause a fatal reaction in persons with a normal defense mechanism. Most of the bacteria that grow at the low temperature at which blood is stored are gram-negative organisms, notably those belonging to the *Pseudomonas*, *Achromobacter*, and coliform groups. When the diagnosis is suspected, the transfusion should be discontinued immediately, and large doses of broad-spectrum antibiotics should be administered intravenously. Gentamicin is currently the antibiotic of choice. Blood volume expanders and dopamine may be useful when shock is present, but steroids should usually be avoided unless shock cannot be effectively managed by every other means available. In experimental animals, a higher frequency of survival can be obtained by steroid treatment of shock produced by gram-negative bacterial endotoxin, but its use in man remains controversial.

ANTI-IgG AND ANTI-IgA REACTIONS

In persons with an inherited deficiency of IgA, the administration of blood containing IgA may elicit antibodies to this protein. Subsequent transfusion may result in an acute anaphylactic reaction. In such patients who require transfusion, the use of washed cells or frozen blood to limit the amount of IgA given to the patient is clearly indicated. Occasional patients who are not deficient in IgA may develop alloanti-IgA antibodies or anti-IgG (anti-Gm) antibodies.

GRAFT VERSUS HOST DISEASE

Transfusions represent a special hazard for patients with the lymphopenic agammaglobulinemias and immunologic deficiencies. These patients are unable to reject allogeneic cells and are therefore vulnerable to graft versus host disease, which may be produced by transfusions of blood, packed red blood cells, platelet packs, or any preparations containing viable lymphocytes. Since patients with this disease often have hematologic abnormalities, transfusions are needed frequently, and fatal graft versus host reactions may be produced. When immunologic deficiencies involving defects of the thymic dependent function must be treated with blood or blood products that might contain immunologically competent lymphocytes, it is best to use frozen cells and irradiate the blood with a minimum of 200 rads prior to the infusion. Blood stored as long as 21 days has been shown to contain viable, immunologically competent lymphocytes. Graft versus host reactions from administration of unirradiated blood to patients immunosuppressed by intensive anticancer treatment are occurring with increasing frequency, and these may be lethal.

TRANSMISSION OF INFECTIOUS DISEASES

The transmission of serum hepatitis or infectious viral hepatitis is a significant transfusion hazard in any medical center. Its occurrence can be reduced by careful and meticulous exclusion of any donor having a past history consistent with hepatitis and by testing for HB_SAg in donor blood with a sensitive test like radioimmunoassay. Unfortunately, there are no good tests that can be applied for routine screening of donors for infection with hepatitis A or C. Administration of gamma globulin is ineffective for preventing serum hepatitis, but the use of hyperimmune globulin appears to be helpful in preventing the disease and minimizing its consequences, if it occurs. Among the more common infectious diseases that may be transmitted through blood transfusions are syphilis, malaria, brucellosis, and cytomega-lovirus infection (CMV). The CMV infection is especially important follow-ing open heart surgery and renal transplantation and in both circumstances is felt to arise primarily as a result of transfusion of blood containing the virus.

Nonimmune Noninfectious Adverse Reactions

Perhaps the most common of these complications is posttransfusion pul-monary insufficiency. This condition is sometimes seen after repeated trans-fusions and may be caused, at least in part, by the transfusion of blood con-taining microaggregates. These microaggregates consist of fibrin strands and clumps of leukocytes and platelets, which increase in amount with the length of the storage of the blood. Administration of many microaggregates causes embolization and blockage of small pulmonary arterioles and capil-laries, a pulmonary alveolar–capillary diffusion defect, and hypoxia. The in-cidence of the complication can be significantly reduced by the routine use of a microporous filter to remove aggregates when any patient is to receive more than two or three units of blood.

Citrate toxicity may occur in rare instances and is usually associated with the presence of liver disease. It may be prevented by the administration of approximately one gram of calcium gluconate for each three units of transfused CPD stored blood. Potassium toxicity can be a significant compli-cation when large amounts of old blood are transfused to patients with renal failure. Deficiencies in clotting factors may occur with multiple massive transfusions (usually more than 20 units), but they can usually be corrected by the administration of fresh frozen plasma and platelet concentrates.

TRANSFUSION OF COMPONENTS

The development of procedures for the separation and storage of various components of the blood has led to revolutionary changes in the practice of hemotherapy. The indications for the use of whole blood are continually decreasing and are now limited primarily to the treatment of acute hemor-rhagic shock or massive blood loss. Table 17–2 lists blood components presently available in most blood centers, with indications for their use.

HEMOLYTIC DISEASE OF THE NEWBORN

Hemolytic disease of the newborn is a classic immunologic condition caused by the accelerated destruction of infant erythrocytes by specific an-tibodies that are derived from the mother by placental transfer. The disease always begins in intrauterine life and may result in death in utero, but it is often diagnosed only after birth. The hemolytic process is maximal at the time of birth and diminishes as the concentration of antibody declines in the

TABLE 17–2. BLOOD COMPONENTS AVAILABLE FOR THERAPY

Component	Approved Shelf Life	Indications for Use
Packed red cells	21 days	Correction of anemia; acute blood loss of minor degree.
Washed cells	24 hours	Sensitization to leukocyte or platelet antigens causing febrile reactions. Patients in whom transfusion of plasma is contra-indicated (such as with T-activated polyagglutinable cells or patients with IgA deficiency).
Frozen cells (deglycerolized)	24 hours	Rare blood types. Extreme sensitization to leukocyte antigens with febrile reactions when given washed cells. Prospective transplant recipients to decrease sensiti-zation to HLA antigens.
Fresh frozen plasma (thawed)	6 hours	Treatment of clotting disorders when specific concentrates are not available or when the precise factor has not been determined.
Single donor plasma (cryoprecipitate removed, thawed)	24 hours	Expansion of blood volume in the treatment of shock secondary to plasma loss. May be useful in selected patients to restore defective opsonins.
Platelet concentrate	72 hours	Treatment or prevention of bleeding from thrombocytopenia. HLA compatible platelets appear to be more effective.
Cryoprecipitate (thawed)	6 hours	Treatment of classical hemophilia, hypo-fibrinogenemia, or von Willebrand's disease.
$Rh_0(D)$ immune globulin	–	Prevention of $Rh_0(D)$ sensitization.
Leukocyte concentrates	24 hours	Treatment of selected patients with severe leukopenia. HLA compatible leukocytes appear to be more effective. Should be given as soon as possible.
Modified whole blood (cryoprecipitate and/or platelets removed)	21 days	Same as whole blood. Has the advantage of fewer microaggregates.

infant's circulation. Since IgG but not IgM is placentally transferred, IgM does not participate in the disease. Any blood group antigen capable of stimulating high levels of IgG may cause the disease. However, classically it has been seen in Rh incompatibility and ABO incompatibility, with the former condition usually being more severe. It was first demonstrated in 1939 that hemolytic disease in the newborn is caused by antibodies passed from mother to fetus, and the nature of the disease was increasingly under-stood in the early 1940s. For practical purposes, RhD and anti-D antibodies are involved. Of all women immunized at pregnancy to Rh antigens, 93 per cent formed anti-D with or without anti-C. Of all infants whose disease was severe enough to require some type of treatment, 99 per cent were D-posi-tive infants born of mothers with anti-D in their serum. Before Rh-immune globulin was routinely administered, approximately 20 per cent of Rh–

women who delivered Rh+ infants formed anti-D. The formation of anti-D during the first pregnancy was around 1 per cent and therefore Rh hemolytic disease of the newborn was unusual in first pregnancies. However, the incidence of serious problems increased progressively in subsequent pregnancies because of the successively greater risk of immunization of the mother by D-positive cells entering the circulation at the time of delivery. In mothers whose serum contained anti-D, the incidence of intrauterine death among Rh-positive fetuses was approximately 29 per cent.

The most severe form of the Rh disease is hydrops fetalis. These infants are often stillborn, or are grossly edematous and severely anemic. Those with less severe forms of the disease develop icterus early in neonatal life, but the degree of the anemia may be variable. Red cells are destroyed by the reticuloendothelial system, and indirect bilirubin levels rise remarkably not only because of the rapid destruction of blood, but also because the newborn's enzymatic systems for degrading bilirubin are not fully developed. As might be expected, prematurity contributes to the problem. Kernicterus is the condition of cerebral damage occurring in affected infants, who become deeply jaundiced, usually with bilirubin levels greater than 20 mg per 100 ml. Irreversible damage in the brain may be caused by brain lipids absorbing unconjugated bilirubin. Treatment of the disease is best accomplished by transfusion of the unborn infant in utero or by exchange transfusions in the newborn before bilirubin levels have reached a dangerous concentration. It is best to use Rh-negative blood that is compatible with the mother. It is well recognized that maternal antibody may remain in the circulation of the newborn for several days or even weeks before it has been completely consumed. Part of the antibody is removed by the exchange transfusion as are many of the infant's Rh-positive red cells. This method of therapy has been of great benefit in treatment of the established disease.

However, Rh-negative prevention is even more impressive. IgG anti-D given within 72 hours of birth to Rh-negative mothers bearing Rh-positive infants will be effective in suppressing sensitization of the mother in approximately 90 per cent of the cases. The possible mechanisms involved are discussed in Chapter 10.

Hemolytic disease of the newborn caused by the transfer from the mother of IgG anti-A, anti-B, or both, is more common but less severe than Rh-related hemolytic disease. It tends to be more severe when incompatibilities occur and the mother has blood type O. Laboratory evidence of hemolytic disease may be present in as many as 1 in 30 births involving a fetal-maternal incompatibility, but disease severe enough to warrant treatment is as rare as 1 in 3000 births. In those patients requiring exchange transfusion, group O red cells are preferable, combined with fresh AB plasma. A more detailed discussion of the therapeutic aspects of hemolytic disease in the newborn is beyond the scope of this text.

18

Allergic Diseases

The basic mechanisms of disease resulting from allergic reactions to extrinsic antigens, usually apart from infections or infestations, will be discussed in this chapter. These disease conditions include atopic allergic reactions, anaphylactic shock, serum sickness, allergic drug reactions, and contact dermatitis.

ATOPIC DISEASES

Diseases of allergy were seen in clinical practice long before an understanding of immunologic mechanisms evolved. Because of this, some of the terminology is out of step with current concepts, but it has become so deeply ingrained that it continues to be used. This is especially true with the atopic diseases, which include allergic rhinitis (hayfever), allergic conjunctivitis, asthma, urticaria, allergic angioneurotic edema, food allergies, and some forms of infantile eczema. These conditions have, as a primary basis, an underlying genetic predisposition to atopic diseases, usually manifested by a positive family history, and a hypersensitivity to certain allergins, mediated by antibodies belonging to the IgE class (reagins). Exposure of a sensitized individual to antigen results in reaction with the corresponding IgE antibody, which is bound to mast cells, to trigger from them the release of histamine and other vasoactive mediators, such as slow reacting substances of anaphylaxis (SRSA). The erythema, swelling, itching, and smooth muscle contraction are all secondary to the effects of these biologically active substances. Since IgE-producing plasma cells are found primarily in the lymphoid tissues of the nasal, tracheobronchial and gastrointestinal mucosa, it is not surprising that these are generally the target organs of atopic allergy.

The specific allergins causing atopic diseases can be determined by a variety of testing procedures (Chapter 12), which include the prick skin test, various provocation tests, and the radioallergosorbent test (RAST), each of which has specific value in various circumstances. Most patients with atopic disorders have elevated levels of IgE in their serum, and many have high eosinophil counts. However, neither is diagnostic. Histamine release from basophils on allergin challenge has also been used successfully to determine sensitization.

In certain patients, there may be an end-organ predisposition to atopic diseases, as they are more common in patients who exhibit dermatographia and may be precipitated by emotional turmoil or physical stress. Other patients with rhinitis and asthma have no demonstrable IgE-mediated hypersensitivity, thus making an imperfect association between atopy and IgE antibody–antigen reactions. However, it has been shown in at least some of these patients that cytotropic antibodies of the IgG class are acting to take the place of IgE in producing the diseases.

ALLERGIC RHINITIS

The syndrome of repeated episodes of rhinorrhea, nasal congestion and itching, and repeated sneezing is highly indicative of allergic rhinitis, although nonspecific irritants and even repeated respiratory infections can produce similar symptoms. In many patients with this atopic disease, there are associated symptoms of allergic conjunctivitis or sinusitis. About one of every eight persons in the United States is affected by allergic rhinitis, but the incidence is most often seasonal or occasional. Allergic rhinitis is usually associated with inhaled allergins, the most common among which are ragweed and other pollens, house dust, molds (spores), and animal dandruff. Symptomatic treatment with antihistaminic drugs is sufficient for control of symptoms in most cases. Inhaling nonspecific irritants such as cigarette smoke or pollutants of combustion should be avoided whenever possible since these intensify the clinical symptomatology.

ASTHMA

Some 2 per cent of the general population have asthma, a condition which is characterized primarily by intermittent bronchial constriction. Since the bronchi normally dilate somewhat during inspiration and constrict during expiration, further constriction leads to a functional expiratory blockade of the air passages, which is associated with typical expiratory wheezes. About two thirds of asthma patients develop the symptoms because of atopic allergy to environmental (usually inhaled) allergins. Typically, the patients have a positive family history for atopic diseases, elevated serum levels of IgE, eosinophilia, positive skin tests, and often an associated history of allergic rhinitis. This form of asthma (extrinsic asthma) often begins in childhood and characteristically before the age of 30. Hyposensitization or immunization is often helpful in control of the condition, but antihistamines are usually of little value. Beta-adrenergic drugs help to control the symptoms by reducing histamine release and by producing direct relaxation of bronchial smooth muscle. Steroids are of value in refractory cases.

Another form of asthma, known as intrinsic asthma, does not seem to be associated with reaginic antibody and allergy. This form usually begins in adulthood, is not associated with a family history of atopy or elevated levels of IgE, is not associated with exposure to specific allergins, and does not respond to hyposensitization. Respiratory infections or nonspecific irritants seem to trigger the onset. Some patients with intrinsic asthma develop severe asthmatic attacks following the ingestion of certain drugs, especially aspirin, but also other analgesics, food dyes, and food preservatives derived from benzoic acid. In some patients, there seems to be a mixture of intrinsic and extrinsic components, and such patients often are diagnosed as having mixed asthma.

The divergent etiologic pathways for the development of clinical asthma point to a common pathway of bronchoconstrictive mediators that can be triggered in a number of ways.

URTICARIA AND ANGIOEDEMA

IgE-mediated allergic reactions of the skin typically cause an initial vasoconstriction, followed by vasodilatation with increased vascular permeability, edema, and itching. Localized edema (wheals) occuring in the dermis is called hives or urticarial lesions. When the process is more generalized and the edema involves deeper tissues with a predilection for sites with thin overlying mucous membranes or skin, it presents clinically as angioedema, typically involving the face, hands, feet, and oropharyngeal cavity. Urticaria and angioedema may usually be controlled by oral antihistaminic agents and avoidance of the allergin, but beta-adrenergic drugs and steroids are sometimes useful in severe or refractory cases. Food allergies and drugs are frequent causes of urticaria and angioedema, but nonallergic mechanisms may also produce this symptom complex. These include exercise, heat, cold, vibration, pressure, sunlight, and emotional stress. Patients with chronic urticaria (longer than 6 to 8 weeks) may have associated underlying diseases, including intestinal parasites, Hodgkin's disease, urticaria pigmentosa, systemic mastocytosis, occult infections, and the presence of cryoglobulins or cold agglutinins.

ANAPHYLAXIS

Anaphylaxis is an acute systemic allergic reaction characterized by shock, angioedema, bronchial constriction, urticaria, itching, diarrhea, nausea, and vomiting. A spectrum from mild to severe forms may exist; when fatal, death is usually caused by shock or laryngeal obstruction from angioedema. The most common precipitating causes are drugs (especially penicillin), insect stings (especially wasps and bees), and occasionally food allergies (such as eggs or shellfish). True acute anaphylaxis is usually an IgE-mediated reaction, but other acute systemic allergic responses involving activation of the complement system may produce a similar clinical picture.

IMMUNOTHERAPY OF ATOPIC DISORDERS

Hyposensitization (desensitization) is a form of empiric treatment in which a sensitive individual is repeatedly injected with increasing amounts of an allergin, generally by the intradermal or subcutaneous route. The effect of such treatment on specific IgE levels has been variable. Often, an initial increase is followed by a subsequent decrease. Some individuals become progressively more sensitized. The most likely explanation of the effectiveness of hyposensitization (when it works) is the development of an IgG-blocking antibody. The mechanism of action of this blocking antibody is not clear, but at least two possibilities exist: it may bind antigen to prevent its interaction with IgE at the mast cell surface or it may serve as a feedback mechanism to decrease the synthesis of specific IgE antibody. It seems likely that both mechanisms operate in some patients.

The potential benefit of passively administered IgG blocking antibody to specific allergins is now being investigated. The material is extracted from the plasma of nonatopic individuals immunized with the appropriate antigen. Another potential method of therapy currently under investigation is the use of synthetic molecules that have a structure similar to the Fc portion of the ϵ heavy chain. These may cause competitive displacement of IgE from the receptor sites of mast cells. Since the synthetic competitive inhibitors have no antibody specificity, degranulation of the mast cells is prevented by inhibition of mast cell sensitization by the immunologically active IgE. The most exciting development in the approach to prophylaxis against allergy has come from the research of Ishizaka and his colleagues. These investigators have been able to stimulate the development of specific helper cells for the IgG system and specific suppressor cells for the IgE system by choosing just the right adjuvant and the right route and timing of immunization in the mouse. If this discovery can be extended to many rather than a few antigens and extrapolated from mouse to man, the possibility of being able to immunize against atopic allergy could be of great benefit in treating those who suffer so much from their hypersensitivity.

SERUM SICKNESS

This condition, once relatively common because of the passive administration of heterologous antitoxins to prevent the development of tetanus, diphtheria, and certain other diseases, is now rarely seen. Perhaps the most common cause for such reactions at the present time is the administration of antilymphocyte globulin in efforts to control allograft rejection or to treat autoimmunities.

The immunologic mechanisms of this disorder are discussed in Chapter 8. Clinical symptoms include fever, rashes, arthralgia, heart disease and renal lesions associated with generalized vascular damage from deposition of antigen-antibody complexes. These especially involve the kidneys and lung. Injection of a foreign protein into a previously sensitized individual may produce anaphylactic shock (discussed in more detail above and in Chapter 8).

Since most of these pathologic changes are complement-mediated, large doses of adrenocortical steroids may be of benefit.

EXTRINSIC ALLERGIC ALVEOLITIS

Extrinsic allergic alveolitis encompasses a group of diseases that have also been called allergic pneumonia, hypersensitivity pneumonia, and interstitial granulomatous pneumonitis. The first recognized example of allergic alveolitis was called farmer's lung since it occurred primarily in farmers as a result of an allergic disease secondary to exposure to the mold spores in hay or other moldy plant products. Since then, the disease has been recognized with increasing frequency to be caused by a wide variety of inhaled allergins (Table 18–1).

The disease may occur in either an acute or chronic form, depending upon the intensity and length of exposure. Fever, malaise, and anorexia or weight loss or both often occur in association with dyspnea and a nonproductive cough. Chest roentgenograms may show patchy or diffuse, usually central, nodular infiltrates. Serum IgA and IgG may be elevated, but elevated levels of IgE are not a prominent feature. Lung biopsy shows inflammation, fibrosis, and granuloma. The condition can be confused with sarcoidosis, pneumoconiosis, eosinophilic granuloma, beryllium disease, and other disorders that cause widespread pulmonary fibrosis. However, the main diagnostic problem with this disease is simply lack of consideration of allergic alveolitis in the differential diagnosis.

Allergic alveolitis is usually caused, at least in a major way, by antigen-

TABLE 18–1. PARTIAL LISTING OF DISEASES OF EXTRINSIC ALLERGIC ALVEOLITIS

DISEASE	SOURCES OF ANTIGENIC PARTICLES
Farmer's lung	Moldy hay or other plant products
Ventilation pneumonitis	Mold or bacteria in air conditioners or humidifiers
Mushroom worker's lung	Post spawning compost
Bagassosis	Moldy sugar cane bagasse
Malt worker's lung	Malt dust or moldy barley
Suberosis	Moldy cork bark
Cheese worker's lung	Mold on cheese
Bird fancier's lung	Proteins in dust from droppings of birds, especially pigeon, budgerigar, parrot, chicken
Wheat weevil's disease	Infected wheat flour
Fishmeal worker's lung	Fishmeal in animal food factories
Pituitary snuff taker's lung	Porcine and bovine pituitary powder

antibody reactions that activate the complement system to produce a localized "complex" disease. However, present evidence also indicates that tissue injury associated with delayed hypersensitivity responses may play a role in the pathogenesis. In a few cases, atopic allergies may occur concurrently. Precipitin tests against the offending allergin are usually positive, but positive tests occur in many exposed individuals who do not develop disease. Inhalation tests may confirm the diagnosis, but must be done with caution.

Avoidance of the allergin is the most obvious and perhaps most effective form of treatment, but steroids can be beneficial, especially in persistent disease.

PULMONARY EOSINOPHILIA

This term refers to a group of conditions in which pulmonary infiltrations are associated with a blood eosinophilia. The infiltrates are often fleeting or migratory, but their resolution may be associated with fibrosis. Occasionally, the disease progresses to or is associated with polyarteritis nodosa. Pulmonary eosinophilia can occur with asthma, extrinsic allergic aleveolitis, exposure to drugs such as penicillin or sulfonamides, or infestation with helminths, including *Ascaris*, *Toxocara*, Bilharzia, microfilaria, and so on. Commonly, however, pulmonary eosinophilia is associated with an allergy to fungus which may reside in the lung, most notably *Aspergillus* but also *Candida*, *Mucor*, *Coccidiomyces*, *Blastomyces*, *Helminthosporium* and *Geotrichium*. In many cases, the cause cannot be found. When pulmonary eosinophilia occurs with asthma, the most common cause is hypersensitivity to *Aspergillus* (80 per cent of cases in England). Sputum plugs with eosinophils and hyphae, and associated proximal bronchiectasis are typical. Pulmonary eosinophilia without asthma is frequently associated with hypersensitivity to drugs, such as penicillin, PAS, nitrofurantoin and the sulfas. However, in tropical countries helminth infections are more common. It appears that nearly all basic forms of immune injury may participate in these conditions, but atopic IgE-mediated and antigen-IgG antibody immune complex mechanisms appear to be involved most often in the pathogenesis. It is usually steroid-responsive.

ALLERGIC CONTACT DERMATITIS

Contact dermatitis may occur either because of a nonspecific irritant effect of an applied substance or because of a well-defined allergic response. Certain substances may be associated with a mixture of the two, but only true allergic contact dermatitis will be considered here.

In the vast majority of occasions allergic contact dermatitis is the result of a T cell-mediated response caused by sensitization to a small molecular weight chemical which becomes attached to normal proteins of the skin and acts as a hapten. In a few instances, antibody-mediated responses seem to predominate while still others show mixed responses. Genetic factors markedly influence the susceptibility to develop the disease. Once sensitization occurs, it is usually long-lasting, and may persist for years or even a lifetime.

The typical pathologic features include dilatation of small capillaries and lymphatics in the dermis, with edema and exudation of inflammatory cells that are predominantly lymphocytes. Focal edema develops in the epidermal prickle cell layer, in which intercellular edema may result in rupture of the epidermis and the formation of vesicles. Hyperkeratosis and parakeratosis may also be seen. Since these reactions are featured by extreme itching, they are regularly scratched, and physical damage of skin, extreme keratosis, and infection are common accompaniments.

The agents that cause allergic contact dermatitis are numerous and varied. Many plants produce such allergins—the best known and clinically most important are poison ivy and poison oak. Numerous industrial compounds, including heavy metals, chromates, and organic solvents, are frequently important. Ingredients in cosmetics and household products may also incite the reaction. In addition, topically applied medications form a large segment of causative agents.

Diagnosis of the condition may be made on clinical and pathologic grounds, but the inciting agent is usually proved only by patch testing or intradermal tests.

Experimentally, intravenous injection of the hapten, combined with a skin test, can produce prolonged unresponsiveness within 24 hours, but this practice is not applicable to man. Instead, clinicians must be content with identifying the allergin and advising patients to avoid it, along with nonspecific topical and systemic therapy. The use of systemic adrenocortical steroids may result in prompt and sometimes dramatic relief of symptoms, but their routine use should be avoided.

ALLERGIC DRUG REACTIONS

Almost every segment of clinical care involves the frequent administration of one or more drugs. Many types of adverse reactions to drugs occur, including toxic effects, allergic reactions, idiosyncrasies, and unwanted but normal side-effects. Several hundred drugs have been proved to be sensitizing agents, and approximately one of every ten persons has developed a drug sensitivity of one sort or another. Since drug reactions may be both lethal and disabling, the prevention, recognition, and management of them is of major consequence. Allergic reactions to penicillin, for example, still account for nearly 100 deaths per year in the United States of America, to say nothing of the extensive suffering resulting from sensitivity to the drug.

PREVENTION

Most serious drug reactions can be avoided by taking a careful history. However, drug reactions can occur in patients with a negative history, and a large percentage of interrogated patients believe that they have experienced some sort of allergic reaction to at least one drug to which they are in fact not allergic. Thorough analysis of the circumstances will often show that the adverse reactions were not likely to have resulted from a drug allergy. At other times, convincing evidence for hypersensitivity is obtained from a person who has received several drugs, and the real offender cannot be identified without rechallenge. Whenever a history suggests hypersensitivity to a drug, that drug should not be administered except in those rare instances when a satisfactory alternative does not exist and the beneficial effect of the drug outweighs the possible risks. Those persons with documented drug allergies should carry authoritative identification that clearly communicates this information.

MECHANISMS

A few therapeutic compounds are of sufficiently high molecular weight to provide an antigenic stimulus without complexing with body proteins, but the majority of allergic reactions to drugs occur to well defined organic compounds with molecular weights of less than 1000. These sensitizing agents, therefore, act as haptens to provide an initial antigenic stimulus only when conjugated to the proteins of the host. A few drugs may combine directly with proteins, but the majority, such as aspirin, barbiturates, and sulfonamides, appear incapable of binding firmly to proteins and undergo partial metabolic degradation before the responsible allergenic structure is obtained.

Allergic reactions to penicillin (Fig. 18–1) have been studied more completely than reactions to any other drug. Although there is still much to be learned, an analysis of these studies provides insight into the mechanisms of allergic drug reactions and emphasizes their complexity. Benzylpenicillin

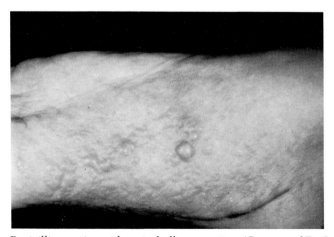

Figure 18–1.   Penicillin reaction with vesicobullous eruption. (Courtesy of Dr. Leon Goldman.)

(penicillin G) may combine with proteins, but there is strong evidence that d-benzylpenicillinic acid and other degradation products are usually the responsible allergins, rather than the intact molecule. The major determinant group which is capable of combining irreversibly with proteins is the benzylpenicilloyl group, and, in addition, there are several minor determinant groups that may be responsible for reactions.

A number of types of allergic responses may be elicited by these immunogenic degradation products of benzylpenicillin. As with other haptens which cause allergy, delayed hypersensitivity reactions appear to be to the specific hapten-protein conjugate, whereas immediate reactions do not require carrier protein specificity. Careful testing demonstrates that the majority of normal adults have serum antibodies specific for the benzylpenicilloyl group, indicating that this is a strong antigen of widespread occurrence. The IgG type of antibody is by far the most common type of antibody found, but it does not seem to participate in allergic reactions to penicillin. Instead, IgG acts as a blocking antibody, preventing allergic reactions in the majority of instances. Immediate allergic reactions appear to occur because of interaction between the IgE type of antibody and minor determinant groups. Late urticarial reactions seem to occur predominantly because of reactions of the IgE type of antibody with specificity for the benzylpenicilloyl group. The genetically determined capacity for the synthesis of IgE antibody appears to by a major factor in the development of such clinical allergic reactions. Whether these are qualitative or quantitative immunologic abnormalities has not yet been established. Interestingly, the presence of IgE antibodies to penicillin does not necessarily indicate that the patient will have an allergic reaction when given the drug. The IgM type of antibody with specificity for the benzylpenicilloyl group may participate in maculopapular and other late reactions. Allergic contact dermatitis to penicillin is a delayed hypersensitivity type of response, which requires the presence and participation of T lymphocytes.

With few exceptions, the drugs that produce allergic reactions do so in a manner entirely similar to other antigens. However, the allergic manifestations of drug sensitivities often have sites of predilection characteristic for a given drug. One likely explanation for such a predilection is that antigenic degradation products of a drug are processed primarily by a given type of cell, or alternatively, the allergenic degradation product may have a particularly strong affinity for binding to a protein found in high concentration in a certain location.

RECOGNITION

Every conceivable type of allergic reaction can be seen with drug hypersensitivities, and both humoral mechanisms and cell-mediated mechanisms appear to be responsible.

Clinical manifestations include fever, urticaria, skin rashes of almost every variety, pruritis, purpura, edema, anaphylaxis, shock, asthma, hematopoietic suppression, hemolytic anemias, serum sickness, vasculitis, renal failure, and autoimmune phenomena. One or more of these may characteristically be associated with the development of hypersensitivity to a given drug, but more often they are not. Autoimmune diseases often appear as a manifestation of drug allergy because sensitivity is directed in part toward carrier protein in the patient's body fluid or cells. Those drug reactions producing severe hematologic disturbances, such as hemolytic anemia, thrombocytopenia, or agranulocytosis, especially seem to depend on an indirect immunologic assault of antigen-antibody complexes directed against the cells and tissues of the body. These are discussed further in Chapter 16.

Drug hypersensitivities should be suspected in any patient who develops allergic symptoms while receiving drugs. Often, a definitive diagnosis of drug allergy can be made only by observing regression of the symptoms on discontinuing the drug and their recurrence when the drug is resumed. This is usually considered to be unacceptable unless the condition is serious and alternative drugs are not available.

In vitro testing for drug sensitivity is often not productive, since the allergin is usually a degradation product rather than the intact drug. When the intermediate allergin is known, such as with the benzylpenicilloyl and minor groups of penicillin, a battery of tests, including skin testing with the antigen, may provide an indication of existing allergy to the drug, but no single test has been entirely foolproof in predicting or diagnosing allergy. The common manifestations of drug hypersensitivity and the common offending drugs most used in clinical practice are shown in Table 18–2.

For the clinician, the allergic manifestations to the antibiotics are of

TABLE 18–2. COMMON MANIFESTATIONS OF HYPERSENSITIVITY TO DRUGS FREQUENTLY USED IN CLINICAL PRACTICE

TYPE OF REACTION	SENSITIZING DRUG
Anaphylaxis	Penicillin, vaccines, heterologous serum, procaine
Serum sickness	Penicillin; sulfa; heterologous serum, especially horse serum
Drug fever	Streptomycin, barbiturates, penicillin, sulfas, quinidines, hydralazine, amphotericin
Skin eruptions, rashes, eczema, exfoliative dermatitis, etc.	Sulfas, penicillin, iodides, many others
Stevens-Johnson syndrome	Dilantin and other hydantoins, sulfonamides, penicillin
Thrombocytopenia	Quinidine, quinine, sulfas, chlorothiazide, sedormid
Agranulocytosis	Aminopyrine, phenothiazines
Acute vasculitis	Vaccines, penicillin, sulfas, thiouracil
Chronic vasculitis	Propylthiouracil, sulfas
Drug-induced lupus	Hydralazine, isonicotinic acid, hydrazide, hydantoins, dione compounds
Drug-induced hemolytic anemia	Quinidine, quinine, PAS, phenacetin, penicillin, sulfonamides, insulin, cephalosporins

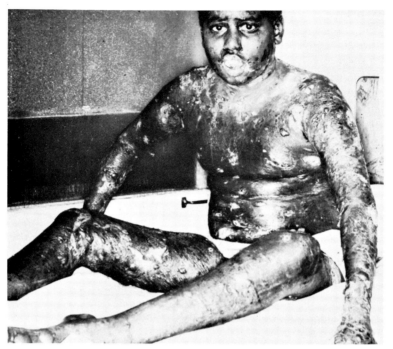

Figure 18–2. Chronic Stevens-Johnson syndrome and pemphigoid lesions due to long-acting sulfa.

relatively great importance. Allergies to penicillin and penicillin derivatives may be both acute and chronic. Anaphylactic reactions, which may occur suddenly and unexpectedly, are dramatic events which are fortunately less common than the other clinical forms of drug allergy. Sulfonamides cause allergic reactions relatively frequently, and these are usually associated with some type of dermatosis (Figs. 18–2 and 18–3). Chloramphenicol can cause inhibition of hematopoiesis, but this complication is not an allergic manifestation.

TREATMENT

In the vast majority of cases, treatment should include discontinuance of the drug. Only if no suitable alternative drug exists and if continued treatment may be important to prevent a clearly unfavorable outcome is it permissible to continue administering a drug to which a patient has proven sensitivity. Usually, the symptoms of hypersensitivity will disappear within a short period of time after an offending drug has been stopped.

Treatment of mild reactions may not be necessary and treatment of some lesions, such as fixed drug eruptions, may be ineffective. Acute but mild reactions such as urticaria, itching, edema, or other histamine-mediated lesions can often be satisfactorily controlled by the administration of an antihistaminic agent.

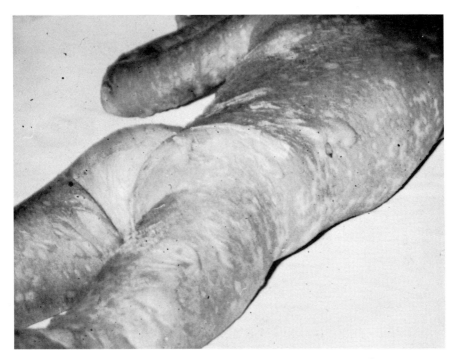

Figure 18–3. Stevens-Johnson syndrome induced by a hydantoin.

The acute, severe reaction of anaphylactic shock usually happens unexpectedly and may terminate fatally if not treated promptly and effectively. To have this complication occur is a sobering experience for both the patient and his physician. Treatment must include maintenance of an adequate airway, by tracheostomy or endotracheal intubation if necessary. Establishment of an intravenous pathway is essential. Epinephrine should be given intravenously for the treatment of the shock and for bronchospasm, and a steroid such as methylprednisolone should be given in large doses to minimize further consequences of the allergic reaction. These basic drugs should be readily available in every area where drugs are given by injection. A tourniquet placed above the site of injection of the allergin often helps to retard entry of the drug into the circulation.

Treatment of severe but more sustained hypersensitivity reactions, such as allergic vasculitis or drug-induced lupus erythematosus, can be quite unrewarding, but large doses of the adrenocortical steroids are usually dramatically beneficial. Recognition of the relationship of these life-threatening reactions to drug treatment and discontinuance of the drug leads to the gradual resolution of vasculitis and associated diseases of the parenchymal organs, such as the kidney and the liver.

Desensitization procedures are occasionally successful, but they may be dangerous and are necessary only in rare circumstances.

19

Immunologic Deficiency Diseases

The importance of individual components of immunologic function to the body economy has been most clearly revealed when isolated deficiencies have given rise to clinical disease. Because such abnormalities can now be so effectively detected and defined by new laboratory methods, diseases of immunodeficiency are being discovered with increasing frequency. Indeed, the combined major primary immunodeficiency disorders appear to occur as frequently as the combined disturbances in hematopoiesis plus the lymphoid malignancies of childhood. Immunodeficiency disorders must be considered in two major categories: the primary, often genetically determined, immunodeficiencies and secondary immunodeficiency states. The latter occur as complications of infections and infestations, gastrointestinal disorders, malnutrition, aging, lymphoid malignancies, other cancers and many other diseases. Immunodeficiency of varying severity is also encountered as a side-effect of many treatment modalities, including radiation therapy and chemotherapy for cancer, and immunosuppressive treatment to prevent allograft rejection or to treat autoimmune diseases. From this perspective, the primary and secondary immunodeficiencies are not rare diseases, but disorders that rank among the most frequent and most serious ailments of man.

PRIMARY IMMUNODEFICIENCIES

The primary immunodeficiency diseases are usually genetically determined and comprise abnormalities of development or inborn errors of metabolism that reflect defects of differentiation, development, or function of classes or subclasses of the lymphoid cells; failure of development or dysplasia of the thymus; defective development of biologic amplification

280

systems, as with abnormalities or deficiencies of the complement system; and faulty development or inborn metabolic errors of the fundamental effector processes involved in immunologic resistance. Increasing knowledge of the immunologic defenses, their interacting cellular and molecular components, the evolving details of sequential stages of cellular differentiation, and the nature and control of the cellular and molecular interactions in immunity permits increasingly precise definitions of the primary immunodeficiency diseases. In turn, much of the expanding understanding of the lymphoid systems and immunologic functions has derived from insights generated by study of the patients who suffer from primary immunodeficiencies. Furthermore, patients with these diseases have provided and will increasingly provide crucial tests of the therapeutic value of our developing knowledge. Thus, as Experiments of Nature, it is the patients with primary immunodeficiencies who have frequently raised the critical questions that have directed fundamental immunologic inquiry and who provide a critical testing ground for the developing science of immunobiology.

Table 19–1 lists the major primary immunodeficiencies and the current views concerning the location and nature of the cellular defects, their genetic basis, and the immunopathology involving the lymphoid apparatus. As

TABLE 19–1.   THE MAJORITY PRIMARY IMMUNODEFICIENCY DISEASES

| TYPE | SUGGESTED CELLULAR DEFECTS | | | INHERITANCE | | |
	B Cells (a)*	B Cells (b)†	T Cells	X-linked	Autosomal Recessive	Other§
X-linked agammaglobulinemia	X	(X)‡		X		
Thymic hypoplasia			X			X
Severe combined immunodeficiency	X	(X)	X	X	X	X
With dysostosis	X	?	X		X	
With adenosine deaminase deficiency	X		X		X	
With generalized hematopoietic hypoplasia	X		X		X	
Selective Ig deficiency						
IgA	?	X	(X)			X
Others		?				X
X-linked immunodeficiencies with increased IgM	X			X		
Immunodeficiency with ataxia telangiectasia	X	X			X?	
Immunodeficiency with thrombocytopenia and eczema (Wiskott-Aldrich syndrome)			X	X		X
Immunodeficiency with thymoma	X		X			X
Immunodeficiency with normo- or hypergammaglobulinemia	X	X	(X)			X
Transient hypogammaglobulinemia of infancy	X					X
Varied immunodeficiencies (largely unclassified and common)	X	X	(X)		(X)	X

* Absent or very low.
† Easily detectable or increased.
‡ Some cases with circulating B lymphocytes without detectable surface Ig have been found.
§ Implies multifactorial or unknown genetic basis or no genetic basis.
(From Good, R. A.: The primary immunodeficiency diseases, in Beeson, P., and McDermott, W., Textbook of Medicine. Philadelphia, W. B. Saunders Company, 1975, p. 105.)

would be expected, these primary immunodeficiency diseases are regularly associated with an increased frequency and severity of infections with bacteria, viruses, fungi, or protozoa. In many of these disorders, so-called autoimmune, vascular, and mesenchymal diseases have occurred with inordinate frequency. In some, malignancies have occurred with abnormal frequency, especially lymphosarcomas and reticulum cell sarcomas involving the lymphoid apparatus itself, central nervous system malignancies, and epithelial malignancies of the stomach, colon, and head and neck region.

X-LINKED AGAMMAGLOBULINEMIA OF BRUTON

This classic form of immunologic deficiency has been named for its discoverer. Patients with this disease of X-linked inheritance usually begin to have recurrent bacterial infections during the second six months of life. Untreated patients develop extraordinary susceptibility to infection with certain extracellular pyogenic pathogens like pneumococcus, streptococcus, hemophilus, and *Pseudomonas*, but infections with other organisms, such as staphylococcus, occasionally occur. Each of the known immunoglobulins is virtually absent from the serum, although IgG can usually be measured in extremely small amounts by sensitive quantitative immunochemical techniques.

These patients often fail completely to produce circulating antibodies after bacterial or virus infections or following immunization with any of many different vaccines. In spite of failure to respond with antibody production, these patients develop the delayed type of allergy normally and can usually reject allografts of skin in a normal or nearly normal fashion. Histologic studies show that their lymph nodes and spleen lack germinal centers, and that plasma cells are absent from their lymph nodes, spleen, bone marrow, and connective tissues, including the lamina propria of the intestine. Tonsils are very poorly developed, if present at all, and lack follicular components. By contrast, these patients have normal or nearly normal levels of circulating lymphocytes, nearly normal numbers of lymphocytes in the thymic dependent regions of lymph nodes and spleen, and a perfectly normal thymus. Figure 19–1 compares tonsil, thymus, and stimulated lymph nodes from a normal person and a patient with the Bruton type of agammaglobulinemia. Such patients clearly have failed to develop that population of lymphoid cells and plasma cells that matures under the influence of the primary gut-associated lymphoid tissues or bone marrow. On the other hand, the population of lymphoid cells that matures under direct thymic influence has developed normally.

These patients are prone to develop connective tissue diseases, such as arthritis, dermatomyositis, and diffuse vasculitis. They also seem unable to resist infections with hepatitis virus, and such infections usually cause either massive liver destruction or chronic active hepatitis with steady progression to complete destruction of the liver. In striking contrast, these patients can resist many virus infections without difficulty even though they appear to produce very little or no antibody to the viruses. For example, they respond

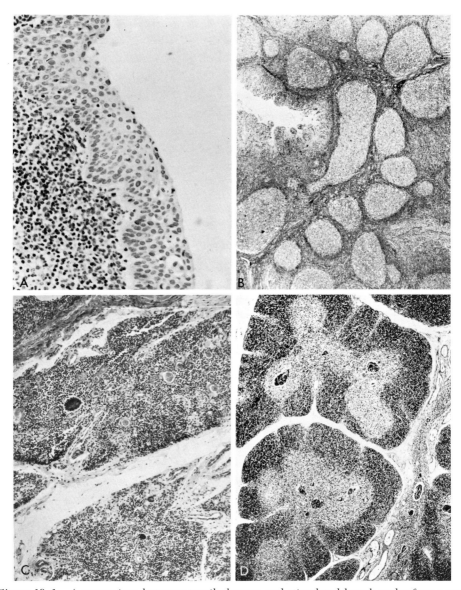

Figure 19–1.   A comparison between tonsil, thymus, and stimulated lymph nodes from a normal person and from a patient with Bruton's agammaglobulinemia. *A*, Tonsil from a patient with Bruton's agammaglobulinemia. *B*, Normal tonsil from a four-year-old patient. *C*, Thymus from a patient with Bruton's agammaglobulinemia. *D*, Normal thymus from a four-year-old child.

Illustration continued on following page

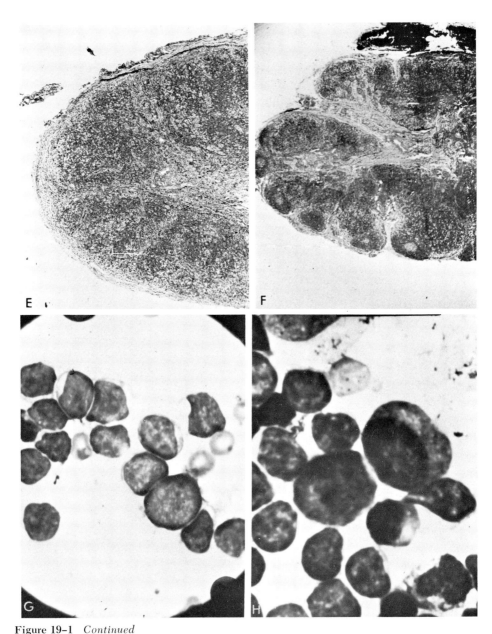

Figure 19-1 *Continued*
E, Microscopic section of a lymph node from a patient with Bruton's agammaglobulinemia. *F*, Microscopic section of a normal lymph node following secondary antigenic stimulation. *G*, Cells from an imprint of a lymph node from a patient with Bruton's agammaglobulinemia after antigenic stimulation. No plasma cells are found. *H*, Lymph node imprint from a normal person following antigenic stimulation. Numerous plasma cells can be found. (From Hoyer, J. R., et al.: Lymphopenic forms of congenital immunologic deficiency diseases. Medicine *47*:201–206, 1968.)

to measles infection normally, recover at the usual time, and even resist rein-
fection. Often no antibody to measles virus can be demonstrated. Similarly,
they develop immunity to vaccinia, varicella, mumps, and several other
viruses, including the common respiratory viruses. Although they fail to develop demonstrable circulating antibodies to mycobacteria, fungi, most en-
terobacteria, staphylococci, and other low-grade pathogens, they resist infections with these agents quite well. Their granulocytes and macrophages can
exercise phagocytic processes normally in vitro if opsonins are added. Their
reticuloendothelial system clears aggregated protein and colloidal particles
promptly from the circulation, and they can develop all of the cell-mediated
immunities normally.

The numbers of T lymphocytes in the blood appear to be within normal
limits or slightly higher than normal, but in most cases B lymphocytes are
completely lacking. The numbers of lymphocytes of the third population,
including K cells, which are nonphagocytic lymphocytes with receptors for
IgG, and the number of cells bearing double markers, e.g., receptors for
sheep red blood cells and receptors for IgG (T_γ cells) or C3, are normal.
Recent studies have shown that some patients with this form of agammaglobulinemia possess lymphocytes in their bone marrow that contain cytoplasmic IgM, a cell which is a likely precursor to the B cell lineage. Thus,
the defect for some of these patients appears to lie developmentally between
the most primitive Ig-producing cell in the marrow and mature B lymphocytes. It is important, however, to recognize that X-linked agammaglobulinemia, like most of the primary immune deficiencies, is a heterogeneous
disease. A family with multiple cases of clearly defined agammaglobulinemia of X-linked inheritance has been described in which numbers of B
lymphocytes were normal. In addition, several cases have been described
with all of the pathologic and immunologic features that have been associated with X-linked agammaglobulinemia in patients with clear evidence
of autosomal inheritance.

Gamma globulin treatment, although very helpful, does not entirely control the disease in these patients, and they often develop persistent respiratory disease with progressive pulmonary inflammation, bronchiectasis, and
pulmonary fibrosis. Some ultimately die from pulmonary failure. The exact
basis of the progressive pulmonary disease is not yet established, but seems
to be related to a deficiency of the local antibody system responsible for
secretory IgA production. Others of this group have ultimately developed
progressive fatal encephalitis, probably attributable to persistent virus infection.

COMMON VARIABLE IMMUNODEFICIENCY (CVI)

Perhaps the most frequently encountered patients with primary immunologic deficiency diseases are those having the late-appearing common variable immunodeficiency syndrome. Clinically apparent immunologic deficiency may appear at any time between the ages of 2 and 80 years. Some of
these patients have a hereditary disease that seems to be transmitted as an

autosomal recessive trait; in others, late appearance of immunologic deficiency seems to be the result of an autosomal dominant inheritance. Thus, their late-appearing clinical disease may represent an abiotrophy, an inherited defect not manifest until later in life. The manifestations of the disease include recurrent pneumococcal pneumonia or infections with other highly virulent bacteria, an inordinate incidence of both lymphoid malignancies and malignancies of other types, and a high frequency of connective tissue diseases, especially rheumatoid arthritis and hematologic disorders.

Immunoglobulin deficiencies are constantly present, but are highly variable from patient to patient and even from time to time in the same patient. These patients regularly possess more IgG than do patients with the sex-linked Bruton's agammaglobulinemia. They may possess normal or increased amounts of IgM in some instances. Some lack mainly IgM and IgA, with normal or nearly normal levels of IgG. Since the patterns of immunoglobulin in these patients are not constant, we prefer not to use the confusing term dysgammaglobulinemia. All have sufficient IgG to permit isolation and study of these interesting proteins, which tend to have restricted electrophoretic mobility, to band like a myeloma protein on electrophoresis in acrylamide gel, and to have unusual ratios of the two different types of light chain. In the aggregated form, IgG from these patients may fix complement poorly.

Deficiency of cellular immunity can often be demonstrated on careful study. Often, the patients do not reject homografts as rapidly as normal, are slow to develop or fail to develop demonstrable cellular immunity, and handle virus infections poorly.

The high frequency of lymphoid malignancy in this population of immunologically defective patients has been a source of much provocative argument. Some consider the immunologic deficiencies to have been secondary to an underlying lymphoid malignancy from the beginning. However, the lymphoid malignancies usually appear long after the immunologic deficiency is known to have been present, sometimes as long as 20 years. In addition, other forms of malignancy also occur with high frequency. A relatively large number of patients with this form of immunologic deficiency disease have an enlarged spleen, enlarged lymph nodes, enlarged tonsils, and sometimes enlarged Peyer's patches along the lower ileum. Their lymphatic tissues sometimes completely lack germinal centers, but may instead contain both excessive numbers and unusually large germinal centers. Most patients with CVI possess normal numbers of B precursor cells in the marrow, and have normal or only slightly reduced numbers of B cells in the circulating blood. Like patients with the Bruton type of agammaglobulinemia, CVI patients often lack plasma cells entirely or have gross quantitative deficiencies of these elements in the lymphoid tissues, bone marrow, and lamina propria of the gastrointestinal tract, but plasma cells are sometimes present in substantial numbers in certain limited locations.

Stimulation of lymphocytes from normal blood with pokeweed mitogen (PMW) results in differentiation of some of the cells to plasmacytoid elements that synthesize and secrete Ig. The differentiating event leading to the appearance of the plasmacytoid cells requires the presence of a subpopulation of helper T cells which have been identified as T cells with receptors for IgM and called Tμ cells. By contrast, stimulation of the blood lymphocytes of CVI patients with PWM usually does not lead to plasma cell development. Furthermore, most patients with CVI have been found to have lymphocytes in their circulation that interfere with the capacity of normal lymphocytes to synthesize and secrete Ig or to develop plasma cell morphology after stimulation with PWM. In some, removal of the T lymphocytes from the peripheral blood leukocytes and replacement with normal T lymphocytes frees the remaining B lymphocytes to differentiate normally to plasma cells that synthesize and secrete Ig. These suppressor lymphocytes are sensitive to irradiation and to high concentrations of adrenal corticosteroids.

The role of a steroid-sensitive suppressor lymphocyte in the pathogenesis of some cases of CVI is consonant with the early description of cases of CVI that responded dramatically to treatment with adrenal corticosteroids. In many patients with CVI, however, removal of the patient's suppressor lymphocytes and their replacement by normal T lymphocytes does not make immunoglobulin synthesis and secretion possible after PWM stimulation. Thus, although recent evidence suggests that the pathogenic basis for some cases of CVI resides in a suppressor T cell, the most frequent pathogenic mechanism seems to reside in an abnormality of B cell development that reflects an arrest in development at a step of differentiation between B cell and plasma cell. Although the molecular basis of the cooperative and nonspecific functions of T cells in the development and differentiation of B cells has not yet been defined in human systems, experimental models for these analyses have been developed which promise early definition.

Patients with CVI are prone to develop both Coombs' test positive and Coombs' test negative hemolytic anemias, gastric atrophy, pernicious anemia, and a variety of other autoimmune diseases and phenomena. They also develop amyloidosis with extraordinary frequency. Treatment with gamma globulin stops the succession of life-threatening pneumococcal infections, but paranasal sinus disease and pulmonary infections persist, often leading to death from pulmonary insufficiency.

TRANSIENT HYPOGAMMAGLOBULINEMIA OF INFANCY

Newborn babies begin life with gamma globulin levels equal to or slightly higher than those of their mothers. During the first few weeks of life, a decline in IgG levels occurs because the baby's ability to synthesize gamma globulin remains relatively inadequate as the IgG of maternal origin is catabolized. With increasing production, the levels of IgG begin to rise, reaching normal adult concentrations at about 1.5 to 2 years of age. Only minute amounts of IgM are normally present in serum at birth, but soon afterward, the levels of IgM begin to rise, and adult levels are reached during the second half of the first year. IgA production does not begin until later, and the levels of these immunoglobulins rise slowly to reach adult concentrations at some time after two years of age.

Children are encountered occasionally who suffer from recurrent bacterial infections that occur primarily between 6 and 18 months of age. These children are hypogammaglobulinemic and immunologically deficient, and except for the fact that their disease is self-limited, they cannot readily be distinguished from patients with primary agammaglobulinemia. They appear to be suffering the consequence of an inordinate delay in developing full immunologic maturity. Transient hypogammaglobulinemia affects children of both sexes, tends to occur in families, and may, at least in some instances, be transmitted as an autosomal recessive trait.

Evidence suggests that some of the children with transient hypogammaglobulinemia of infancy do not become completely normal even though gamma globulin levels and immunologic capacity improve dramatically with time. Thus far, detailed definition of this syndrome in terms of T cell numbers, B cells numbers, and in vitro responses of these cells has not been accomplished.

Isolated Absence of a Single Immunoglobulin

Until very recently, only one of the immunologic deficiencies seemed to be associated with defective development of a single type of immunoglobulin molecule — the isolated deficiency of IgA. This disorder is not uncommon, occurring in 1 of 1000 persons. The defect is probably transmitted as an autosomal recessive trait. The patients may be clinically well, or they may have recurrent gastrointestinal infections and a spruelike syndrome, or recurrent respiratory disease. Although secretory IgA is normally a component of saliva and respiratory secretions, it is of interest that patients with isolated absence of IgA often have not suffered from recurrent respiratory disease. However, many seem to be troubled with it almost constantly. In certain diseases, like ataxia-telangiectasia, absence of IgA along with other immunologic defects is clearly correlated with recurrent sinopulmonary disease. Many patients who lack IgA have one of a variety of mesenchymal disease, such as rheumatoid arthritis, lupus erythematosus, and tenosynovitis. They may also suffer from central nervous system disease, especially convulsive disorders. Recent studies in Switzerland and England have linked IgA deficiency to convulsive disorders and also have linked Dilantin treatment to a dramatic reduction in circulating IgA levels.

Studies of many children who suffered from recurrent sinusitis, middle ear infections, recurrent pulmonic infections and progressive pulmonary damage have revealed a selective lack of circulating levels of IgA. Some of these patients also lack IgE, but others possess normal or even increased amounts of IgE. This latter relationship may be a reflection of the general principle, stated earlier, that when one component of the immune system is deficient, the remaining systems may be excessively stimulated. In this instance, excessive stimulation of the local IgE immune system when the IgA system is lacking or deficient may give rise to increased atopic-type allergic reactions and serious or annoying symptomatology involving both upper and lower respiratory systems. An attempt has been made to link defective early development of the IgA system with development of severe atopic disease in families in whom severe allergy is a problem. While observations suggest that retarded development of IgA may favor atopic IgE responses, confirmation of this postulate has been slow to develop. Further definitive study is needed on this important point.

Studies of patients with isolated deficiency of IgA have clarified another important point. These patients regularly possess circulating and tissue B lymphocytes with IgA at their surface. In one study with appropriate helper T lymphocytes plus PWM stimulation, the patients' IgA-bearing B cells became able to be differentiated into IgA-producing plasmacytoid cells. These investigations establish clearly that the structural gene functions for α chain synthesis are present and in some patients can be activated to synthesize and secrete IgA. Several patients who lack demonstrable circulating IgA but have secretory IgA have been described. At least one patient who possessed circulating IgA and IgA-producing cells in lymphoid tissue and lamina propria of the GI tract, but lacked secretory IgA, has been studied at the National Institutes of Health. The patient appeared to be deficient in the ability to produce the so-called transport or secretory component of IgA. This component is coupled to IgA in the intestinal or glandular epithelial cells, and may be involved in the transport of dimeric IgA from the lamina propria to the gut lumen. The patient suffered from an increased frequency of respiratory and gastrointestinal disease. Patients with IgA deficiency have been described who have suppressor T cells selective for the IgA system.

ASSOCIATION OF DEVELOPMENT OF IgA SECRETION TO THE DEVELOPMENT OF THYMUS

In several human conditions, as well as in experimental animals, extreme T cell deficiencies may sometimes be associated with failure to develop the capacity to produce IgA. This is thought to reflect an essential or important role for a subpopulation of T lymphocytes in development of full potential of the plasma cell system for IgA synthesis and secretion. In the nu/nu mouse in which the thymus fails to develop normally, IgA as well as a subclass of IgG is regularly absent from both blood and secretions. This deficiency can be corrected by providing either well-tolerated syngeneic lymphoid cells from heterozygote nu/+ donors or by transplantation of thymus or thymus anlage from neonatal or embryonic normal donors. More studies are needed to define the precise relationship of differentiation of IgA-producing cells to the development of thymic dependent cell populations, but the existence of an important interrelationship of the thymus and T cell system and IgA development seems to have been established.

Since it is probable that other patients will be discovered with immunologic deficiencies based on an isolated inability to synthesize different types of heavy chains or light chains of the immunoglobulin molecule, it is important to search for these defects.

III AND IV PHARYNGEAL POUCH SYNDROME OF DiGEORGE

The thymus develops from epithelial anlagen derived from the third and fourth pharyngeal pouches, as do the parathyroids, some of the clear cells of the thyroid, and the ultimobranchial body. A syndrome characterized by congenital absence of the parathyroids and thymus, and abormalities of the aortic structure that is derived from the fourth pharyngeal arch, has been recognized in infants for many years. Abnormalities of the appearance of the mouth and the pinnae of the ears have also been associated with this condition; these children consequently have typical facies (Fig. 19–2).

Infants present with tetany of the newborn, but they are unable to survive long primarily because they lack the capacity to develop and express cell-mediated immune responses. Circulating lymphocyte counts are usually near normal at birth, but soon decline to a significantly low level, and the patients defend themselves poorly against certain fungus and virus infections. In contrast, the levels of their immunoglobulins are usually normal; plasma cells are present in normal numbers in the lymphoid tissues, connective tissues and marrow; and the B lymphocyte regions of the lymph nodes and spleen are preserved. The thymic dependent deep cortical areas of lymph nodes and thymic dependent lymphoid regions of spleen are grossly depleted or almost devoid of cells (Fig. 19–3A). Development of delayed allergy, allograft rejection, the number of T lymphocytes, and proliferative responses to the plant lectins PHA and Con A are usually very grossly deficient. The numbers of B lymphocytes of all classes are sometimes markedly increased over the normal, but differentiation of these B lymphocytes to plasma cells after pokeweed mitogen stimulation is defective unless normal T lymphocytes are also provided.

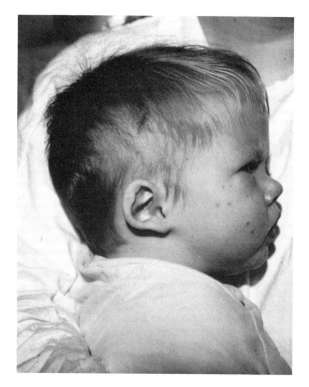

Figure 19–2. A patient with DiGeorge syndrome.

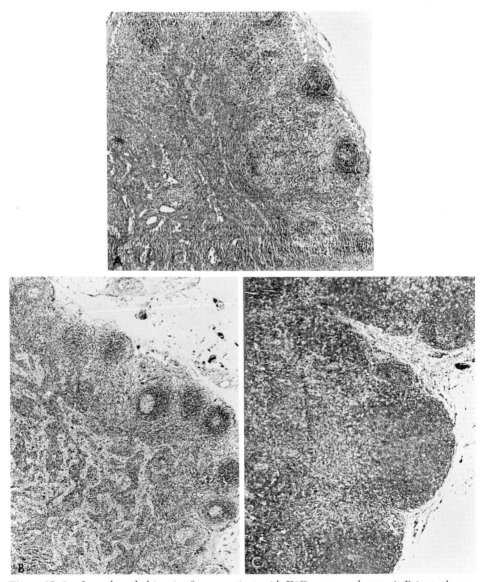

Figure 19–3. Lymph node biopsies from a patient with DiGeorge syndrome. *A*, Prior to thymus transplant. *B*, One month following thymus transplant. *C*, Six months following thymus transplant.

Patients with the immunodeficiency associated with the DiGeorge syndrome clearly have an immunologic deficit consequent to failure of normal development of the thymus. Strong support for this concept of the pathogenesis in this form of immunodeficiency disease comes from the observation that transplantation of embryonic thymic tissue has corrected this immunodeficiency on six separate occasions. Figure 19–3 (B and C) shows the correction of lymph node morphology by thymic transplant in such a case.

T Cell Deficiencies Other Than the DiGeorge Syndrome

As methods have become available for identifying and enumerating the subclasses of the lymphoid cells, several patients with selective deficiencies of the T cell populations have been identified. These patients either lack or are grossly deficient in the lymphocytes that form rosettes with SRBC. They cannot develop or express delayed allergy or reject skin allografts normally, and they have lymphocyte populations which do not respond by proliferating normally in response to in vitro stimulation with PHA or Con A. The circulating and tissue lymphocytes also fail to respond normally upon stimulation with allogeneic lymphocytes in mixed leukocyte cultures, and they do not respond normally to in vitro stimulation by bacterial or fungal antigens. B lymphocyte numbers are sometimes greatly increased, but on other occasions their numbers have been only moderately increased, associated with an increase of blood lymphocytes lacking markers by which B and T cells are identified (so-called null cells). In several instances, this apparent T cell deficiency has appeared to be corrected by transplantation of embryonic thymus.

While these patients do not have the other physical stigmata of the DiGeorge syndrome, they do have a similar increased susceptibility to infections with low grade bacterial pathogens, fungi, and certain viruses. That these forms of T cell deficiency reflect a heterogeneous group of disorders is indicated by the findings that IgA levels have sometimes been normal and sometimes low. Many more clinical and immunologic analyses will be necessary before the selective immunodeficiencies based on defects of normal development of the several T lymphocyte populations have been defined.

Severe Combined Immunodeficiency (SCID)

Two years before Bruton described agammaglobulinemia, Glanzman and Riniker in Switzerland described a familial disease which leads to death in infancy from infection and is characterized by gross deficiency or absence of lymphocytes in the circulation. Plasma cells often fail to develop in the bone marrow and lymphoid tissue, and the lamina propria of the gastrointestinal tract contains few or no lymphoid or plasma cells. This disease was later found to be associated with agammaglobulinemia and the lack of ability to express all types of adaptive immune responses. Severe combined immunodeficiencies are now known to comprise an extremely heterogeneous group of disease with differences in genetic basis, pathogenesis, lymphoid cellular development, and therapy.

Autosomal Recessive SCID without Recognized Enzyme Deficiency. In one form of the disease, the inheritance is autosomal recessive, and the parents appear to be immunologically normal with normal lymphoid tissue. Both B and T cells are almost completely absent in the blood, lymph nodes, and spleen of the affected patients. The thymus is present, but very small, being generally 1 to 2 gm in weight instead of the normal 20 to 25 gm, and it shows unmistakable evidence of failure to develop normally. Hassall's corpuscles are lacking, the veins and arteries are small, and the organ has little or no excess of fat. The epithelial stroma is present and well developed into lobes and lobules, appearing strikingly like an early embryonic thymus. Thymic humoral factors like Bach's *hormone thymique* may be present in the circulation but thymopoietin levels are low. Figure 19–4 illustrates the lymphoid tissue from a patient with this form of SCID.

These infants lack all of the immunologic functions present in a normal infant. They fail to reject homografts, they do not develop delayed allergy or produce antibodies, they possess only small amounts of IgG, and they usually completely lack IgM and IgA.

Since the defect in these patients involves the B cell line of lymphoid cells and plasma cells, as well as the thymic dependent line of lymphocytes, the abnormality of the thymus could not account entirely for the observed immunologic deficiency. Instead, one must postulate the existence either of a defect at the lymphoid stem cell stage or some more general influence on differentiation of lymphoid cells. Since a pituitary control mechanism may be essential for development of the lymphoid tissue, it is remotely possible that some forms of this disease are related to a defective development of that influence.

With such a broadly based immunologic deficiency, the patients with SCID cannot survive. They generally succumb during their first year of life to low grade opportunistic pathogens such as *Pseudomonas, Staphylococcus,* Enterobacteriaceae, *Pneumocystis carinii,* or *Candida.* If exposed, they may die of a characteristic giant cell pneumonia (Hecht's pneumonia) produced by the measles virus, from varicella infection, or with progressive and generalized vaccinia. Usually, they do not show the characteristic rash of measles. Cytomegalovirus infection has also repeatedly produced fatal infections.

Since they cannot reject foreign cells and since, like neonatally thymectomized animals, they are inordinately susceptible to the ravages of graft-versus-host reaction, they often die following blood transfusion or attempted treatment with immunologically competent cells. The generalized disease produced in them by transfer of immunologically competent cells includes a characteristic skin rash, hepatosplenomegaly, hemolytic anemia, aregenerative anemia, fever, toxicity, and rapid wasting. Instances have been described in which chronic graft-versus-host reaction has occurred in such patients on the basis of transfer of immunologically competent lymphocytes from the mother through the placenta.

This disease has now been treated successfully on repeated occasions

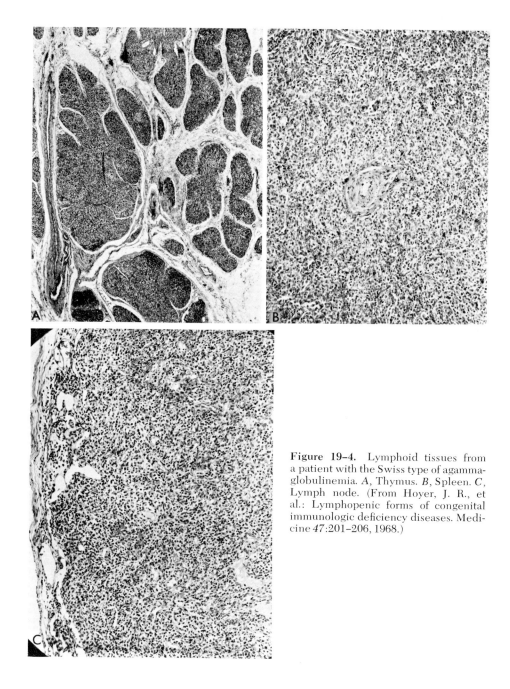

Figure 19–4. Lymphoid tissues from a patient with the Swiss type of agamma-globulinemia. *A*, Thymus. *B*, Spleen. *C*, Lymph node. (From Hoyer, J. R., et al.: Lymphopenic forms of congenital immunologic deficiency diseases. Medicine *47*:201–206, 1968.)

by bone marrow transplantation, using marrow from a well-matched sibling donor. When HLA- and MLC-matched sibling marrow has been used, neither fatal GVH nor persistent chronic GVH reactions have been observed. Full restoration of immunologic function accomplished by marrow transplantation is attributable to cells derived from the host's marrow, but in some cases the correction appears to involve the bone marrow stem cells, while in others a more peripheral reconstruction has probably been accomplished.

Severe Combined Immunodeficiency Associated with Deficient or Abnormal Enzymes in the Purine Metabolic Pathway. Severe combined immunodeficiency has also been recognized as a disease of autosomal recessive inheritance that may involve deficiency of adenosine deaminase (ADA) or nucleoside phosphorylase (NP). Parents of the patients tend to have values for these enzymes in the red cells or leukocytes that are approximately one half those observed in normal persons. Figure 19–5 indicates the metabolic pathways that appear to be involved in these disorders. Immunologic and cellular defects, although probably more variable than those observed in the Glanzman-Riniker syndrome discussed above, usually involve both B and T cell systems, and immunologic reconstitution of these patients has repeatedly been accomplished by bone marrow transplantation. A state of mixed chimerism deriving from successful bone marrow transplantation has been shown to exist, in which the patient's red blood cells lack ADA while the lymphocytes contain normal amounts of ADA. Approximately 15 to 20 per cent of patients with SCID at present have identifiable defects of ADA. Usually, these have been described as absence of the enzyme, but several cases have been studied in whom ADA appeared to be present, but there was an inhibitor capable of blocking its activity. Abnormalities of thymic development are regularly associated. T cell deficiencies and abnormal

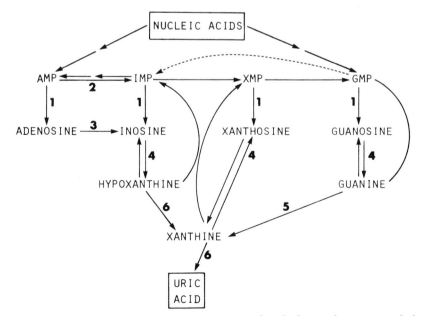

Figure 19–5. Metabolic pathways in SCID, associated with abnormal purine metabolism.

lymphoid tissue at all sites have been described in some cases, and in these both T cell and B cell function and numbers have been deficient. In other cases, B cell numbers have approached normal. Correction of this variant has also been repeatedly achieved by marrow transplantation, using marrow from a matched sibling donor. One patient with this form of immunodeficiency, who did not have a matched relative who could give bone marrow, has been treated with repeated transfusions of red blood cells from donors having normal levels of ADA, resulting in rather striking functional improvement.

Patients with severe immunodeficiency involving both T and B cell functions, but especially with deficient development of T lymphocyte populations, have been found to lack the closely related enzyme nucleoside phosphorylase (NP). The fact that lack of this enzyme can be associated with failure of development, especially of the thymus and T cell system, provides strong evidence that the metabolic pathway in which both ADA and NP operate is vital to T cell development, and perhaps to all lymphoid development. Inosine phosphorylase deficiency has also produced this disease.

Variants of SCID. Families in which SCID has been found to be transmitted as an X-linked recessive trait have been extensively studied. Cases in which an autosomal recessive disease is associated with severe skeletal abnormalities are described, and there are patients in whom T cells were poorly developed and B cell numbers were normal though with grossly defective functions. From the genetic analysis, it is clear that these different variants must represent at least four different disease entities. It seems virtually certain, however, that as our methods for analyses become more and more definitive, ultimately extending to complete biochemical definition, it will be established that there are a number of different genetically or environmentally based pathogeneses of SCID. If, however, a matched sibling donor or a well-matched relative is available in the immediate family, this disease in all the forms thus far described seems readily correctable by bone marrow transplantation.

Treatment of SCID by Transplantation of Cultured Thymus or Fetal Liver. Recently, a patient with SCID that involved failure of normal development of both B and T lymphocyte populations was dramatically corrected by transplantation of thymus from a normal infant, which had been kept in culture for approximately three weeks. This approach to therapy did not induce GVH reaction; the B cell population seemed better reconstructed than the T cell population. However, thymic transplantation, using either fresh or cultured thymus, has not been beneficial to other patients with SCID, which again argues for the heterogenicity of the diseases that are classified as SCID.

When a matched sibling donor or relative is not available, successful reconstruction has also been accomplished using early (under 12 weeks) fetal liver alone or together with thymus transplants from the same or other fetuses. Finally, in one patient, the immunodeficiency syndrome of SCID was corrected using marrow from an HLA-B and HLA-D-matched donor found in the general population.

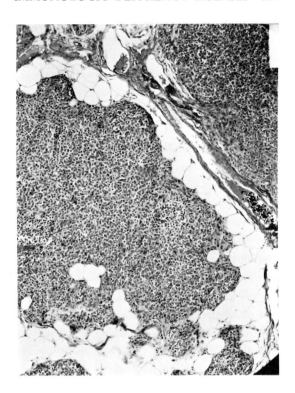

Figure 19–6. Thymus of patient with ataxia telangiectasia.

IMMUNODEFICIENCY WITH ATAXIA TELANGIECTASIA

A severe and complex immunodeficiency is a regular concomitant of the ataxia-telangiectasia syndrome of Louis-Bar. Deficient thymic development (Fig. 19–6), absence of Hassall's corpuscles, decreased numbers and functions of T cells, absent or deficient IgA, and, sometimes, absent or deficient IgE and defective ability to develop or express delayed allergy and allograft rejection are characteristically observed in these patients. The children seem quite normal at birth, but usually immunologic defects are observed as early as they can be studied. They develop progressive cerebellar ataxia, usually between 1 and 2 years of age, which is associated with pathologic changes in the Purkinje cells of the cerebellum. The vascular component of the disease appears in the form of telangiectasis in sclerae, eyelids, and the antecubital and popliteal spaces. This progressive vascular abnormality develops when the children are between 1.5 and 5 years of age and is accompanied by progeric changes of skin and hair. The ovaries in females and testicles in males fail to develop normally. Alpha-fetoprotein is present in inordinately high concentrations in most patients. Increased susceptibility to sinusitis, otitis, and upper and lower respiratory infections may be a major problem.

Malignancy is a very frequent complication, which may appear in more than 10 per cent of the patients. These are predominately lymphoreticular neoplasms, but brain tumors and cancers of the stomach and upper GI tract also occur with increased frequency. Figure 19–7 illustrates a lymphosarcoma which developed in one of our patients with the AT syndrome. This

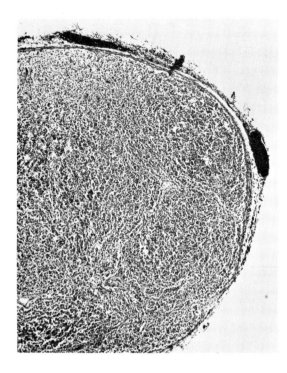

Figure 19–7. Malignancy from a patient with ataxia telangiectasia.

lymphosarcoma proved highly resistant to the efforts of a chemotherapeutic program for non-Hodgkin's solid tissue lymphoma being used at that time. Irradiation treatment and chemotherapy, especially with alkylating agents, is very poorly tolerated by these patients. The predisposition to certain cancers has been attributed both to the immunodeficiency and to a chromosomal instability. The patients regularly show abnormalities of the 14th chromosome reflected in ring chromosome formation, and it has been thought best to classify them among the groups of patients with chromosomal instability syndrome. The disease is probably transmitted as an autosomal recessive trait, and a very high proportion of family members, some 30 to 40 per cent, have died of cancer. Like the patients, family members seem to have instability of their chromosomes, and also like the patients, they have cells highly susceptible to damage by X-irradiation in culture.

The nature of the underlying metabolic or enzymatic defect responsible for the complex syndrome is unknown. Recent studies using cell complementation in vitro seem to indicate that several different metabolic defects may underlie the same clinical and pathologic syndrome. Heroic efforts to correct the disease have been made by surgeons in the Soviet Union, by transplantation of fetal thymus and sternum with its bone marrow. However, these efforts have not yet been of clear benefit.

WISKOTT-ALDRICH SYNDROME

The Wiskott-Aldrich syndrome is a sex-linked recessive disease that is associated with extraordinary immunologic defects. Patients with this disease suffer from thrombocytopenia, eczema, and marked susceptibility to many infections (Fig. 19–8). Few have been able to survive to adult life. They develop an enigmatic, progressive, secondary depletion of lymphocytes in the peripheral blood and a deficiency of lymphocytes in the thymic dependent regions of lymphatic tissues (Fig. 19–9), but the thymus seems to be normal morphologically in most cases. These changes are associated with a progressively severe deficiency of the cellular immunities.

Patients with Wiskott-Aldrich syndrome fail to develop the normal isohemagglutinins and hemolysins, and they fail to respond to the polysaccharide antigens which have been tried. By contrast, they may show quite normal responses to certain protein antigens. Reduced responses to certain other primary protein antigens are also seen, which reflect a defect in the afferent limb of the immune response. However, deficiencies in responses to protein antigens are never as severe as the defects involving polysaccharide antigens. Like the patients with ataxia telangiectasia, those with Wiskott-Aldrich syndrome are prone to develop lymphoreticular malignancies. The malignancies may rapidly become widespread and seem to have a great propensity to invade the central nervous system.

It has seemed to us that the basic defect in these patients involves the afferent limb of the immune response and perhaps resides primarily in macrophage function. Recent studies appear to support this view since it has been shown that the blood monocytes of patients with the W-A syndrome have defective monocyte-mediated antibody-dependent cytotoxicity despite normal numbers of monocytes. Whether this is the fundamental cellular defect in these patients still seems questionable at this time. Recent evidence suggests that these patients, like those with ataxia telangiectasia, may have chromosomal instability.

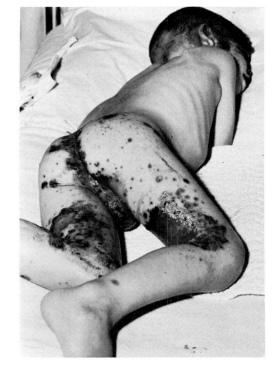

Figure 19–8. A patient with Wiskott-Aldrich syndrome with disseminated herpes simplex infection.

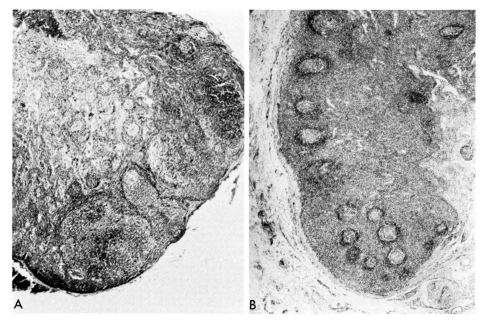

Figure 19–9. A, Lymph node from a patient with Wiskott-Aldrich syndrome early in the course of the disease. B, Lymph node taken late in the course of Wiskott-Aldrich syndrome.

Treatment of these patients has been woefully inadequate. They may die from infection as a consequence of the immunologic deficiency, from hemorrhage secondary to thrombocytopenia, or from the malignant tumors. A child with the W-A syndrome has been successfully treated at the University of Wisconsin with massive doses of cyclophosphamide, plus transplantation of bone marrow from a healthy female sibling who was well-matched at the HLA-A, HLA-B, and HLA-D loci. The child became chimeric in marrow and blood and developed the ability to form isohemagglutinins and platelets much better than before the transplant was made. This patient has been healthy and continues to be chimeric nine years after the original transplant was done, although his platelets continue to be abnormal with a count of 35,000 to 75,000. The platelet abnormality is not associated with bleeding. Thus, a dramatic improvement in the clinical course, largely attributable to correction of the immunodeficiency, accompanied establishment of a chimeric state. Others have advocated using transfer factor in treatment of this rather desperate disease, and objective improvements in cellular immunity have been produced in some patients by such therapy. However, some of these patients have developed Coombs' positive acute and subacute hemolytic anemia, and controlled trials have not yet been reported. A recent complete correction of the hematologic and immunologic abnormalities by bone marrow transplantation is encouraging.

THYMOMA WITH IMMUNODEFICIENCY

Numerous patients in whom thymoma and immunodeficiency with hypogammaglobulinemia are reported have now been studied. The first of these provoked the extensive studies that established the major role of the thymus in developmental immunology. In these patients, the numbers of B cells are grossly deficient and even the B cell precursor in the bone marrow has seemed to be lacking. They may develop a progressive lymphopenia, including decline in the numbers of T lymphocytes in some instances. Susceptibility to a wide spectrum of pathogens is a major clinical problem.

The thymoma-agammaglobulinemia syndrome may sometimes be associated with defective erythropoiesis, and the latter hematopoietic disorder often occurs with thymoma in patients who do not show defects of B cell function. Removal of the thymic tumor, composed of abnormal spindle-shaped epithelial cells, does not correct the immunodeficiency. The precise relationship of the immunodeficiency disease to the thymic tumors is not yet clear. Analysis of thymic humoral factors, which is now becoming possible, may clarify these relationships. Patients with thymoma-agammaglobuline-mia, like those with X-linked infantile agammaglobulinemia and like many with common variable immunodeficiency, often have suppressor lympho-cytes in their blood that are capable of inhibiting plasma cell differentiation and development, but that do not seem to be crucially involved in the pathogenesis of the immunodeficiency syndrome. Experimental evidence indicates that high concentrations of thymopoietin may inhibit early steps in B cell development. Perhaps the thymic tumors produce thymopoietin in amounts large enough to exert such an influence. A few patients with thymoma-agammaglobulinemia have developed striking eosinopenia, but the basis for this interesting association is enigmatic.

ANTILYMPHOCYTE AUTOANTIBODY AS A BASIS FOR IMMUNOLOGICAL DEFICIENCY

A number of patients have been described in recent years who have immunologic deficiencies, primarily but not exclusively of cellular immunities, which are associated with the presence of serum autoantibodies directed against lymphocytes. They appear to be able to develop primary antibodies quite well but exercise immunologic memory poorly. Lymphocytopenia, particularly of small lymphocytes, is striking, but these patients may have normal levels of immunoglobulins and plasma cells. The thymus is normally developed, but shows involutional changes. This is a clinical disease in which the patients seem to be making their own antilymphocyte globulin. It is associated with an increased susceptibility to infection and with immune deficits, especially of cellular immunity.

CHRONIC GRANULOMATOUS DISEASE (CGD)

The first of the primary immunodeficiency disorders of phagocytic cells to be discovered was chronic granulomatous disease of childhood, also called chronic septic granulomatosis, fatal granulomatous disease, and dys-phagocytosis with lipochrome histiocytosis. In this disease, the monocytes

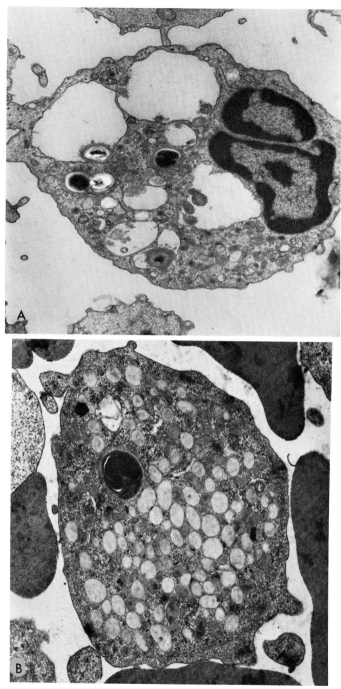

Figure 19–10. *A*, Electron micrograph of a neutrophil from a normal person after phagocytosis. Note the paucity of lysosomal granules in the immediate vicinity of the phagocytic vacuoles. *B*, Electron micrograph of a neutrophil from a patient with fatal granulomatous disease of childhood. Note the relative lack of degranulation in the vicinity immediately surrounding the ingested bacteria. (Courtesy of Dr. J. G. White.)

and granulocytes of the host can ingest bacteria normally, but fail to kill catalase-positive bacteria after their ingestion (Fig. 19–10). Variants of this syndrome based on different pathogeneses have been described and are classified as four separate entities: (1) A sex-linked recessive CGD, in which multiple enzymatic abnormalities are expressed after phagocytosis; there appears to be a fundamental membrane defect associated with absence of the surface antigen called KX. (2) An autosomal recessive CGD associated with deficiency of glutathione reductase activity in the phagocytic cells. (3) An autosomal recessive form of CGD, in which complete absence of glucose 6-phosphate dehydrogenase is characteristic. (4) An autosomal recessive form with no deficiency of glutathione reductase or glucose 6-phosphate dehydrogenase. Type 1, the most frequent form of CGD, was the first to be discovered, and may be considered to be the prototype. This X-linked recessive disorder has been of major help in defining the crucial role of phagocytic cells in the bodily defense.

Certain microorganisms, including staphylococci, *Serratia marcescens*, many fungi, and several enteric bacteria, are phagocytized well by the leukocytes of these patients, but are not killed effectively. Defective killing by neutrophils and monocytes renders these patients inordinately susceptible to infection by pathogens that are oridinarly of low grade virulence for normal persons. The most striking clinical feature is frequent purulent and granulomatous types of infection which involve skin, bones, lung, lymphatic tissues, and liver. The patients seem to deal with infections caused by low grade pyogenic pathogens in a manner similar to that expressed by normal persons infected with mycobacteria, brucella, or *Listeria,* and granuloma formation regularly occurs for reasons which are still poorly understood. The defective killing of ingested bacteria does not involve every type of microorganism. Streptococci and pneumococci are readily killed by the leukocytes of these patients, and infections with these bacteria are uncommon and cause litle problem.

Accompanying the ingestion of bacteria by these abnormal leukocytes is a constellation of biochemical abnormalities. The leukocytes show normal increases in lipid membrane synthesis, glycolysis, glycogenolysis, lactic acid synthesis, and Krebs cycle activity following phagocytosis, but they fail to show the normal increase in O_2 consumption, hexose monophosphate pathway activity, and formate oxidation. NADH and NADPH oxidase activities do not increase normally, although the levels of these enzymes are normal in the resting cells, and the cells fail to generate superoxide (O_2^-), singlet oxygen $('O_2)$, and OH— radicals normally. Thus, the cells of these patients fail to halogenate the ingested microorganisms and fail to attack their membranes with the radicals that normal cells use to destroy such organisms. The cells of these patients can kill streptococci, pneumococci and certain other organisms very well because the latter generate H_2O_2, which facilitates halogenation.

Recently, an exciting set of studies has shown that the leukocytes of patients with the X-linked variety regularly lack an antigen normally expressed on the cell surface. We postulate that it is the surface abnormality of the neutrophils and monocytes that constitutes the fundamental anomaly in this disease and that, in some way as yet undetermined, the internalization of the

TABLE 19–2. THE RELATION OF Kx SURFACE ANTIGEN TO CGD

Normal healthy persons have Kx on their RBC in trace amounts, but strongly present on their leukocytes. Kx is in some manner essential to generation of Kell antigens.

In the rare McLeod variant, Kx is on granulocytes but there is no Kx on RBC — neutrophils phagocytize and kill normally.

In the common CGD (Kell-positive CGD patients), Kx is absent on granulocytes, but present on RBC.

In the uncommon CGD (Kell-negative CGD patients), Kx is absent on both granulocytes and RBC.

(Data from Marsh, W. L., Uretsky, S. C., and Douglas, S. D.: J. Pediatr. 87:1117, 1975.)

membranes of normal cells that possess this determinant trips a metabolic chain of events resulting in the efficient killing of the catalase-positive microorganisms. Table 19–2 summarizes present knowledge of the Kx antigen that is lacking on CGD patients' cells. These findings establish that the membranes of the cells are abnormal in CGD. Such an abnormality might be related to an enzyme defect in the membrane itself that is essential to initiating the sequence of metabolic events triggered by phagocytosis. Such an enzyme could be the intramembranous NADH recently described as being deficient in CGD. Confirmation of the intramembranous enzyme defect is awaited because the full definition of CGD requires such an analysis. None of the several enzyme defects of whole granulocytes described up to this time have been confirmable.

CHEDIAK-HIGASHI ANOMALY

A generalized defect in lysosomal structure is associated with pigment dilution in patients with Chediak-Higashi anomaly. The same association has been found in Aleutian mink, certain roan Hereford cattle, beige mice, and even a killer whale which showed pigment dilution. The generalized abnormality of lysosomal development is associated with an increased susceptibility to certain infections, especially those caused by enteric bacteria. Skin and bowel infections are particular problems during infancy in this disease. The morphologically abnormal neutrophils (Fig. 19–11) do not phagocytize normally, nor do they kill ingested organisms efficiently. All of the immunoglobulins are present in normal amounts, and both cellular and humoral immunities seem to be normal.

If these children survive long enough, they characteristically develop widely disseminated malignancies of the lymphoid system, which invade both the central and peripheral nervous systems with great regularity. During the malignant phase, these children's leukocytes may contain many virus particles, often as many as 10,000 to 20,000 per cell. It has not been established that these viruses are causative for the lymphoreticular malignancy because they are not consistently present in the cancer cells, and the possibility of a passenger virus seems likely. Recent studies establish that the microtubular structure of these patients' leukocytes is lacking. The latter defect is corrected by treating the cells with ascorbate, which lowers cyclic AMP and induces the appearance of normal microtubules. This treatment corrects the functional abnormality of the leukocytes. Whether such treatment

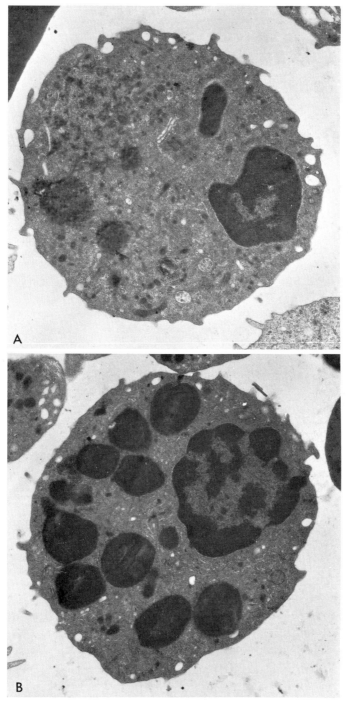

Figure 19–11. *A*, Electron micrograph of a neutrophil from a patient with Chediak-Higashi syndrome. *B*, Electron micrograph of an eosinophil from a patient with Chediak-Higashi syndrome. (Courtesy of Drs. J. G. White and C. C. Clawson.)

will cure the disease associated with Chediak-Higashi syndrome remains to be determined.

Myeloperoxidase Deficiency

An autosomal recessive phagocytic defect in which the host's monocytes and neutrophilic leukocytes lack myeloperoxidase has been associated with *Candida* sepsis. However, most cases of *Candida* septicemia occur in patients whose neutrophils and monocytes are numerically deficient, but who have normal amounts of myeloperoxidase. On the other hand, only two of six patients with myeloperoxidase deficiency have had evidence of candidal sepsis, and it seems likely that this infectious complication occurs when other concomitant immunologic defects are also present.

Chronic Mucocutaneous Candidiasis

Persistent infection of the skin and mucous membranes by *Candida albicans* is one of the most distressing diseases of man. This is sometimes accompanied by profound endocrinopathy, including parathyroid deficiency, thyroid disease, diabetes, and Addison's disease. The endocrinopathy is often associated with other autoimmune phenomena and is thought to have an autoimmune pathogenesis. Numerous defects in the inflammatory processes caused by T cell–mediated immune reactions have been described in association with chronic mucocutaneous candidiasis and these have been proposed as the basis of the disease. The defects have included deficient numbers of T lymphocytes, deficient or abnormal mediator production by T lymphocytes, and deficient responses of the monocyte-macrophage system to products of the stimulated lymphocytes. Cutaneous anergy to candidal antigens has been a frequent accompaniment of these immunologic defects. In some instances the anergy has been limited to candidal antigens, but often the anergy involves many other antigens, sometimes extending to all antigens studied. In some instances it is thought that circulating antigen-antibody complexes or other specific suppressor molecules present in the serum are inhibiting effective cell-mediated immunity.

Treatment of chronic mucocutaneous candidiasis guided by these concepts has been tried, with variable success. For example, approximately 50 to 60 per cent of patients will respond to repeated administration of transfer factor prepared from lymphocytes of normal persons. Truly dramatic results have been reported in individual cases. In our own investigations of this therapeutic modality, transfer factor has frequently resulted in conversion of the delayed allergic reaction to candidal antigens from negative to positive. The fact that transfer factor may act in some way nonspecifically to enhance delayed allergic responses to many antigens provides the basis for further study to define these important clinical observations in more specific terms. Levamisole, which also appears to act as a nonspecific immunopotentiator, has seemed to be of value in some cases in uncontrolled studies. In other cases, persistent and vigorous antifungal therapy which eliminates the candidal infection has seemed to reverse the selective immunodeficiency.

DEFICIENCIES OF THE COMPLEMENT SYSTEM

Over the past 25 years, the complement system in man and guinea pig has been almost completely defined in molecular terms. This great achievement has made it possible to identify primary immunodeficiencies attributable to inborn errors of metabolism, resulting in deficiencies or abnormalities of the individual complement components. As one would predict from the fact that the complement system has presumably been a stable system over several hundred millions of years, deficiencies of most of the complement components have often been associated with serious disease. Autoimmune diseases, serious mesenchymal disease, vascular disease, and increased susceptibility to infection of the lungs, skin, bowel, and respiratory tract have all been recognized as concomitants of deficiencies or abnormalities of the individual complement components. Listed in Table 19–3 are the defects of the complement system thus far described—they comprise genetically determined deficiencies of each of the proteins in the classical complement cascade (except C9), plus defects of at least three inhibitors or modulators of complement components.

TABLE 19–3.   HEREDITARY DEFICIENCIES OF THE   COMPLEMENT SYSTEM IN MAN

C COMPONENT	DISEASE
C1s	Systemic lupus erythematosus (SLE)
C1s	Lupus-like syndrome
C1s IN	Hereditary angioneurotic edema (HANE)
C1s IN	HANE—renal disease
C1s IN	HANE—SLE-like disease, two affected male children in a kindred
C1s IN	HANE—discoid lupus in two unrelated individuals
C1r	Recurrent infection and chronic glomerulonephritis
C1r	LE-like syndrome, necrotizing skin lesions, skin infection, arthritis and infections
C3	Recurrent infections (severe)
C3	Recurrent infections (mild)
C3	Fevers, skin rash, arthralgias
C4	Four unrelated, apparently healthy individuals, no family history
C4	LE-like syndrome
C5	SLE and recurrent infections
C5 dysfunction	Leiner's syndrome, gram-negative skin and bowel infection
C6	Mild Raynaud phenomenon; otherwise healthy
C6	Recurrent meningococcal meningitis
C6	Recurrent meningococcal infections
C6	Meningococcal infections
C7	Raynaud's phenomenon
C7 (inactivator)	Healthy
C7	Renal disease
C8	Prolonged disseminated gonococcal infection
C8	Xeroderma pigmentosum, no obvious complement-related disease
C8	Lupus-like disease (healthy)
C3b IN	Recurrent infection
C8	Lupus-like syndrome and chronic glomerulonephritis

Some deficiencies occur with rather striking frequency. Indeed, the C2 null gene occurs with a frequency of 1 to 2 per cent in the general population. Others represent uncommon and much more severe disease. Deficiencies of C2 and C4 appear to be linked to the major histocompatibility complex (MHC), as is a polymorphism for factor B of the alternative pathway. Other complement components and their deficiencies do not appear to be related to the major histocompatibility system.

Association of C2 Deficiency with Disease. When C2 deficiency was first discovered, it appeared in healthy scientists. It was thus natural to think that this complement component could be absent without producing disturbance in health. Indeed, this experience caused some to question whether the complement system was important to the body's defense at all. However, from phylogenetic considerations, it seemed likely that the complement system was of major importance. Further, it was soon found that isolated C2 deficiency occurred in association with chronic progressive glomerulonephritis. About the same time, a case of C1 esterase inhibitor deficiency which produces secondary C4 and C2 deficiency also occurred in conjunction with similar progressive renal disease, and, shortly thereafter, a case of isolated C1 deficiency appeared in a patient who developed progressive glomerulonephritis. These findings prompted a search for diseases associated with C2 deficiency. The associated diseases now include lupus, lupus-like syndrome, frequent infections, especially of the respiratory tract, anaphylactoid purpura, infections, autoimmune phenomena and disease, mesenchymal diseases, renal diseases, lethal dermatomyositis, and many others that are seen with extraordinary frequency in C2-deficient patients (Table 19–4).

Deficiencies of Other Complement Components. Throughout the complement deficiency diseases listed in Table 19–3, a preponderance have associated infection and vascular and mesenchymal diseases. C3 deficiencies and conditions such as absence of the inactivator of C3b (which leads to gross depletion of C3) are most strikingly associated with an increased susceptibility to infection, but C5 abnormality and C6, C7, and C8 deficiencies are also sometimes associated with infections. By contrast, one case of apparent absence of C3 has not been associated with such obvious susceptibility to infection.

Measures are already being developed to correct the immunodeficiencies based on complement component defects. The most obvious approach has been substitution therapy, and plasma therapy has in part aborted or minimized the severity of attacks of hereditary angioneurotic edema, prevented the fungal and gram-negative bacterial skin and bowel infections in Leiner's syndrome associated with C5 abnormality, and prevented the frequent infections in C3 deficiency or deficiency of C3b inhibitor. Kidney transplantation corrected the complement component deficiency in a patient with C1r deficiency, and marrow transplantation has repeatedly corrected the deficiency of C1q that accompanied some cases of SCID. Normal plasma has also been used to treat some of the deficiencies of the later-acting components during infection. Perhaps the most dramatic therapeutic and pro-

TABLE 19-4. ASSOCIATION WITH CLINICAL DISEASE OF INHERITED C2 DEFICIENCY IN MAN

AUTHOR	PROPOSITUS AGE	CLINICAL DISEASE	FUNCTIONAL C2 (% of normal)
Silverstein, 1960	49	Healthy	4–10
Klemperer et al., 1966			
Ruddy et al., 1970	–	Healthy	<1
Klemperer et al., 1967	–	Healthy	4
Cooper et al., 1968	7	Synovitis	<1
Pickering et al., 1971	12	Membranous glomerulonephritis	<1
Day et al., 1973		SLE	
Agnello et al., 1972	55	SLE-like syndrome	<1
Sussman et al., 1973	10	Anaphylactoid purpura	<1
Leddy et al., 1975	59	Fatal dermatomyositis	<1
Douglas et al., 1976	24	Discoid lupus	<1
Osterland et al., 1975	18	SLE, Hemolytic anemia	<1
Alper et al., 1974°	–	Purpura	–
Leddy et al.°	22	Mild membranoproliferative glomerulonephritis	<1
Day et al., 1973†	20	Healthy	<1
Stern et al., 1976	–	Discoid lupus	<1
Wild et al.	38	Discoid lupus	<1
Day et al., 1976	26	Hodgkin's disease	<1
	28 sib.	Hypertension, recurrent septic meningococcal infection	<1
Wolski et al., 1975	17	SLE-like syndrome	<1
Becker°		CLL and dermatitis herpetiformis	<1

°Personal communication.
†Unpublished observation.
(From Day, N. K., and Good, R. A.: Inherited deficiencies of the complement system, *in* Day, N. K., and Good, R. A. (eds.), Biological Amplification Systems. New York, Plenum Press, in press.)

phylactic accomplishment in diseases due to defective complement system is the recent finding that anabolic steroids will almost completely prevent attacks of hereditary angioneurotic edema that are associated with absence of C1 esterase inhibitor from the blood. Not only were the recurrent attacks of edema prevented, but also the treatment seems to have induced the production or decreased the degradation of the C1 esterase inhibitor, since concentrations of C1 esterase inhibitor increased and approached normal after the steroid treatment. This dramatic achievement suggests that recessive genes may be induced to expression as a means of treating diseases of dominant inheritance.

Our ability to analyze, identify, and define the nature of many immunodeficiencies has made great strides, and it is anticipated that many new immunodeficiencies will be discovered and that those we now recognize will be better understood. Substitution therapies and prophylactic regimens have already corrected some of the immunologic defects, and a few have been corrected by thymic, bone marrow, or fetal liver transplantation. This approach to cellular engineering, although only recently available, holds great promise for dealing with the more frequent immunodeficiencies and hematologic disorders. A number of otherwise fatal diseases, including aplastic anemia, chronic granulomatous disease, Wiskott-Aldrich syndrome, four genetically distinct forms of SCID, the DiGeorge syndrome, and other T cell deficiency syndromes have already been effectively treated by this means.

As progress toward effective cellular engineering is made, knowledge of the control mechanism for normal differentiation and function of blood and lymphoid cells should appear rapidly. With it, new drugs and a true immunopharmacology can be developed for manipulating, restoring, and modulating the immune system when it is faulty.

SECONDARY IMMUNODEFICIENCIES

As methods are being refined to recognize, diagnose, dissect, treat, and prevent the primary immunodeficiencies, they provide the basis to recognize and analyze secondary immunodeficiencies. Major secondary immunodeficiencies are encountered with acute and chronic malnutrition; during bacterial, viral, fungal, protozoal, and helminthic infections; in association with autoimmune disease; following trauma; during the course of and as a consequence of thymic involution and perturbation of the cellular environment associated with aging. Indeed, the commonest diseases of man are likely to produce immunodeficiencies or are associated with them. Secondary immunodeficiencies are present in all branches of medical practice, and must be defined more precisely and manipulated more effectively than is done in present day medical practice. Many of the conditions associated with secondary immunodeficiency are discussed in Chapters 9, 13, 14, 15, 16, 17, and 20.

20

Nutrition and Immunity

Pestilence and famine have had an undeniable association since the earliest times of recorded history. With the rapid advances in medicine of modern times, however, many physicians in developed countries tend to forget that this association still exists even in the best equipped and most advanced hospitals in which the highest quality of care is available. In less well developed countries, malnutrition and infection continue to assume an ever present and alarming threat. It has been recently estimated that problems involving the interaction of malnutrition and infection still affect three fourths of the world's inhabitants and account for the majority of deaths. Because of the ever increasing population and a limited worldwide capacity to produce food, malnutrition promises to be a major concern for clinicians for the foreseeable future.

Not only can malnutrition lead to an increased susceptibility to infection, but also infection can result in an increased requirement for nutrients by hypercatabolism and increased losses of body constituents. Often, there is additionally a decreased dietary intake, and together, these can result in precipitation of acute deficiency states in persons who were marginally compensated before the infection. A vicious cycle can be started which, if not promptly and properly treated, can end in death. The state of nutrition can also affect the immune response in other diseases, including cancer and autoimmunity and, as with infection, the presence of these diseases can affect the nutritional state.

Only in recent years has there been significant progress in understanding the role of nutrition in maintenance or alteration of a normal immune response, partly because of problems in methodology and partly because the interactions are so complex and involve so many variables. Even our present knowledge is fragmentary, but it is rapidly expanding to provide some clear insights and concepts of increasing importance in patient management.

PROTEIN-CALORIE MALNUTRITION

Protein-calorie malnutrition (PCM) is actually improperly named since individuals with this condition also have vitamin and mineral deficiencies to a varying degree. The best studies of immune function in PCM have been done in children with kwashiorkor and marasmus, but it is apparent that the same findings apply to many forms of chronic and subacute undernutrition, including those associated with hypercatabolic states. Children with kwashiokor have diets low in protein, fats, vitamins, and trace minerals. They develop large fatty livers, muscle wasting, edema of the trunk and extremities, and extremely low total serum proteins. In contrast, patients with marasmus usually have a more balanced but grossly insufficient diet, the onset is triggered by acute disease (especially diarrhea), they do not have a fatty liver or edema, and have only slightly reduced serum proteins. The alterations of immunologic function are similar for both types of PCM, as well as for other forms of marked undernutrition in adults, and every major component of immunologic function may be affected.

EFFECTS ON THE LYMPHOID ORGANS

PCM is associated with marked thymic atrophy and reduction of the lymphoid mass in the spleen, lymph nodes, Peyer's patches, appendix, and tonsils. The thymic dependent areas are especially affected. Germinal centers are usually reduced in number, but occasionally are normal or even increased.

EFFECT ON B CELL FUNCTION

B cell numbers in the peripheral circulation may be normal or increased. Hypogammaglobulinemia has usually been demonstrated to be associated with severe uncomplicated PCM, but children with PCM may have elevated levels of gamma globulin as a consequence of repeated infections. In general, IgM levels are higher than age-matched normal controls. IgA levels have been variable, but often elevated with concomitant infection, and IgE levels are frequently markedly elevated as a result of parasitic infection.

The responses of children with PCM to antigenic stimulation have been studied by several investigators with variable results depending somewhat on the antigen. Primary antibody responses are usually depressed to most of the antigens, especially those requiring T cell–B cell cooperation, and secondary responses are usually less affected. When the protein or protein-calorie deficiency is imposed very early in life, inability to develop the immunoglobulin-synthesizing system normally may be reflected in extreme hypogammaglobulinemia or even agammaglobulinemia.

EFFECT ON T CELL FUNCTION

Circulating T cell numbers are frequently reduced in PCM, and the response of the remaining ones to PHA may be reduced with the more severe forms of malnutrition. Delayed hypersensitivity responses to recall antigens are almost always depressed, and the response to DNCB sensitization is regularly impaired.

CHANGES IN COMPLEMENT ACTIVITY

Hemolytic activity of serum, Factor B levels, and all of the components of the classical complement pathway except C4 have been found to be reduced in PCM, especially in children with severe kwashiorkor.

NEUTROPHIL FUNCTION

The phagocytic process is usually normal in neutrophils from patients with PCM, but intracellular killing of ingested bacteria may be significantly impaired. Associated with this defect are metabolic changes showing depression of glycolytic pathway activity and reduction of NADPH oxidase activity. Also, chemotactic activity and NBT reduction may be reduced by severe PCM.

OTHER FORMS OF PCM IN HUMANS

Chronic or subacute starvation in adults appears to produce changes similar to some of the forms of PCM seen in children, especially when associated with hypercatabolism. In particular, patients with major thermal injury and other severe forms of trauma develop immunologic abnormalities which resemble those seen in kwashiorkor in virtually every respect (Table 20–1). At first it was felt that the immunologic abnormalities following burn injury were a result of the injury itself. Certainly, the hypercatabolic state may contribute to the problem, but it is now clear that most of the recorded changes in years past had nutritional deficits as their underlying basis, and most of them can be prevented or corrected by aggressive nutritional therapy (Chapter 13). Likewise, most of the acquired immunologic abnormalities in hospitalized patients, not associated with infection or immunosuppressive drug therapy, now appear to have undernutrition as their primary cause. It is of utmost importance to realize that restoration of the immune responses to normal by nutritional support will prevent the majority of life-threatening and fatal infections in such patients (Chapter 13).

TABLE 20-1. COMPARISON OF IMMUNOLOGIC ABNORMALITIES IN KWASHIORKOR AND SEVERE THERMAL INJURY

IMMUNOLOGIC VARIABLE	KWASHIORKOR	SEVERE THERMAL INJURY
Gamma globulin	Low, may be elevated with infection	Low at first, usually becomes elevated later but may remain low with massive burns or continued under-nutrition
Response to an antigenic stimulus	Normal to decreased	Normal to decreased
Delayed hypersensitivity response to recall antigens	Decreased	Decreased
T cell response to PHA	Decreased	Decreased
Chemotactic response of neutrophils	Decreased	Decreased
Inflammatory response to skin abrasion	Decreased	Decreased
Phagocytosis by neutrophils	Normal	Normal or increased
Intracellular killing of bacteria by neutrophils	Decreased	Decreased
Glycolytic pathway activity of neutrophils	Decreased	Decreased

ANIMAL MODELS OF PCM

The observed changes in immunologic function in humans with PCM can be duplicated by controlled reduction in dietary intake of proteins and calories in experimental animals. The results of such experiments depend greatly upon the kind, duration, and degree of deprivation and the experimental animal, but do not differ appreciably from the human experience when appropriate experiments are performed. Selective protein deficiencies and their effect on the immune system will be discussed in more detail below.

EFFECT OF DIETARY REPLETION IN PCM

Surprisingly rapid restoration of immunologic function can be achieved by dietary supplementation of chronically starved individuals, and virtually all of the observed abnormalities can be corrected. In fact, dietary repletion often results early in higher than normal levels of both immunoglobulins and complement components. The rapidity of the restoration depends upon both the degree and length of undernutrition and the amount and type of dietary supplementation. Essential amino acids seem to be crucial.

VITAMIN AND MINERAL DEFICIENCIES

No nutritional deficiency has consistently been more synergistic with infectious disease than vitamin A deficiency. Paradoxically, vitamin A deficiency has only a minimal effect on antibody responses, but may affect phagocytic function and properdin levels to a limited degree. Therefore, this deficiency may often reflect an underlying PCM.

In contrast, pyridoxine (B6) deficiency impairs nucleic acid synthesis and depresses antibody formation, delayed hypersensitive responses, and the ability of phagocytes to kill bacteria. Pantothenic acid deficiency also causes impaired antibody formation.

Vitamin C deficiency probably increases the incidence of infection, primarily by an influence on reparative processes, but several studies suggest that such deficiencies may also have an adverse effect on phagocytic function. Whether large amounts of vitamin C are beneficial in preventing infection remains a topic of considerable controversy.

Deficiencies of the other vitamins either have not been studied sufficiently for their influence on the immune response or have a variable effect.

Iron deficiency has been reported to be associated with diminished antibacterial functions of neutrophils. However, other nutritional defects were not excluded in these patients. Conversely, iron deficiency may actually protect against bacterial infection, and the administration of iron during active infections can markedly worsen the disease because many bacteria require iron for their growth. It is certainly clear that iron supplementation should almost never be given during the acute phase of bacterial infection. The effect of other mineral and trace metal deficiencies remains a matter of speculation, but the special relationship of zinc to development and normal function of the T cell system requires comment.

Zinc deficiency, which may occur when losses are excessive and intake minimal, has been associated with profound T cell deficiency. The recent discovery that treatment with zinc will correct the entire syndrome of acrodermatitis enteropathica and its associated severe T cell deficiency seems most pertinent. Further treatment with zinc has repeatedly corrected T cell deficiencies in malnourished patients and patients with exudative enteropathy. These findings make it imperative to consider deficiencies of zinc when correcting immunodeficiencies by nutritional manipulation. Other trace metals may play equally important roles in immunologic functions that have not yet been elucidated. It seems certain that much remains to be learned from carefully controlled studies in animals and critical clinical observations in man about the influence of trace metals and vitamins on differentiation and function of the immune systems.

EFFECT OF INFECTION AND STRESS ON NUTRITIONAL REQUIREMENTS

Infections consistently worsen the nutritional status, particularly compounding the problem in malnourished individuals. The mechanisms include increased loss of nutrients (as with diarrhea or from open wounds), decreased dietary intake because of anorexia or misdirected management, decreased absorption from the GI tract, alterations in metabolism, or increased requirements caused by the infection. In septic patients, there may be an increase in basal metabolic expenditure of 20 to 40 per cent or even more. In severe injury with associated sepsis, such as a large infected burn, the metabolic requirements may be doubled. Endogenous fuel stores are rapidly consumed, first depleting glycogen and then protein, but the changes associated with stress prevent effective utilization of fat as a source of energy. Serum glucagon, insulin, and catecholamine levels are characteristically increased, and a peripheral resistance to insulin may develop, causing poor utilization of glucose. Negative nitrogen balance is a consistent feature of severe infections, and fever causes additional urinary nitrogen loss, often to a marked degree. Protein repletion therefore requires intakes well above basal requirements to prevent a negative balance, and therapy to prevent or correct acquired abnormalities of immune defense must be extremely aggressive in the patient who was previously marginally malnourished.

ANIMAL STUDIES OF THE EFFECT OF SELECTIVE DIETARY MANIPULATION ON THE IMMUNE RESPONSE

Acute deprivation of protein with or without caloric restriction increases antibody synthesis and neutrophil antibacterial functions but may depress T cell immune responses. Severe chronic restriction of protein or protein-calories results in severe depression of T cell responses and diminishes B cell responses. Sometimes phagocytic functions are also diminished, but usually to a lesser extent. On the other hand, moderate degrees of chronic protein restriction (4 to 12 per cent of caloric intake) with normal caloric intake have resulted in enhanced T cell function and depressed B cell function concurrent with an increased resistance to the growth of transplanted tumor cells in most instances. The effect on tumor growth has been found in part to be a result of decreased synthesis of blocking antibody. Such diets may also reflect a greater sensitivity of suppressor T cells to moderate degrees of protein depletion than of helper cells. Underfeeding has also been shown to delay the appearance of spontaneous and carcinogen-induced tumors in a variety of animal systems. Conversely, overfeeding has resulted in accelerated appearance and growth rate of malignant tumors.

The effect of dietary influence on the development of autoimmunity in NZB mice is equally impressive. Mice fed an 11 per cent fat–17 per cent protein diet had far greater autoimmune reactions than did animals fed a 4.5 per cent fat–23 per cent protein diet. Moderate protein deprivation slowed development of autoimmunity and inhibited the involution of immunologic functions that usually occurs with age in these animals. In B/W hybrid mice, the life span was doubled when calories were restricted, and in such animals, dietary restriction from the time of weaning significantly influenced the development and involution of immune responses later in life. Renal disease, vascular disease, autoimmunity, immunologic involution, and the development of spontaneous suppressor cells that appear with aging was prevented by giving the animals low caloric intake from the time of weaning. Thus, major diseases associated with aging may be influenced favorably by moderate lifelong caloric restriction.

The far-reaching implications of such studies and their potential application to the control of human disease are just now beginning to be evaluated. At the present time, nutritional therapy has its major impact on medicine through the control of infection by preventing and correcting acquired abnormalities of immune defense.

21

HLA and Disease

Early attempts at clinical transplantation of the kidney quickly revealed that genetic relationships were important in determining the success of immunosuppressive regimens. Methods for testing histocompatibility were soon developed so that a reasonably large data base began to accumulate, and the techniques were quickly applied to analysis of disease associations. This analytic direction was stimulated by the demonstration of an importance of H2 antigenic phenotype in the development of leukemia and certain virus diseases in mice. Now, a large variety of human diseases has been found to arise more often in persons with certain HLA antigens.

The basic organization of the HLA system has been discussed in Chapter 15, and the genetic linkages are represented diagrammatically in Figure 15–5.

ASSOCIATIONS OF HLA AND DISEASE

HLA-B and HLA-D antigens seem to be more closely associated with disease than are antigens of the HLA-A and HLA-C series. While the basis for this association is not entirely clear, it seems probable from current evidence that their proximity to the genes of the Ir region is partly responsible, for the Ir genes appear to control many immune responses. Certainly, these genes control the ability to respond to many antigens, including the formation of IgE upon exposure to ragweed pollen, and they have been shown to regulate cytotoxic activity of lymphocytes. It is unfortunate that the Ia antigens (coded for by Ir genes) remain so poorly defined in man at the present time, since such a strong relationship to disease is apparent. Most of the conditions associated with HLA are thought to be of an autoimmune nature, further sugesting a link to altered immune responsiveness.

Some of the associations between single HLA antigens and disease are shown in Table 21–1. Among these, only the association between ankylosing spondylitis and HLA-B27 has diagnostic significance at the present time. In some instances the association of two antigens (haplotypes) is more significant than are single antigens. Associations in the HLA-D locus include DW2 with multiple sclerosis and C2 deficiency, DW3 with juvenile onset (insulin

318

TABLE 21-1. ASSOCIATIONS BETWEEN HLA AND SELECTED DISEASES

ANTIGEN	DISEASE	FREQUENCY OF ANTIGEN (%)	
		Controls	Patients
HLA-A1	Celiac disease	21	41
HLA-A2	Chronic glomerulonephritis	54	63
HLA-A3	Multiple sclerosis	24	41
	Idiopathic hemochromatosis	31	69
HLA-B7	Multiple sclerosis	26	35
HLA-B8	Idiopathic Addison's disease	24	67–69
	Graves' disease	21–24	47–53
	Insulin dependent diabetes	24	39–45
	Myasthenia gravis	24	52–58
	Chronic hepatitis	24	53
	Celiac disease	24	45–78
	Dermatitis herpetiformis	24–27	57–62
	Hodgkin's disease	24	26–29
	Acute lymphatic leukemia	24	29
HLA-B13	Psoriasis vulgaris	4	16–18
HLA-B27	Ankylosing spondylitis	8	88–90
	Reiter's syndrome	8	76–79
	Psoriatic arthritis	8	31
	Acute anterior uveitis	8	55–74
HLA-BW15	Insulin dependent diabetes	18	33–40
HLA-BW16	Psoriasis	5	15
HLA-BW17	Psoriasis vulgaris	8	29

dependent) diabetes mellitus and idiopathic Addison's disease, and DW4 with adult rheumatoid arthritis. It is interesting that the relative risk of most of these disease associations is high, 4 to 10× for most and as much as 120× for the association between HLA-B27 and ankylosing spondylitis, compared to the relative risk of blood group O with duodenal ulcer (1.3×). In contrast to these rather strong associations for many nonmalignant diseases, the risk factors between HLA and malignant diseases are thus far rather weak (less than 2×), the best associations being with Hodgkin's disease (A1, B8, B5, and B18) and acute lymphatic leukemia (A2, B8, and B12).

As knowledge of disease process increases and as definition of the major histocompatibility systems becomes more complete, the associations of the HLA system with human disease may become far more precise. Cogent examples are seen in the diseases of multiple sclerosis and dermatitis herpetiformis. An interesting association between HLA-A3 and HLA-B7 and multiple sclerosis was first recognized that statistically linked the HLA-A3-B7 haplotype to this poorly understood disease. With the discovery of the method of analyzing the HLA-D antigens using homozygous test cells, the DW2 allele, which is in genetic disequilibrium with HLA-A3 and B7, was found to be much more frequently associated with multiple sclerosis than either HLA-A3 or HLA-B7. Finally, using antisera which seem to recognize an Ia antigen on the B lymphocyte, the association of the HLA system and multiple sclerosis has climbed to more than 90 per cent in some studies. Thus, with increasing knowledge of the major histocompatibility region, multiple slcerosis has been progressively identified to be associated with the HLA system and now can be linked as closely to HLA as can ankylosing spondylitis.

The poorly understood skin disease called dermatitis herpetiformis has been associated with the B8 allele of the HLA system. Recently, it was found that many, but not all, cases of apparent dermatitis herpetiformis show deposits of IgA in the skin at the sites of their bullous skin lesions. When only those dermatitis herpetiforms patients who had demonstrable IgA deposits in their skin lesions were considered, the association with the B8 allele rose to more than 85 per cent. The most likely interpretation of these findings is that dermatitis herpetiformis is heterogeneous and that the form in which IgA antibodies are involved in the pathogenesis is linked intimately to the B8 allele of the HLA system, while forms that have other pathogenesis are not.

The frequent association of HLA-B8 with a number of diseases may indicate a common pathogenic pathway which is as yet unclear, but may involve linkage to an Ir gene. On the other hand, association of a single disease with two or more HLA antigens suggests multiple predisposing factors acting by different mechanisms. The precise mechanisms by which associations occur remain unclear, and as mentioned before, many may be associated more with Ir products than HLA antigens. However, two explanations have been advanced that seem to have major importance. The first of these, molecular mimicry, may result in cross-tolerance to an infecting organism and its antigenic component that is similar to the associated HLA antigen. This relationship might result in prolonged or persistent infection. On the other hand, loss of self-tolerance caused by an immune response to antigens of an infecting microbe that bear similarity to the associated HLA antigen might initiate an autoimmune reaction and lead to autoimmune disease. A second explanation for the association between HLA and disease is that HLA antigens may influence receptor function, permitting virus adherence or penetration, alteration of cell-to-cell interactions, and formation of antigen-antibody complexes on the cell membrane.

It is apparent that the major histocompatibility complex has importance in clinical medicine far exceeding its role in transplantation. Nonetheless, our knowledge of this role remains fragmentary at present. Without doubt, within the next few years, immunogenetics involving immune responsiveness will become increasingly important in both diagnosis and prognosis, and probably in therapy.

REFERENCES

TEXTS

Ascher, M. S., Gottlieb, A. A. and Kirkpatrick, C. H.: Transfer Factor: Basic Properties and Clinical Applications. Academic Press, New York, 1976.

Barrett, J. T. (ed): Basic Immunology and Its Medical Application. C.V. Mosby Co., St. Louis, 1976.

Bellanti, J. A. (ed): Immunology. W. B. Saunders Co., Philadelphia, 1971.

Benacerraf, B.: Immunogenetics and Immunodeficiency. MTP, St. Leonard's House, Lancaster, England, 1975.

Bloom, B. R. and David, J. R.: In Vitro Methods in Cell-Mediated and Tumor Immunity. Academic Press, New York, 1976.

Brent, L. and Holborow, J. (eds): Progress in Immunology. II, Vol. 1–5, American Elsevier Publishing Co., New York, 1974.

Burnet, F. M.: Immunology; Readings from Scientific American, W. H. Freeman and Co., San Francisco, 1975.

Chirigos, M. A.: Modulation of Host Immune Resistance in the Prevention or Treatment of Induced Neoplasias. Fogarty International Center Proceedings No. 28, DHEW Publications, Washington, D.C., 1977.

Cline, M. J. (ed): The White Cell. Harvard University Press, Cambridge, Mass., 1975.

Day, N. K. and Good, R. A. (eds): Biological Amplification Systems in Immunology. (Comprehensive Immunology, Vol. 2.) Plenum Publishing Corp., New York, 1977.

Dumonde, D. C.: Infection and Immunology in the Rheumatic Diseases. Blackwell Scientific Publications, Oxford, 1976.

Finch, C. E. and Hayflick, L.: Handbook of the Biology of Aging. Van Nostrand Reinhold Co., New York, 1977.

Freedman, S. O. and Gold, P. (eds): Clinical Immunology. Second Edition. Harper and Row, Hagerstown, Md., 1976.

Friedman, H., Escobar, M. R. and Reichard, S. M.: The Reticuloendothelial System in Health and Disease. Advances in Experimental Medicine and Biology Series. Vol. 73B. Plenum Press, New York, 1976.

Fudenberg, H. H., Stites, D. P., Caldwell, J. L. and Weils, J. V. (eds): Basic and Clinical Immunology. Lange Medical Publications, Los Altos, Cal., 1976.

Gell, P. G. H., Coombs, R. R. A. and Lachmann, P. J. (eds): Clinical Aspects of Immunology. Third Edition. Blackwell Scientific Publications, Oxford, 1975.

Golub, E. S.: Cellular Basis of the Immune Response. Sinauer Associates, Inc., Sunderland, Mass., 1977.

Hamashima, Y.: Immunohistopathology. J. B. Lippincott Co., Philadelphia, 1976.

Hanna, M. G., Jr. (ed): Contemporary Topics in Immunobiology. Vols. 1–5. Plenum Press, New York, 1972–1976.

Hobart, M. J. and McConnell, I. (eds): The Immune System: A Course on the Molecular and Cellular Basis of Immunity. Blackwell Scientific Publications, Oxford, 1975.

Jankovic, B. D. and Isakovic, K. (eds): Microenvironmental Aspects of Immunity. Plenum Press, New York, 1973.

Jerne, N. K.: The Harvey Lectures. Series 70. Academic Press, New York, 1976.

Katz, D. H., Benacerraf, B.: The Role of Products of the Histocompatibility Gene Complex in Immune Responses. Academic Press, New York, 1976.

Koprowski, C. and Koprowski, H.: Viruses and Immunity. Academic Press, New York, 1975.

Makinodan, T. and Yunis, E. (eds): Immunology and Aging. (Comprehensive Immunology, Vol. 1.) Plenum Publishing Corp., New York, 1977.

Marchalonis, J. J.: Immunity in Evolution. Harvard University Press, Cambridge, Mass., 1977.

Mestecky, J. and Lawton, A. R. (eds): The Immunoglobulin A System. Advances in Experimental Medicine and Biology Series. Vol. 45. Plenum Press, New York, 1974.

Miescher, P. A. and Muller-Eberhard, H. J.: Textbook of Immunopathology. Vol. II. Grune and Stratton, New York, 1976.

Murphy, G. P., Cohen, E., Fitzpatrick, J. E. and Pressman, D.: HLA and Malignancy. Alan R. Liss, Inc., New York, 1977.

Nowotny, A. (ed): Cellular Antigens. Springer-Verlag, New York, 1972.

Olsen, R. E.: Protein-Calorie Malnutrition. Academic Press, New York, 1975.

Park, B. H. and Good, R. A. (eds): Principles of Modern Immunobiology: Basic and Clinical. Lea and Febiger, Philadelphia, 1974.

Porter, R. R. and Ada, G. L. (eds): Contemporary Topics in Molecular Immunology. Vol. 6. Plenum Press, New York, 1977.

Rajka, O. and Korossy, S. (eds): Immunological Aspects of Allergy and Allergic Diseases. Vols. 1 and 2. Plenum Press, New York, 1974.

Rockstein, M. and Sussman, M. L.: Nutrition, Longevity and Aging. Academic Press, New York, 1976.

Roitt, I. M. (ed): Essential Immunology. Second Edition. Blackwell Scientific Publications, Oxford, 1974.

Rose, N. R. and Friedman, H.: Manual of Clinical Immunology. American Society for Microbiology, Washington, D.C., 1976.

Rozing, J.: B Lymphocyte Differentiation in the Mouse. Drukkerij J. H. Pasmans, 'S-Gravenhage, Rotterdam, 1977.

Salton, M. R. J.: Immunochemistry of Enzymes and Their Antibodies. Wiley Medical Publications, New York, 1977.

Samter, M. (ed): Immunological Diseases. Second Edition. Little, Brown and Company, Boston, 1971.

Stutman, O.: Contemporary Topics in Immunobiology. Vol. 7, T Cells. Plenum Press, New York, 1977.

Tomasi, T. B.: The Immune System of Secretions. Prentice-Hall, Englewood Cliffs, N.J., 1976.

Weir, D. M.: Handbook of Experimental Immunology. Blackwell Scientific Publications, Oxford, 1967.

Weiser, R. S., Myrvik, Q. N. and Pearsall, N. N.: Fundamentals of Immunology for Students of Medicine and Related Sciences. Lea and Febiger, Philadelphia, 1969.

Weiss, D. W.: Immunological Parameters of Host-Tumor Relationships. Vol. IV. Academic Press, New York, 1976.

JOURNALS

Cohn, Z. A., Kunkel, H. G., Hirsch, J. G. and McCarty, M. (eds): Journal of Experimental Medicine. The Rockefeller University Press, New York.

Eichwald, E. J. (ed): Transplantation. Williams and Wilkins Co., Baltimore.

Feldman, J. (ed): Journal of Immunology. Williams and Wilkins Co., Baltimore.

Glynn, L. E. (ed): Immunology. (Official journal of the British Society for Immunology.) Blackwell Scientific Publications, Oxford.

Lawrence, H. S. (ed): Cellular Immunology. Academic Press, New York.

Myrvik, Q. N. (ed): Journal of the Reticuloendothelial Society. Reticuloendothelial Society, Winston-Salem, N. Car.

Neter, E. (ed): Infection and Immunity. American Society for Microbiology, Washington, D.C.

Rapaport, F. T. (ed): Transplantation Proceedings. Grune and Stratton, Inc., New York.

CONTINUING REVIEW SERIES

Bach, F. H. and Good, R. A. (eds): Clinical Immunobiology. Academic Press, New York.

Dixon, F. J. and Kunkel, H. G. (eds): Advances in Immunology. Academic Press, New York.

Kallos, P. (ed): Progress in Allergy. S. Karger, Basel.

Möller, G. (ed): Transplantation Reviews. Munksgaard, Copenhagen.

Chapter 2

Cooper, M. D. and Lawton, A. R.: The development of the immune system. Sci. Am. 231:59–72, November. 1974.
Cooper, M. D., Peterson, R. D. A. and Good, R. A.: The development of the immune system in the chicken. *In* Smith, R. T., Miescher, P. A. and Good, R. A. (eds): Phylogeny of Immunity. University of Florida Press, Gainesville, 1966.
Good, R. A.: Immunodeficiency in developmental perspective. Harvey Lect., Series 67:1–107, 1973.
Good, R. A. and Gabrielsen, A. E. (eds): The Thymus in Immunobiology. Hoeber Division, Harper and Row, New York, 1964.
Good, R. A. and Papermaster, B. W.: Ontogeny and phylogeny of adaptive immunity. *In* Dixon, F. J., Jr. and Humphrey, J. W. (eds): Advances in Immunology. Vol. 4. Academic Press, New York, 1964, pp. 1–115.
Makinodan, T. and Yunis, E. (eds): Immunology and Aging. (Comprehensive Immunology, Vol. 1.) Plenum Press, New York, 1977.
Old, L. J. and Boyse, E. A.: Current enigmas in cancer research. Harvey Lect., Series 67:273–315, 1973.
Porter, R. and Knight, J. (eds): Ontogeny of Acquired Immunity. CIBA Foundation Symposium. American Elsevier Publishing Co., New York, 1972.
Smith, R. T., Good, R. A. and Miescher, P. A. (eds): Ontogeny of Immunity. University of Florida Press, Gainesville, 1967.
Šterzl, J. and Silverstein, A. M.: Developmental aspects of immunity. *In* Dixon, F. J., Jr. and Humphrey, J. W. (eds): Advances in Immunology. Vol. 6. Academic Press, New York, 1967, pp. 337–459.
Walford, R. L. (ed): The Immunologic Theory of Aging. Munksgaard, Copenhagen, 1969.

Chapter 3

Ascher, M. S., Gottlieb, A. A. and Kirkpatrick, C. H. (eds): Transfer Factor; Basic Properties and Clinical Applications. Academic Press, New York, 1976.
Eijsvoogel, V. P., Roos, D. and Zeijlemaker, W. P. (eds): Leukocyte Membrane Determinants Regulating Immune Reactivity. Academic Press, New York, 1976.
Elves, M. W. (ed): The Lymphocytes. Second Edition. Year Book Medical Publishers, Chicago, 1972.
Feldman, M. and Globerson, A. (eds): Immune Reactivity of Lymphocytes: Development, Expression and Control. Plenum Press, New York, 1975.
Ford, W. L.: Lymphocyte migration and immune responses. Prog. Allergy 19:1–59, 1975.
Rosenthal, A. S. (ed): Immune Recognition. Academic Press, New York, 1975.
Sprint, J.: Recirculating lymphocytes. *In* Marchalonis, J. J. (ed): The Lymphocyte: Structure and Function. Marcel Dekker, Inc., New York, 1975.
Turk, J. L. (ed): Delayed Hypersensitivity. Second Edition. American Elsevier Publishing Co., New York, 1975.
Weiss, L. (ed): The Cells and Tissues of the Immune System: Structure, Function, Interactions. Prentice-Hall, Inc., Englewood Cliffs, N.J., 1972.

Chapters 4 and 5

Bellanti, J. A. and Dayton, D. H. (eds): The Phagocytic Cell in Host Resistance. Raven Press, New York, 1975.
Metcalf, D. and Moore, M. (eds): Haemopoietic Cells. American Elsevier Publishing Co., New York, 1971.
Metchnikoff, E. (ed): Immunity in Infective Diseases (translated by Binnie, F. G.). University Press, Cambridge, England, 1907.
Murphy, P. (ed): The Neutrophil. Plenum Press, New York and London, 1976.
Nelson, D. S. (ed): Immunobiology of the Macrophage. Academic Press, New York, 1976.
Pearsall, N. N. and Weiser, R. S. (ed): The Macrophage. Lea and Febiger, Philadelphia, 1970.
Stossel, T. P.: Phagocytosis: recognition and ingestion. Semin. Hematol. 12:83–116, 1975.
Suter, E. and Ramseiar, H.: Cellular reactions in infection. *In* Dixon, F. J., Jr. and Humphrey, J. H. S. (eds): Advances in Immunology. Vol. 4. Academic Press, New York, 1964, pp. 117–173.

vanFurth, R. (ed): Mononuclear Phagocytes in Immunity, Infection and Pathology. Blackwell Scientific Publications, Oxford, 1975.

Volkman, A.: Disparity in origin of mononuclear phagocyte populations. J. Reticuloendothel. Soc. 19:249–268, 1976.

Williams, R. C., Jr. and Fudenberg, H. H. (eds): Phagocytic Mechanisms in Health and Disease. Intercontinental Medical Book Corp., New York, 1972.

Chapter 6

Atassi, M. Z. (ed): Immunochemistry of Proteins. Vol. 1. Plenum Publishing Corp., New York, 1976.

Day, E. D. (ed): Advanced Immunochemistry. Williams and Wilkins, Baltimore, 1972.

Litman, G. and Good, R. A. (eds): Immunoglobulins. *In* Comprehensive Immunology Series. Plenum Press, New York, 1977.

Ritzman, S. E. and Daniels, J. C. (eds): Serum Protein Abnormalities: Diagnostic and Clinical Aspects. Little, Brown and Co., Boston, 1975.

Tamari, T. B. (ed): The Immune System of Secretions. Prentice-Hall, Inc., Englewood Cliffs, N.J., 1976.

Williams, C. A. And Chase, M. W. (eds): Methods in Immunology and Immunochemistry. Academic Press, New York, 1971.

Chapter 7

Wolstenholme, G. E. W. and Knight, J. (eds): CIBA Foundation Symposium on Complement. Little, Brown and Co., Boston, 1965. (Symposium by many authorities.)

Many reviews in general references.

Chapter 8

Lawrence, H. S. and Landy, M. (eds): Mediators of Cellular Immunity. Academic Press, New York, 1969.

Movat, H. Z. (ed): Inflammation, Immunity and Hypersensitivity. Harper and Row, New York, 1971.

Sell, S. (ed): Immunology, Immunopathology and Immunity. Second Edition. Harper and Row, New York, 1975.

Chapter 9

Dresser, D. W. and Mitchison, N. A.: The mechanism of immunological paralysis. *In* Dixon, F. J., Jr. and Kunkel, H. G. (eds): Advances in Immunology. Vol. 8. Academic Press, New York, 1968, pp. 129–181.

Gabrielsen, A. E. and Good, R. A.: Chemical suppression of adaptive immunity. *In* Dixon, F. J., Jr. and Kunkel, H. G. (eds): Advances in Immunology. Vol. 6. Academic Press, New York, 1967, pp. 91–229.

Good, R. A., Martinez, C. and Gabrielsen, A. E.: Progress toward transplantation of tissues in man. *In* Levine, S. Z. (ed): Advances in Pediatrics. Vol. XIII. Year Book Medical Publishers, Chicago, 1964, pp. 93–127.

Gorman, J. G., Freda, V. J., Pollack, W. J. and Robertson, J. G.: Protection from immunization in Rh-incompatible pregnancies: A progress report. Bull. N.Y. Acad. Med. 42:458–473, 1966.

Landy, M. and Braun, W. (eds): Immunological Tolerance; A Reassessment of Mechanisms of the Immune Response. Academic Press, New York, 1969.

McConnell, R. B.: The prevention of Rh haemolytic disease. *In* DeGraff, A. C. (ed): Annual Review of Medicine. Vol. 17. Annual Reviews, Inc., Palo Alto, 1966, pp. 291–306.

Rosenthale, M. E. and Mansmann, H. C. (eds): Immunopharmacology. Spectrum Publications, Inc., New York, 1975.

Schwartz, R. S.: Specificity of immunosuppression by antimetabolites. Fed. Proc. 25:165–168, 1966.

Uhr, J. W. and Moller, G.: Regulatory effect of antibody of the immune response. *In* Dixon, F. J., Jr. and Kunkel, H. G. (eds): Advances in Immunology. Vol. 8. Academic Press, New York, 1966, pp. 81–127.

Weigle, W. O. (ed): Natural and Acquired Immunologic Unresponsiveness. World Publishing Co., Cleveland, 1967.

Chapter 10

Audibert, F., Chédid, L., LeFrancier, P. and Choay, J.: Distinctive adjuvanticity of synthetic analogs of mycobacterial water-soluble components. Cell. Immunol. 21:243–249, 1976.

Castro, J. E.: The effect of *Corynebacterium parvum* on the structure and function of the lymphoid system in mice. Eur. J. Cancer 10:115–120, 1974.

Christie, G. H. and Bomford, R.: Mechanisms of macrophage activation by *Corynebacterium parvum*. I. In vitro experiments. II. In vivo experiments. Cell. Immunol. 17:141–155, 1975.

Floc'h, F. and Werner, G. M.: Increased resistance to virus infections of mice inoculated with BCG (Bacillus Calmette-Guerin) Ann. Immunol. (Paris) 127:173–186, 1976.

Freund, J.: Effect of paraffin oil and Mycobacteria on antibody formation and sensitization. Am. J. Clin. Pathol. 21:645, 1951.

Hadden, J. W., Coffey, R. G., Hadden, E. M., Lopez-Corrales, E. and Sunshine, G. H.: Effects of levamisole and imidazole on lymphocyte proliferation and cyclic nucleotide levels. Cell. Immunol. 20:98–103, 1975.

Howard, J. G., Scott, M. T. and Christie, G. H. (eds): Cellular mechanisms underlying the adjuvant activity of *Corynebacterium parvum*: Interactions of activated macrophages with T and B lymphocytes. *In* Immunopotentiation. CIBA Foundation Symposium, No. 18. American Elsevier Publishing Co., New York, 1973.

Jordan, G. W. and Merigan, T. C.: Enhancement of host defense mechanisms by pharmacological agents. Annu. Rev. Pharmacol. 15:157, 1975.

Laucius, J. F., Bodurtha, A. J., Mastrangelo, M. J. and Creech, R. H.: Bacillus Calmette-Guerin in the treatment of neoplastic disease. J. Reticuloendothel. Soc. 16:347–373, 1974.

Oettgen, H. F., Pinsky, C. M. and Delmonte, L.: Treatment of cancer with immunomodulators, *Corynebacterium parvum* and levamisole. Med. Clin. North Am. 60:511–537, 1976.

Pabst, H. F. and Crawford, J.: L-Tetramisole enhancement of human lymphocyte response to antigen. Clin. Exp. Immunol. 21:468–473, 1975.

Reed, C. E., Benner, M., Lockey, S. D., Enta, T., Makino, S. and Carr, R. H.: On the mechanism of the adjuvant effect of *Bordetella pertussis* vaccine. J. Allergy Clin. Immunol. 49:174–182, 1972.

Regelson, W.: Host modulation of resistance to infection and neoplasia. Annu. Reports Med. Chem. 8:160–171, 1973.

Wagner, W. H. and Hahn, H. (eds): Activation of Macrophages. Proceedings of a Workshop. American Elsevier Publishing Co., New York, 1974.

White, R. G.: The adjuvant effect of microbial products on the immune response. Annu. Rev. Microbiol. 30:579–600, 1976.

Wolstenholme, G. E. W. and Knight, J. (eds): Immunopotentiation. CIBA Foundation Symposium No. 18 (new series). American Elsevier Publishing Co., New York, 1973.

Chapters 11 and 12

Ackroyd, J. F. (ed): Immunological Methods. F. A. Davis Co., Philadelphia, 1964.

Kabat, E. A. and Mayer, M. M. (eds): Experimental Immunochemistry. Second Edition. Charles C Thomas, Springfield, Ill., 1961.

Kwapinski, J. B. (ed): Methodology of Immunochemical and Immunological Research. Wiley-Interscience, New York, 1972.

Landsteiner, K. (ed): The Specificity of Serological Reactions. Harvard University Press, Cambridge, 1945.

Litwin, S. D., Christian, C. L. and Siskind, G. W. (eds): Clinical Evaulation of Immune Function in Man: Proceedings of the Third Irwin Strasburger Memorial Seminar on Immunology. Grune and Stratton, New York, 1976.

Rajka, E. and Korossy, S. (eds): Immunological Aspects of Allergy and Allergic Diseases. Vols. 1 and 2. Plenum Press, New York, 1974.

Rose, N. R. and Bigazzi, P. E. (eds): Methods in Immunodiagnosis. J. Wiley and Sons, New York, 1973.

Rose, N. R. and Friedman, H. (eds): Manual of Clinical Immunology. Am. Soc. Microbiol., Washington, D.C., 1976.

Vyas, G. N., Stites, D. P. and Brecher, G. (eds): Laboratory Diagnosis of Immunologic Disorders. Grune and Stratton, New York, 1975.

Weir, D. M. (ed): Handbook of Experimental Immunology. Vols. 1, 2, 3. Second Edition. Blackwell Scientific Publications, Oxford, 1973.

Chapter 13

Allen, J. C. (ed): Infection and the Compromised Host. Williams and Wilkins, Baltimore, 1976.

Altemeier, W. A. and Alexander, J. W.: Surgical infection and choice of antibiotics. *In* Sabiston, D. C., Jr. (ed): Christopher's Textbook of Surgery. 11th Edition. W. B. Saunders Co., Philadelphia, 1977.

Brown, I. N.: Immunological aspects of malaria infection. Adv. Immunol. 11:267–349, 1969.

Dubos, R. J. and Hirsch, J. G. (eds): Bacterial and Mycotic Infections of Man. Fourth Edition. J. B. Lippincott Co., Philadelphia, 1965.

Dunlop, R. H. (ed): Resistance to Infectious Disease; Proceedings of an International Symposium, July 3 and 4, 1969. Modern Press, Saskatoon, 1970.

Geraldes. A. (ed): Effects of Interferon on Cells, Viruses and the Immune System. Academic Press, New York, 1975.

Guze, L. B. (ed): Microbial Protoplasts, Spheroplasts and L-forms. Williams and Wilkins Co., Baltimore, 1968.

Horsfall, F. L., Jr. and Tamm, I. (eds): Viral and Rickettsial Infections of Man. Fourth Edition. J. B. Lippincott Co., Philadelphia, 1965.

Larsh, J. E. and Weatherly, N. F.: Cell-mediated immunity in certain parasitic infections. Curr. Top. Microbiol. Immunol. 67:113–137, 1974.

Nahmias, A. J. and O'Reilly, R. J. (eds): Immunology of Human Infection. Plenum Publishing Corp., New York. In press.

Notkins, A. L. (ed): Viral Immunology and Immunopathology. Academic Press, New York, 1975.

Wilson, G. S. and Miles, A. (eds): Topley and Wilson's Principles of Bacteriology, Virology and Immunity. Sixth Edition. Williams and Wilkins Co., Baltimore, 1975.

Chapter 14

Baldwin, R. W.: Tumour-specific immunity against spontaneous rat tumours. Int. J. Cancer 1:257, 1966.

Becker, F. F. (ed): Biology of Tumors: Surfaces, Immunology, and Comparative Pathology. (Cancer—A Comprehensive Treatise: Vol. 4.) Plenum Press, New York, 1975.

Bekesi, J. G., Holland, J. F., Cuttner, J. et al.: Immunotherapy in acute myelocytic leukemia (AML) with neuraminidase (N'ASE)-treated allogeneic myeloblasts with or without MER. Proc. Am. Assoc. Cancer Res. 17:184, 1976 (abstract).

Bhattacharya, M. and Barlow, J. J.: Immunologic studies of human serous cystadenocarcinoma of the ovary—demonstration of tumor-associated antigens. Cancer 31:588, 1973.

Carswell, E. A., Wanebo, H. J., Old, L. J. et al.: Immunogenic properties of reticulum cell sarcomas of SJL/J mice. J. Natl. Cancer Inst. 44:1281, 1970.

Clarkson, B., Dowling, M. D., Gee, T. S. et al.: Treatment of acute leukemia in adults. Cancer 36:775, 1975.

Crispen, R. G. (ed): Neoplasm Immunity: Theory and Application. Proceedings of a symposium sponsored by the University of Illinois, Sept. 11, 1974. ITR, Chicago, 1975.

Gross, L.: Intradermal immunization of C3H mice against a sarcoma that originated in an animal of the same line. Cancer Res. 3:326, 1943.

Gutterman, J. U., Mavligit, G. M., Blumenshein, G. et al.: Immunotherapy of human solid tumors with Bacillus Calmette-Guérin: Prolongation of disease-free interval and survival in malignant melanoma, breast, and colorectal cancer. Ann. N.Y. Acad. Sci. 277:135, 1976.

Harris, J. E. and Sinkovics, J. G. (eds): The Immunology of Malignant Disease. C. V. Mosby Co., St. Louis, 1970.

Harris, J. E. and Sinkovics, J. G. (eds): The Immunology of Malignant Disease. Second Edition. C. V. Mosby Co., St. Louis, 1976.

Hewitt, H. B., Blake, E. R. and Walder, A. S.: A critique of the evidence for active host defense against cancer, based on personal studies of 27 murine tumours of spontaneous origin. Br. J. Cancer 33:241, 1976.

Homburger, F. (ed): Immunological Aspects of Neoplasia. Vol. 13. Progress in Experimental Tumor Research. S. Karger, Basel, 1970.

Homburger, F. (ed): Immunology of Cancer. Vol. 19. Progress in Experimental Tumor Research. S. Karger, Basel, 1974.

Israel, L.: Preliminary results of nonspecific immunotherapy for lung cancer. Cancer Chemother. Rep. 4(3):283, 1973.

Israel, L. and Halpern, B.: Le *Corynebacterium parvum* dans les cancers avancés. Première évaluation de l'activité thérapeutique de cette immuno-stimuline. Nouv. Presse Med. 1:19, 1972.

Kitagawa, M. and Yamamura, Y. (eds): Cancer Immunology: Immune Surveillance and Specific Recognition of Tumor Antigen. University Park Press, Baltimore, 1974.

Klein, E., Holtermann, O., Milgram, H. et al.: Immunotherapy for accessible tumors utilizing delayed hypersensitivity reactions and separated components of the immune system. Med. Clin. North Am. 60:389, 1976.

Lewis, M. G. and Phillips, T. M.: The specificity of surface membrane immunofluorescence in human malignant melanoma. Int. J. Cancer 10:105, 1972.

Mathé, G. and Weiner, R. (eds): Investigation and Stimulation of Immunity in Cancer Patients. Springer-Verlag, New York, 1974.

McKneally, M. F., Maver, C. and Kausel, H.: Regional immunotherapy of lung cancer with intrapleural BCG. Lancet 1:377, 1976.

Oettgen, H. F. and Rapp, H. J.: Immunotherapy of tumors in animals — II. Prog. Immunol. 3:403, 1974.

Old, L. J. and Boyse, E. A.: Current enigmas in cancer research. Harvey Lect. 67:273, 1973.

Prehn, R. T.: Tumor progression and homeostasis. Adv. Cancer Res. 23:203, 1976.

Rojas, A. F., Feierstein, J. N., Mickiewicz, E. et al.: Levamisole in advanced human breast cancer. Lancet 1:211–215, 1976.

Schultz, J. and Leif, R. C. (eds): Critical Factors in Cancer Immunology: Proceedings of the Miami Winter Symposia, Jan. 13–17, 1975. Academic Press, New York, 1975.

Siskind, G. W., Christian, C. L. and Litwin, S. D. (eds): Immune Depression and Cancer: Proceedings of the Second Irwin Strasburger Memorial Seminar on Immunology. Grune and Stratton, New York, 1975.

Symposium: Immunology and Cancer. University of Ottawa Press, Ottawa, 1973.

Chapter 15

Calne, R. Y. (ed): Immunological Aspects of Transplantation Surgery. John Wiley and Sons, New York, 1974.

Munster, A. M. (ed): Surgical Immunology. Grune and Stratton, New York, 1976.

Rapaport, F. T. (ed): Transplantation Proceedings. Grune and Stratton, New York. (Largely a compilation of proceedings from conferences sponsored by the Transplantation Society).

Rapaport, F. T. and Dausset, J. (eds): Human Transplantation. Grune and Stratton, New York, 1968.

Russell, P. S. and Monaco, A. P.: The Biology of Tissue Transplantation. Little, Brown and Co., Boston, 1965.

Chapter 16

Beers, R. F., Jr. and Basset, E. (eds): The Role of Immunological Factors in Infectious, Allergic and Autoimmune Processes. Raven Press, New York, 1976.

Burnet, F. M. (ed): Auto-immunity and Auto-immune Disease; A Survey for Physician or Biologist. F. A. Davis, Philadelphia, 1972.

Shulman, S. (ed): Tissue Specificity and Autoimmunity. Springer-Verlag, New York, 1974.

Chapter 17

Issitt, P. D. and Issitt, C. H.: Applied Blood Group Serology. Second Edition. Spectra Biologicals, Oxnard, Cal., 1975.

Mollison, P. L. (ed): Blood Transfusion in Clinical Medicine. Blackwell Scientific Publications, Oxford, 1972.

Race, R. R. and Sanger, R. (eds): Blood Groups in Man. Sixth Edition. Blackwell Scientific Publications, Oxford, 1975.
Rosenfield, R. E. (ed): Immunohematology Syllabus. Intercontinental Medical Book Corp. New York, 1974.

Chapter 18

Alexander, H. L. (ed): Reactions with Drug Therapy. W. B. Saunders Co., Philadelphia, 1955.
Criep, L. H. (ed): Allergy and Clinical Immunology. Grune and Stratton, New York, 1976.
Criep, L. H. (ed): Dermatologic Allergy: Immunology, Diagnosis, Management. W. B. Saunders Co., Philadelphia, 1967.
Levine, B. B.: Immunochemical mechanisms of drug allergy. In de Graff, A. C. and Creger, W. P. (eds): Annual Review of Medicine, Vol. 17. Annual Reviews, Inc., Palo Alto, Cal., 1966, pp. 23–38.
Levine, B. B., Redmond, A. P., Fellner, M. J. et al.: Penicillin allergy and the heterogeneous immune responses of man to benzylpenicillin. J. Clin. Invest. 45:1895–1906, 1966.
Parker, C. W.: Drug reactions. In Samter, M. (ed): Immunological Diseases. Little, Brown and Co., Boston, 1965, pp. 665–681.

Chapter 19

Benacerraf, B. (ed). Immunogenetics and Immunodeficiency. University Park Press, Baltimore, 1975.
Bergsma, D., Good, R. A., Finstad, J. and Paul, N. W. (eds): Immunodeficiency in Man and Animals. Proceedings. Sinauer Associates, Inc., Sunderland, Mass., 1975. (Birth Defects: Original Article Series, Vol. XI, No. 1, 1975.)

Chapter 20

Alexander, J. W.: Nutrition and surgical infections. In Ballinger, W. F. et al. (eds): Manual of Surgical Nutrition. W. B. Saunders Co., Philadelphia, 1975, pp. 386–395.
Faulk, W. P., Mata, L. J. and Edsall, G.: Effects of malnutrition on the immune response in humans: a review. Trop. Dis. Bull. 72:89–103, 1975.
Hansen, M. A., Fernandes, G., Yunis, E. J., Cooper, W. C., Jose, D. G., Kramer, T. and Good, R. A.: Infection in the special host: the severely malnourished host. In Nahmias, A. J. and O'Reilly, R. (eds): Immunology of Human Infection. Plenum Press, New York. In press.
Latham, M. C.: Nutrition and infection in national development. Science 188:561–565, 1975.
Mata, L. J.: Malnutrition-infection interactions in the tropics. Am. J. Trop. Med. Hyg. 24:564–574, 1975.
Scrimshaw, N. S., Taylor, C. E. and Gordan, J. E. (eds): Interactions of Nutrition and Infection. Monograph Series, No. 57. World Health Organization, Geneva, 1968.
Stinnett, J. D. and Alexander, J. W.: Nutrition as related to host defense and infection. In Richards, J. R. and Kinney, J. M. (eds): Nutritional Aspects of the Care of the Critically Ill. Churchill Livingstone, Edinburgh, Scotland. In press.
Suskind, R. M. (ed): Malnutrition and the Immune Response. Kroc Foundation Series, Vol. 7. Raven Press, New York, 1977.
Wolstenholme, G. E. W. and O'Connor, M. (eds): Nutrition and Infection (In honour of Professor R. Nicolaysen.) CIBA Foundation Study Group No. 31, London. Little, Brown and Co., Boston, 1967.
Worthington, B.: Effect of nutritional status on immune phenomena. J. Am. Diet. Assoc. 65:123–129, 1974.

Chapter 21

Katz, D. H. and Benacerraf, B. (eds): The Role of Products of the Histocompatibility Gene Complex in Immune Responses. Academic Press, New York, 1976.
McDevitt, H. O. and Bodmer, W. F.: HL-A, immune response genes and disease. Lancet 1: 1269–1275, 1974.
Moller, G. (ed): HLA and Disease. Transplantation Reviews. Vol. 22. Munksgaard, Copenhagen, 1975.
Ryder, L. P., Staub Nielsen, L. and Svejgaard, A.: Associations between HL-A histocompatibility antigens and non-malignant diseases. Humangenetik 25:257–264, 1974.
Svejgaard, A., Hauge, M., Jersild, C., Platz, P., Ryder, L. P., Staub Nielsen, L. and Thomsen, P.: The HLA system; An Introductory Survey. Monographs in Human Genetics. Vol. 7. S. Karger, Basel, 1975.

INDEX

Page numbers in italics indicate illustrations. Page numbers followed by (t) indicate tables.